# Emergency Medicine: Diagnosis and Management

# Emergency Medicine: Diagnosis and Management

Edited by **Abby Cusack**

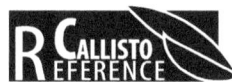

R CALLISTO REFERENCE

New York

Published by Callisto Reference,
106 Park Avenue, Suite 200,
New York, NY 10016, USA
www.callistoreference.com

**Emergency Medicine: Diagnosis and Management**
Edited by Abby Cusack

International Standard Book Number: 978-1-63239-758-4 (Hardback)

Printed in the United States of America.

# Contents

# Preface

The main aim of this book is to educate learners and enhance their research focus by presenting diverse topics covering this vast field. This is an advanced book which compiles significant studies by distinguished experts. This book addresses successive solutions to the challenges arising in the area of application, along with it; the book provides scope for future developments.

This book outlines the processes and applications of emergency medicine in detail. It includes the fundamental as well as modern approaches of this discipline. Emergency medicine refers to the practice of providing immediate care, treatment and medical assistance to patients in order to prevent death and further disability. The aim of emergency physicians is to give urgent stabilization, evaluation, recognition and disposition at the time of emergency. This book strives to provide a fair idea about this discipline and to help develop a better understanding of the latest advances associated with emergency medicine. It also includes contributions of experts and scientists which will provide innovative insights into this field. It will help students, physicians, surgeons, researchers and all those interested in this area to keep pace with the rapid changes in this field.

It was a great honour to edit this book, though there were challenges, as it involved a lot of communication and networking between me and the editorial team. However, the end result was this all-inclusive book covering diverse themes in the field.

Finally, it is important to acknowledge the efforts of the contributors for their excellent chapters, through which a wide variety of issues have been addressed. I would also like to thank my colleagues for their valuable feedback during the making of this book.

**Editor**

# Out-of-Hospital Perimortem Cesarean Section as Resuscitative Hysterotomy in Maternal Posttraumatic Cardiac Arrest

**Francesca Gatti,**[1] **Marco Spagnoli,**[1] **Simone Maria Zerbi,**[1]
**Dario Colombo,**[2] **Mario Landriscina,**[1] **and Fulvio Kette**[3]

[1] *Anaesthesia and Intensive Care Unit 2, Sant'Anna Hospital, San Fermo della Battaglia, 22020 Como, Italy*
[2] *Anaesthesia and Intensive Care Unit 1, Sant'Anna Hospital, San Fermo della Battaglia, 22020 Como, Italy*
[3] *Bergamo 118 Operative Dispatch Center, Azienda Regionale Emergenza Urgenza (AREU), Via Campanini 6, 20124 Milan, Italy*

Correspondence should be addressed to Simone Maria Zerbi; smzerbi@gmail.com

Academic Editor: Serdar Kula

The optimal treatment of a severe hemodynamic instability from shock to cardiac arrest in late term pregnant women is subject to ongoing studies. However, there is an increasing evidence that early "separation" between the mother and the foetus may increase the restoration of the hemodynamic status and, in the cardiac arrest setting, it may raise the likelihood of a return of spontaneous circulation (ROSC) in the mother. This treatment, called Perimortem Cesarean Section (PMCS), is now termed as Resuscitative Hysterotomy (RH) to better address the issue of an early Cesarean section (C-section). This strategy is in contrast with the traditional treatment of cardiac arrest characterized by the maintenance of cardiopulmonary resuscitation (CPR) maneuvers without any emergent surgical intervention. We report the case of a prehospital perimortem delivery by Caesarean (C) section of a foetus at 36 weeks of gestation after the mother's traumatic cardiac arrest. Despite the negative outcome of the mother, the choice of performing a RH seems to represent up to date the most appropriate intervention to improve the outcome in both mother and foetus.

## 1. Introduction

Traumatic cardiac arrest is a life threatening situation with a negligible survival rate [1–3].

A traumatic cardiac arrest in pregnant women is even more challenging condition due to physiological changes which may further limit the generation of an adequate cardiac output (CO). During manual chest compressions cardiac output achieves approximately 30% of the normal CO. In a late term pregnant woman this is further compromised because the aorto-caval compression by the gravidic uterus hampers the venous return and the CO generated by precordial compression is no greater than 10% [4–6].

CPR is often performed only via the standard maneuvers characterized by assisted ventilation and chest compression in left lateral tilt with the aid of a wedge (Cardiff wedge) or via a manual uterus displacement aimed to facilitate the venous return. The evidence of a temporal relationship between emptying the uterus in order to reduce the aorto-caval compression and the increase in CPR effectiveness has suggested that an early C-section may be the most appropriate intervention to improve the outcome in both mother and foetus. Katz and other authors recently pointed out the potential effectiveness of such emergent surgical intervention, although they also emphasized that there is still a cultural and psychological gap in managing correctly these situations [5, 6]. Lack of knowledge, skills and refusal of an aggressive and highly invasive treatment have been recognized as the main determinant of failed emergent C-section [5–9].

The more recent American Heart Association (AHA) and European Resuscitation Council (ERC) Guidelines on CPR provided recommendations on resuscitation in special circumstances such as traumatic cardiac arrest and pregnancy. These recommendations, however, are mainly based on reviews, anecdotal reports, and *in vitro* studies [4, 7].

According to the suggested strategy, we wish to report on a case of a traumatic cardiac arrest in which an emergent delivery was performed on the site of a car crash by the emergency physician while CPR was still ongoing.

## 2. Case Presentation

The 1-1-8 Emergency Medical Service (EMS) Operative Centre (O.C.) was activated on August 17, 2010, following a traffic accident involving two cars in a high-energy, head-on collision. The O.C. referred seven people involved, two of whom were apparently unconscious and trapped in their car.

EMS dispatched three ambulances with certified basic life support and defibrillation (BLSD) rescuers and one advanced life support (ALS) team. This is constituted by a physician, mainly an anaesthesiologist, by a registered nurse certified in out-of-hospital intervention, and by a car driver certified in BLSD maneuvers.

The first ambulance team confirmed cardiac arrest in a woman who was at the 36th gestational week and begun immediately CPR maneuvers. The ALS team arrived soon after and begun standard advanced resuscitation. The rhythm monitoring confirmed a pulseless electrical activity (PEA) with a heart rate (HR) of 30 beats per minute (bpm). Three milligrams (mg) atropine and eight mg epinephrine were administered intravenously. Oral tracheal intubation was successfully performed at the first attempt despite the presence of blood into the pharynx and the patient was manually ventilated at 1.0 inspired oxygen fraction ($FiO_2$).

The clinical examination highlighted head trauma, a facial cyanosis, thoracic trauma with reduced left expansion in the setting of a global severe chest trauma, and an abdominal seat-belt hematoma. According to the clinical findings it was hypothesized that head and/or thoracic trauma could have been the most reliable causes of cardiac arrest. This led the physician to introduce a chest needle for an initial treatment of a potential hypertensive pneumothorax, but the maneuver was uneventful.

The suspect of an abdominal massive hemorrhage led also to the infusion of a volume of about two liters of crystalloids through a left subclavian cannulation. Unfortunately, the lack of ultrasound did not allow the possible recognition of such life threatening condition.

End-tidal $CO_2$ monitoring was not performed because of the lack of the device.

Twelve minutes after cardiac arrest, the EMS physician decided to carry the patient on the spinal board into the ambulance and to proceed with a Perimortem Caesarean Section (PMCS), in agreement with the 1-1-8 O.C. physician and the gynaecologist on duty.

After a quick disinfection, a deep umbilical-pubic laparotomy was performed. There were no signs of bleeding. The uterus was gestational and cut with a lengthwise incision. The head of the foetus was free from the umbilical cord. There was no evidence of meconium.

A female foetus was extracted 3 minutes after onset of the procedure. At the first minute the Apgar score was 3 (the HR was 60 beats per minute, the breathing activity was absent, the muscular tone was flaccid, the corneal reflexes were absent, there was no grimace, and the skin was pink-coloured).

Newborn life support, consisting of airways aspiration and orotracheal intubation with uncuffed tube was performed. The baby was wiped, dried, and warmed up. An intraosseous needle was placed because of lack of vein cannulation.

The Apgar score at the 5th minute was 6, the HR was higher than 100 bpm, and the skin was pink-coloured; the reflexes were absent, there was no grimace, and there was spontaneous but irregular respiratory drive.

Maternal life support was continued by the nurse. After PMCS the hemodynamic condition did not change. Nevertheless, both mother and baby were carried to the hospital. The mother was declared deceased soon after arrival at the emergency department (ED) whereas the newborn was handed over by the neonatologist and admitted to the neonatal intensive care unit (NICU).

Subsequent anatomical findings revealed that the mother deceased because of amniotic pulmonary embolism associated with additional minor traumatic injuries. No major bleeding was identified.

At a distance of four years from the event the baby had a neurological development slightly reduced with a slower language acquisition and a normal physical growth.

## 3. Discussion

Historically a postmortem foetus extraction was described as early as 715 before Christ when the Roman King Numa Pompilius decreed that no child should be buried within his mother (for religious reasons) since some foetus was found still alive [5].

One of the first positive case report of PMCS was described by De Pace and coworkers in 1982 where a woman developed cardiac arrest (CA) during fiberoscopy. After 20 minutes of CPR, PMCS was performed and ROSC was soon achieved in the mother while the baby recovered uneventfully. Both had a full long term neurological survival [10].

The true incidence of cardiac arrest during pregnancy has been estimated to be about 1 over 30,000 pregnancies [11].

Despite the direct deaths in the UK account for less than 50% of the total maternal deaths, there are "indirect" deaths related to psychiatric disease which lead to attempted suicides during pregnancy. These deaths account for 20% of worldwide maternal deaths [12].

Although resuscitation algorithms during cardiac arrest are the same for pregnant patients as for non-pregnant patients, the anatomical and physiological modifications of the late term pregnant woman impose more aggressive interventions such as advanced airway management and the attention to left lateral tilt or lateral displacement of the uterus. The ALS guidelines point out the possible use of a PMCS as soon as a pregnant woman develops cardiac arrest [4, 7].

The striking decision to intervene with a PMCS relied on the four "gold points": the stay and play strategy, the Katz's paradox, the four-minute rule, and the surgical techniques.

According to the stay and play strategy our decision was chosen by judging the difficulty to maintain adequate coronary and cerebral perfusion via manual chest compressions due to the lack of both a mechanical chest compressor and a Cardiff wedge [5, 13, 14]. We estimated that transportation would have dramatically worsened the overall hemodynamic conditions due to the poor perfusion generated by our chest compressions. Yet, the lack of the end-tidal $CO_2$ monitoring impeded us to adequately detect the effectiveness of cardiac compressions. The further reduction of the already low cardiac output by the aorto-caval compression induced us to empty the uterus according to the Katz's principle. Accordingly, the uterus should be emptied and the baby delivered to achieve an improved hemodynamic status during both non-cardiac and cardiac arrest condition even when the foetus is dead in the attempt to save at least the mother [5]. This concept was based on previous physiopathological evidence by Kerr as far as in 1965 when the effects of vena cava compression and the reduction of venous return by the gravidic uterus were demonstrated [15].

As per the four-minute rule, emergency Cesarean section should be performed when the gravidic uterus is considered to be the cause of maternal hemodynamic impairment due to aorto-caval compression regardless of fetal viability [13, 15–19]. The "emergency hysterotomy" is recommended to be initiated within four minutes of maternal cardiopulmonary arrest if ALS maneuvers are unsuccessful, although this is a class IIb intervention with a level of evidence (LOE) C [4]. According to Bloomer, the term "resuscitative hysterotomy" should be preferred instead of Perimortem Cesarean Section as it better represents a way to reverse cardiac arrest rather than simply being a last chance of resuscitative efforts [20, 21].

The issue on the best timing within which the procedure should be performed is still debated. Indeed, it is widely recognized that emergency hysterotomy should be performed as early as possible preferentially after two cycles of CPR (after four minutes after cardiac arrest), without wasting time to perform ultrasonography or Doppler foetal heart sound examination [4, 22, 23].

The surgical technique may represent another option to speed up an emergency C-section. Under these conditions the preferred surgical laparotomy consists of a vertical umbilical-pubic incision which differs from the classical Pfannenstiel incision used in the in-hospital setting [5, 24]. Our surgical procedure was kept as simple as possible, considering the limited expertise of the emergency physician. In fact, although the experts suggest that the placenta should be removed from the uterus as well, we just left it in situ and packed the opened abdomen. Indeed Draycott and the TOSTI study demonstrated that introduction of obstetric emergencies training courses was associated with a significant increase of team work and reduction in low 5-minute Apgar scores and hypoxic-ischemic encephalopathy [6, 25].

In our case this intervention did not have positive effects on the mother but rather on the baby. The subsequent autopsy showed posttraumatic amniotic fluid embolism (AFE) [26] as the main cause of the death rather than massive abdominal hemorrhage. The deceleration of the mother's body inside the vehicle during the impact could be involved in the mechanism of injury, as demonstrated by Crosby and coworkers as far as 1968 [27]. The AFE was the likely reason why ROSC could not be achieved even though the C-section was performed on the scene within 20 minutes without maternal ALS interruption. This time frame was not a limitation since a complete neurological recovery after 30 minutes of CPR was documented in women who experienced cardiac arrest due to traumatic events [28].

Despite the positive outcome we recognized that this case has some limitations: lack of adequate $ETCO_2$ monitoring and ultrasound, absence of circulatory supporting devices, and limited experience. Nevertheless our report represents an unusual case of emergency delivery performed in a mother victim of traumatic cardiac arrest in which the C-section led to a full neurological recovery of the baby at a distance of four years from the event.

By confirming the fortuity of our result, we wish to point out that the key to salvage a pregnant woman in cardiac arrest is to separate the maternal-foetal unit according to the Katz's principle and to emphasize what the AHA guidelines report: "*This strategy seems to be the best way to manage the serious impairment in pregnancy (>24 weeks). The hysterotomy also allows access to the infant so the newborn resuscitation can begin*" [4, 7].

## Consent

The family provided consent to use this information.

## Conflict of Interests

The authors state the absence of any conflict of interests.

## References

[1] G. D. Perkins, S. Brace, and S. Gates, "Mechanical chest-compression devices: current and future roles," *Current Opinion in Critical Care*, vol. 16, no. 3, pp. 203–210, 2010.

[2] S. Huber-Wagner, R. Lefering, M. Qvick et al., "Outcome in 757 severely injured patients with traumatic cardiorespiratory arrest," *Resuscitation*, vol. 75, no. 2, pp. 276–285, 2007.

[3] J. J. Pickens, M. K. Copass, and E. M. Bulger, "Trauma patients receiving CPR: predictors of survival," *Journal of Trauma: Injury Infection & Critical Care*, vol. 58, no. 5, pp. 951–958, 2005.

[4] T. L. V. Hoek, L. J. Morrison, M. Shuster et al., "Part 12: cardiac arrest in special situations: 2010 American Heart Association guidelines for cardiopulmonary resuscitation and emergency cardiovascular care," *Circulation*, vol. 122, no. 3, pp. S829–S861, 2010.

[5] V. L. Katz, "Perimortem cesarean delivery: its role in maternal mortality," *Seminars in Perinatology*, vol. 36, no. 1, pp. 68–72, 2012.

[6] A. Dijkman, C. M. A. Huisman, M. Smit et al., "Cardiac arrest in pregnancy: increasing use of perimortem caesarean section due to emergency skills training?" *BJOG: An International Journal of Obstetrics & Gynaecology*, vol. 117, no. 3, pp. 282–287, 2010.

[7] J. Soar, G. D. Perkins, G. Abbas et al., "European Resuscitation Council guidelines for resuscitation 2010 section 8. Cardiac arrest in special circumstances: electrolyte abnormalities,

poisoning, drowning, accidental hypothermia, hyperthermia, asthma, anaphylaxis, cardiac surgery, trauma, pregnancy, electrocution," *Resuscitation*, vol. 81, no. 10, pp. 1400–1433, 2010.

[8] S. E. Cohen, L. C. Andes, and B. Carvalho, "Assessment of knowledge regarding cardiopulmonary resuscitation of pregnant women," *International Journal of Obstetric Anesthesia*, vol. 17, no. 1, pp. 20–25, 2008.

[9] T. Draycott, T. Sibanda, L. Owen et al., "Does training in obstetric emergencies improve neonatal outcome?" *BJOG: An International Journal of Obstetrics & Gynaecology*, vol. 113, no. 2, pp. 177–182, 2006.

[10] N. L. de Pace, J. S. Betesh, and M. N. Kotler, ""Postmortem" cesarean section with recovery of both mother and offspring," *The Journal of the American Medical Association*, vol. 248, no. 8, pp. 971–973, 1982.

[11] G. Lewis, "CEMACH, Department of health, Welsh office, Scottish Office, Department of Health and social services, Northern Ireland, Why mothers die. Report on enquiries into maternal deaths in the United Kingdom," Registered Charity no. 213280, 2004.

[12] G. Lewis, *The Confidential Enquiry into Maternal and Child Health CEMACH. Saving Mothers' Lives: Reviewing Maternal Deaths to Make Motherhood Safer 2003–2005. The Seventh Report on Confidential Enquirers into Maternal Deaths in the United Kingdom*, CEMACH, London, UK, 2007.

[13] V. Katz, K. Balderston, and M. Defreest, "Perimortem cesarean delivery: were our assumptions correct?" *American Journal of Obstetrics & Gynecology*, vol. 192, no. 6, pp. 1916–1921, 2005.

[14] C. Ellington, V. L. Katz, W. J. Watson, and F. J. Spielman, "The effect of lateral tilt on maternal and fetal hemodynamic variables," *Obstetrics & Gynecology*, vol. 77, no. 2, pp. 201–203, 1991.

[15] M. G. Kerr, "The mechanical effects of the gravid uterus in late pregnancy," *The Journal of obstetrics and gynaecology of the British Commonwealth*, vol. 72, pp. 513–529, 1965.

[16] V. L. Katz, D. J. Dotters, and W. Droegemueller, "Perimortem cesarean delivery," *Obstetrics & Gynecology*, vol. 68, no. 4, pp. 571–576, 1986.

[17] J. H. Bamber and M. Dresner, "Aortocaval compression in pregnancy: the effect of changing the degree and direction of lateral tilt on maternal cardiac output," *Anesthesia & Analgesia*, vol. 97, no. 1, pp. 256–258, 2003.

[18] A. P. L. Goodwin and A. J. Pearce, "The human wedge: a manoeuvre to relieve aortocaval compression during resuscitation in late pregnancy," *Anaesthesia*, vol. 47, no. 5, pp. 433–434, 1992.

[19] G. F. Marx, "Cardiopulmonary resuscitation of late-pregnant women," *Anesthesiology*, vol. 56, no. 2, p. 156, 1982.

[20] V. L. Katz, S. R. Wells, J. A. Kuller, W. F. Hansen, M. J. McMahon, and W. A. Bowes Jr., "Cesarean delivery: a reconsideration of terminology," *Obstetrics & Gynecology*, vol. 86, no. 1, pp. 152–153, 1995.

[21] R. Bloomer, C. Reid, and R. Wheatley, "Prehospital resuscitative hysterotomy," *European Journal of Emergency Medicine*, vol. 18, no. 4, pp. 241–242, 2011.

[22] R. Kue, C. Coyle, E. Vaughan, and M. Restuccia, "Perimortem Cesarean section in the helicopter EMS setting: a case report," *Air Medical Journal*, vol. 27, no. 1, pp. 46–47, 2008.

[23] P. M. Brun, H. Chenaitia, I. Dejesus, J. Bessereau, L. Bonello, and B. Pierre, "Ultrasound to perimortem caesarean delivery in prehospital settings," *Injury*, vol. 44, no. 1, pp. 151–152, 2013.

[24] Q. Warraich and U. Esen, "Perimortem caesarean section," *Journal of Obstetrics and Gynaecology*, vol. 29, no. 8, pp. 690–693, 2009.

[25] J. van de Ven, S. Houterman, R. A. J. Q. Steinweg et al., "Reducing errors in health care: cost-effectiveness of multidisciplinary team training in obstetric emergencies (TOSTI study); a randomised controlled trial," *BMC Pregnancy and Childbirth*, vol. 10, article 59, 2010.

[26] C. Thongrong, P. Kasemsiri, J. P. Hofmann et al., "Amniotic fluid embolism," *International Journal of Critical Illness and Injury Science*, vol. 3, no. 1, pp. 51–57, 2013.

[27] W. M. Crosby, R. G. Snyder, C. C. Snow, and P. G. Hanson, "Impact injuries in pregnancy. I. Experimental studies," *The American Journal of Obstetrics and Gynecology*, vol. 101, no. 1, pp. 100–108, 1968.

[28] G. Capobianco, A. Balata, M. C. Mannazzu et al., "Perimortem cesarean delivery 30 minutes after a laboring patient jumped from a fourth-floor window: baby survives and is normal at age 4 years," *The American Journal of Obstetrics and Gynecology*, vol. 198, no. 1, pp. e15–e16, 2008.

# Lazy Lips: Hyperkalemia and Acute Tetraparesis—A Case Report from an Urban Emergency Department

Christian T. Braun,[1] David S. Srivastava,[1] Bianca Maria Engelhardt,[2]
Gregor Lindner,[3] and Aristomenis K. Exadaktylos[1]

[1] *Department of Emergency Medicine, Inselspital, University Hospital Bern, Freiburgstrasse, 3010 Bern, Switzerland*
[2] *Department of Surgery, Inselspital, University Hospital Bern, Freiburgstrasse, 3010 Bern, Switzerland*
[3] *Department of Respiratory and Critical Care Medicine, Otto Wagner Hospital, Baumgartner Höhe 1, 1140 Vienna, Austria*

Correspondence should be addressed to Christian T. Braun; christian.braun@insel.ch

Academic Editor: Kalpesh Jani

A 58-year-old male patient was admitted to our emergency department at a large university hospital due to acute onset of general weakness. It was reported that the patient was bradycardic at 30/min and felt an increasing weakness of the limbs. At admission to the emergency department, the patient was not feeling any discomfort and denied dyspnoea or pain. The primary examination of the nervous system showed the cerebral nerves II–XII intact, muscle strength of the lower extremities was 4/5, and a minimal sensory loss of the left hemisphere was found. In addition, the patient complained about lazy lips. During ongoing examinations, the patient developed again symptomatic bradycardia, accompanied by complete tetraplegia. The following blood test showed severe hyperkalemia probably induced by use of aldosterone antagonists as the cause of the patient's neurologic symptoms. Hyperkalemia is a rare but treatable cause of acute paralysis that requires immediate treatment. Late diagnosis can delay appropriate treatment leading to cardiac arrhythmias and arrest.

## 1. Introduction

Hyperkalemia is common in emergency department patients with a prevalence rate of about 9%. About 3/4 of cases of hyperkalemia in emergency department patients were described to be caused by either acute or chronic renal failure or medications linked to this condition [1]. Hyperkalemia often appears clinically asymptomatic, and most often the electrolyte disorder gets only symptomatic when hyperkalemia is severe. Clinical features range from mild to life-threatening manifestations such as weakness to malign cardiac arrhythmias. We present the rare case of a severe neurologic manifestation of profound hyperkalemia.

## 2. Case Presentation

A 58-year-old patient was admitted to the Emergency Department of the Inselspital, University Hospital Bern, by the Swiss air ambulance service.

At arrival it was reported that the patient felt an increasing weakness of the limbs for 3 days. On the day of admission, the weakness had intensified to such a high level that the patient called an ambulance.

He had usually a treatment for high blood pressure with aldosterone antagonists.

When asymptomatic bradycardia of 30 beats/min was diagnosed by the ambulance team, they suspected an acute coronary syndrome and treated the patient with P2Y12 receptor inhibitors, heparin, and aspirin. During transport, epinephrine needed to be administered to stabilize the now instable blood pressure. At arrival in the emergency department, the patient was not feeling any discomfort and denied dyspnoea or pain; the blood pressure was 154/58 mmHg, the heart rate was mildly bradycardic with 54 beats/min, tachypnea with a rate of 20/min was present, oxygen saturation was 100% with high-flow oxygen, temperature was 36.5°C, and the patient showed 15/15 points on the Glasgow Coma Scale (GCS) examination.

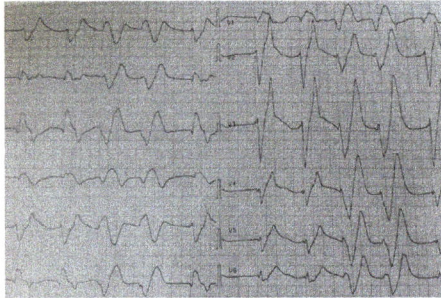

FIGURE 1: The electrocardiogram showing tall and peaked T waves, flattened and broadened P waves, and widened QRS complexes.

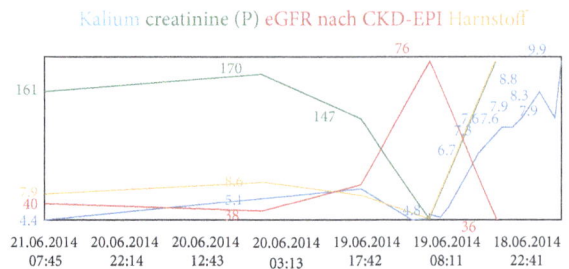

FIGURE 2: Trends of the laboratory parameters from admission to the emergency department until 2 days before discharge of the hospital: potassium, creatinine, GFR CKD-EPI, and urea.

In the physical examination on arrival he showed a normal cardiovascular and gastrointestinal system; the examination of respiratory system was normal except for slight tachypnea.

The nervous system showed the cerebral nerves II–XII intact, the muscle strength of the lower extremities was 4/5, and a minimal sensory loss of the left hemisphere was observed. In addition, the patient complained about lazy lips.

The electrocardiogram showed abnormalities, including tall and peaked T waves, flattened and broadened P waves, and widened QRS complexes (Figure 1). Because myocardial infarction could not be ruled out at that point, an emergency echocardiography study was conducted, which showed a normal result, especially normal left and right ejection fraction, no pericardial effusion, and a normal kinetic of the heart.

During this examination the patient developed a symptomatic bradycardia, accompanied by complete tetraplegia. The reevaluation of the neurologic system revealed a conscious and oriented patient with now areflexic paralysis of both lower and upper limbs.

Power in lower and upper limbs was 0 of 5; the Babinski sign was negative. There was hypoesthesia of the extremities, accentuated at the left side.

Continuously, the patient's vigilance declined to a GCS below 8, so that the patient was intubated for airway protection. Atropine was administered during the episode of bradycardia with low output and pending pulseless electric activity (PEA).

The laboratory analysis, which was available 1 hour after arrival of the patient in the emergency department, showed a serum potassium level of 9,9 mmol/L and sodium of 128 mmol/L, the chloride was 114 mmol/L, and the pH was 7,161 (pCO$_2$ 25 mmHg, bicarbonate 10 mmol/L). Serum creatinine, without known chronic renal failure, was 167 $\mu$mol/L with an estimated glomerular filtration rate of 38 mL/min. Fractional excretion of urea was 12%, which hinted towards prerenal failure.

After getting results on serum electrolytes, the patient was initially treated with calcium gluconate 10% and 8.4% sodium bicarbonate for membrane stabilization followed by 10 IE insulin within 50 mL glucose 40% given for 30 minutes for shifting of serum potassium into the cells and loop diuretics for renal potassium elimination [2, 3].

These therapeutic procedures stabilized the cardiac output and the general condition of the patient but were not therapeutic options for a longer period, so that the patient was transferred to the intensive care unit for hemodialysis for slow correction of hyperkalemia.

One day after correction of hyperkalemia, the patient was extubated and referred to the department of nephrology for further treatment.

During dialysis, the potassium and the arterial blood pH decreased to normal values, but the renal parameters stayed elevated (Figure 2). We assumed this to a prior existing renal insufficiency.

During the hospital stay, the antihypertensive therapy was changed to ACE-inhibitors and prior spironolactone therapy was stopped.

## 3. Discussion

Hyperkalemia often appears without any clinical symptoms, despite diagnostic signs like ECG changes including tall and peaked T waves, flattened and broadened P waves, and widened QRS complexes. Clinically, these patients often present with either bradycardia or tachycardia [2, 3]. Neurological symptoms like paresthesia/tetraparesis seem to appear only with extremely elevated potassium levels [4] and therefore appear quiet rarely [5, 6]. However, electrolyte disorders are common in emergency department patients and often cause unspecific symptoms. Thus, ordering an electrolyte panel or point of care testing should be standard in almost all patients presenting to an emergency department due to the potentially harmful effects of electrolyte disorders on patients outcome.

## Conflict of Interests

The authors declare that there is no conflict of interests regarding the publication of this paper.

## References

[1] C. A. Pfortmüller, A. B. Leichtle, G. M. Fiedler, A. K. Exadaktylos, and G. Lindner, "Hyperkalemia in the emergency department: etiology, symptoms and outcome of a life threatening electrolyte disorder," *European Journal of Internal Medicine*, vol. 24, no. 5, pp. e59–e60, 2013.

[2] L. S. Weisberg, "Management of severe hyperkalemia," *Critical Care Medicine*, vol. 36, no. 12, pp. 3246–3251, 2008.

[3] T. Phiri, T. J. Allain, and G. Dreyer, "Acute confusion and ataxia in the emergency department with an unexpected underlying diagnosis," *Malawi Medical Journal*, vol. 25, no. 2, pp. 33–35, 2013.

[4] K. Panichpisal, S. Gandhi, K. Nugent, and Y. Anziska, "Acute quadriplegia from hyperkalemia: a case report and literature review," *Neurologist*, vol. 16, no. 6, pp. 390–393, 2010.

[5] M. Delgado-Alvarado, E. Palacio-Portilla, A. L. Pelayo-Negro, P. Lerena, and J. Berciano, "From ileostomy to sudden quadriplegia with electrocardiographic abnormalities: a short and unfortunate path," *Neurological Sciences*, vol. 34, no. 8, pp. 1471–1473, 2013.

[6] A. Wahab, R. B. Panwar, V. Ola, and S. Alvi, "Acute onset quadriparesis with sine wave: a rare presentation," *The American Journal of Emergency Medicine*, vol. 29, no. 5, pp. 575.e1–575.e2, 2011.

# An Unusual Cause of Pulmonary Nodules in the Emergency Department

**Ryan Yu[1] and Melanie Ferri[2]**

[1]*Department of Pathology and Molecular Medicine, McMaster University, Hamilton, ON, Canada L8S 4L8*
[2]*Department of Diagnostic Imaging, Juravinski Hospital and Cancer Centre and McMaster University, Hamilton, ON, Canada L8V 5C2*

Correspondence should be addressed to Ryan Yu; ryan.yu@medportal.ca

Academic Editor: Chih Cheng Lai

We report a 51-year-old woman who presented to the emergency department with left-sided pleuritic chest pain 2 weeks after subtotal hysterectomy and bilateral salpingo-oophorectomy for a leiomyomatous uterus. Computed tomography scan of the chest revealed bilateral pulmonary nodules. Biopsy showed cytologically bland spindle cells without overt malignant features. Immunohistochemistry confirmed smooth muscle phenotype, in keeping with a clinicopathologic diagnosis of benign metastasizing leiomyoma (BML). BML does not frequently come to the attention of the emergency physician because it is rare and usually asymptomatic. When symptomatic, its clinical presentation depends on the site(s) of metastasis, number, and size of the smooth muscle tumors. Emergent presentations of BML are reviewed.

## 1. Introduction

Benign metastasizing leiomyoma (BML) is an entity in which benign-appearing uterine smooth muscle tumors are associated with similar-appearing tumors at distant sites [1]. The lung is the most common site of involvement and usually shows multiple, occasionally solitary, well-circumscribed nodules, ranging in diameter from a few millimeters to several centimeters [2]. The finding of multiple pulmonary nodules raises a broad differential diagnosis, including primary or secondary neoplasms, vasculitis, collagen vascular disease, and granulomatous diseases. BML does not frequently come to the attention of the emergency physician because it is rare and usually asymptomatic. However, BML may exhibit a range of clinical presentations, some emergent, depending on the site of involvement, number, and size of the smooth muscle tumors (leiomyomas). We report a patient with benign metastasizing leiomyoma who presented in the emergency department with pleuritic chest pain.

## 2. Case Report

A 51-year-old woman, gravida 2 para 2, presented to the emergency department with a 2-day history of left-sided pleuritic chest pain. Two weeks prior, she underwent subtotal hysterectomy and bilateral salpingo-oophorectomy for a leiomyomatous uterus which was approximately the size of a 12-week gravid uterus. Ten years prior, she underwent a hysteroscopic myomectomy for a submucous leiomyoma. Her medical history was further remarkable for endometriosis, primary biliary cirrhosis, chronic cholecystitis, hypertension, hypercholesterolemia, and transient ischemic attack. On physical examination in the emergency department, she was afebrile with a blood pressure of 150/87, heart rate 60/min, respiratory rate 18/min, and oxygen saturation 99% on room air. She had a BMI of 33, normal heart sounds, and clear chest on auscultation. ECG was normal. ABG showed pH 7.41 and $pCO_2$ 39 mmHg. She had a normal complete blood count, basic metabolic panel, and troponin. D-dimer was 1.2 $\mu$g/mL FEU (reference: less than 0.5 $\mu$g/mL FEU). Chest radiograph showed a 1.3 cm nodule in the left lower lobe (Figure 1) compared with a chest radiograph performed 4 years earlier which was clear. CT pulmonary angiogram (CTPA) showed bilateral, well-circumscribed, noncalcified, and noncavitated pulmonary nodules (Figures 2(a) and 2(b)) concerning for metastatic deposits. The nodules were not present on a chest CT performed 8 years earlier for the same indication. She was referred for thoracic surgery consultation.

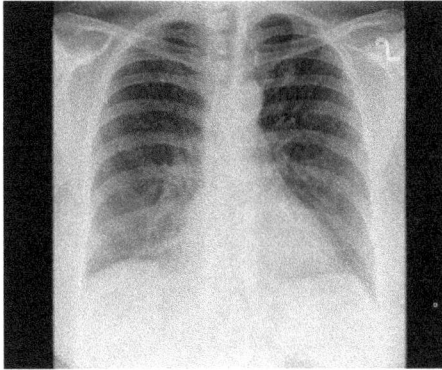

FIGURE 1: PA chest radiograph: there is a 1.3 cm nodule within the left lower lobe (arrow), projected lateral to the left cardiac border.

Subsequent mammogram and CT scan of the abdomen, pelvis, and head showed no other deposits or suggestion of a primary malignancy. She was taken to the operating room for diagnostic wedge resection of one of the nodules by VATS and a hilar lymph node biopsy. She tolerated the procedure well and was discharged from hospital on the third postoperative day without any complications. Microscopic examination of the resected nodule showed a a well-circumscribed, nonencapsulated tumor with a smooth pushing border to the surrounding lung parenchyma (Figure 3(a)). The tumor was composed predominantly of intersecting fascicles of bland smooth muscle cells without cytological atypia (Figure 3(b)). There was no necrosis and less than 1 mitotic figure per 10 high-power fields. On immunohistochemistry, the tumor cells showed strong, diffuse staining for $\alpha$-smooth muscle actin ($\alpha$-SMA) (Figure 3(c)), desmin (Figure 3(d)), and estrogen receptor. There was weak, diffuse staining for progesterone receptor. The Ki67 proliferation index was less than 1%. The findings were consistent with leiomyoma. The hilar lymph node showed reactive changes. In the context of bilateral pulmonary nodules and previously diagnosed uterine smooth muscle tumors, the clinical diagnosis was in keeping with benign metastasizing leiomyoma. Because the patient had a bilateral salpingo-oophorectomy, further growth of the nodules was not anticipated and she opted for periodic monitoring. She was well at 8-month follow-up from presentation in the emergency department, at which time repeat chest CT showed no interval change in the number or size of the pulmonary nodules.

## 3. Discussion

BML is rare, despite the high incidence of uterine leiomyomas in the general population. It occurs in women at an average age of 47 years, most of whom have undergone hysterectomy or myomectomy for uterine leiomyomas [3]. The clinical presentation of BML depends largely on its site of involvement, of which the lung is most frequent. BML involving the lung is usually asymptomatic and found incidentally on imaging, such as during staging workup for unrelated malignancies [4]. The nodules are usually found after hysterectomy or after myomectomy at durations of 3 months to 20 years [3].

BML may also be found concurrently at diagnosis of uterine leiomyomas in patients who present with leiomyoma symptoms (i.e., vaginal bleeding and abdominal or pelvic pain) [5] or in the perioperative period [6]. Uncommonly, BML involving the lung presents with a nonproductive cough or mild chest/back pain. Shortness of breath is also uncommon and tends to present late in patients when the number or size of the nodules begins to compromise lung function. Respiratory failure secondary to a large leiomyoma of the left lower lung that extended and obstructed the right mainstem bronchus has been reported [7]. Rarely, BML presents with hemoptysis [8], pneumothorax associated with lung cysts [5], hemothorax [9], or empyema [10]. Further, BML may have extrapulmonary manifestations including a systolic murmur by right ventricular metastasis [11]; abdominal pain by pelvic metastasis [12]; jaundice by metastasis to the pancreatic head [13]; arm and shoulder pain by metastatic compression of the infraclavicular brachial plexus [14]; severe low back pain and saddle anesthesia by metastasis to the S2 vertebral body with expansion into the spinal canal [15]; and abducens and hypoglossal nerve palsy by metastasis to the posterior cranial fossa [15].

BML lung nodules typically do not calcify or enhance after intravenous contrast administration [5]. They may cavitate [16] and raise additional diagnostic considerations on imaging. Pathologic examination of a BML nodule is necessary to establish the diagnosis, because it allows confirmation of a smooth muscle phenotype by immunohistochemistry (SMA-positive tumor cells). In the clinical context of a concurrent or previously diagnosed uterine smooth muscle tumor(s), a presumptive diagnosis of BML may be rendered. In the absence of history or evidence of a uterine smooth muscle tumor(s), the presumptive diagnosis is multiple fibroleiomyomatous hamartoma, which is histologically indistinguishable from BML. Definitive diagnosis requires molecular analysis of the uterine and pulmonary tumors [17], which is not performed in most cases.

The exact pathogenesis of BML is unknown. Three hypotheses have been proposed [17]: (1) BML represents proliferation of smooth muscle that is native to the lungs; (2) BML gains venous access from the trauma of myomectomy or hysterectomy; (3) BML represents a very low-grade leiomyosarcoma. The first two hypotheses are problematic because BML may involve extrapulmonary sites and may occur in the absence of uterine surgery, respectively. The third hypothesis is most widely accepted and likely reflects sampling error on grossing of the uterine smooth muscle tumor(s).

Investigation and management in the emergency department must be tailored to the particular BML presentation. As mentioned, BML involving the lung is usually asymptomatic. Its presentation as pleuritic chest pain is uncommon and invokes a broad differential diagnosis [18], the most critical of which include pneumothorax, myocardial infarction, and pulmonary embolus (PE) (Figure 4). In this case, the patient's risk of PE was low/intermediate by Wells score [19]. Without evidence of PE on CTPA, her elevated D-dimer most likely reflects the normal process of recovery after hysterectomy. In current practice, a normal D-dimer (i.e., below a cut-off value of 500 $\mu$g/L) may allow the exclusion of PE. However,

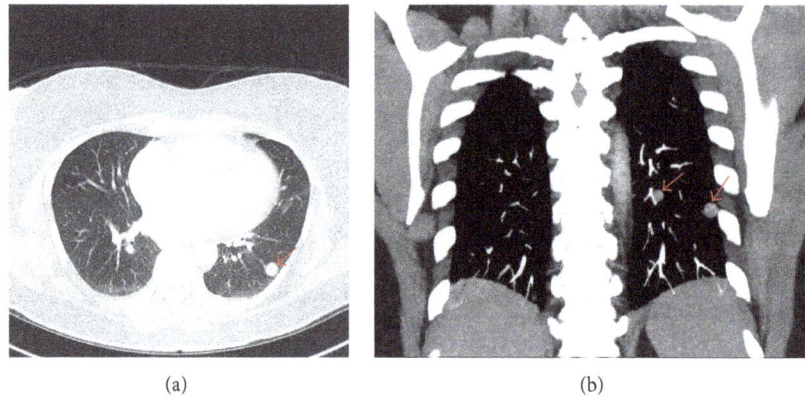

(a)     (b)

Figure 2: CT pulmonary angiogram performed the same day as the chest radiograph. (a) Axial image (lung windows): left lower lobe soft tissue nodule corresponding to the abnormality on the CXR (arrow) demonstrates no internal calcification or cavitation. Six other similar-appearing nodules of varied sizes were scattered throughout the lungs. (b) Coronal MIP image (soft tissue windows): two well-circumscribed left lower lobe nodules (arrows).

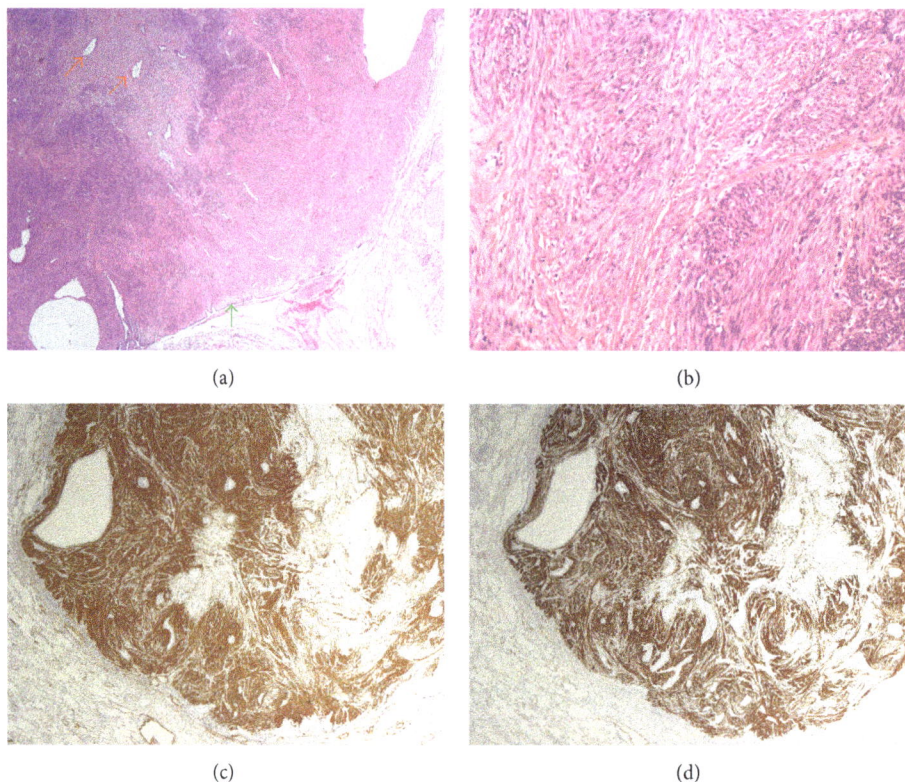

(a)     (b)

(c)     (d)

Figure 3: (a) A well-circumscribed tumor with a pushing border to the lung parenchyma (green arrow) (H&E, 40x). Note entrapped bronchiolar epithelium encircled by collagen (red arrows). (b) Bland smooth muscle cells without cytological atypia (H&E, 100x). (c) Diffuse staining (brown) for SMA (12.5x). Note negative staining (white) of collagen and bronchiolar epithelium in the tumor. (d) Diffuse staining (brown) for desmin (12.5x). There was negative tumor cell staining for p16, p53, WT-1, CD10, CD31, HMB-45, CD117/c-kit, and ALK-1 (not shown).

alternative D-dimer cut-offs may exclude PE more reliably in clinical settings where D-dimer may be elevated for another reason(s), such as older patients [20, 21], postsurgery, and malignancy.

Suspected lung metastases of unknown primary should be referred for biopsy. There is no standardized management approach for lung involvement by BML. Because most lesions stay constant in size for a long time, a wait-and-see strategy consisting of periodic serial imaging is usually reasonable. This strategy also allows detection of lesions suspicious for lung adenocarcinoma, which may be present concurrently among the BML nodules [22] or develop in the course

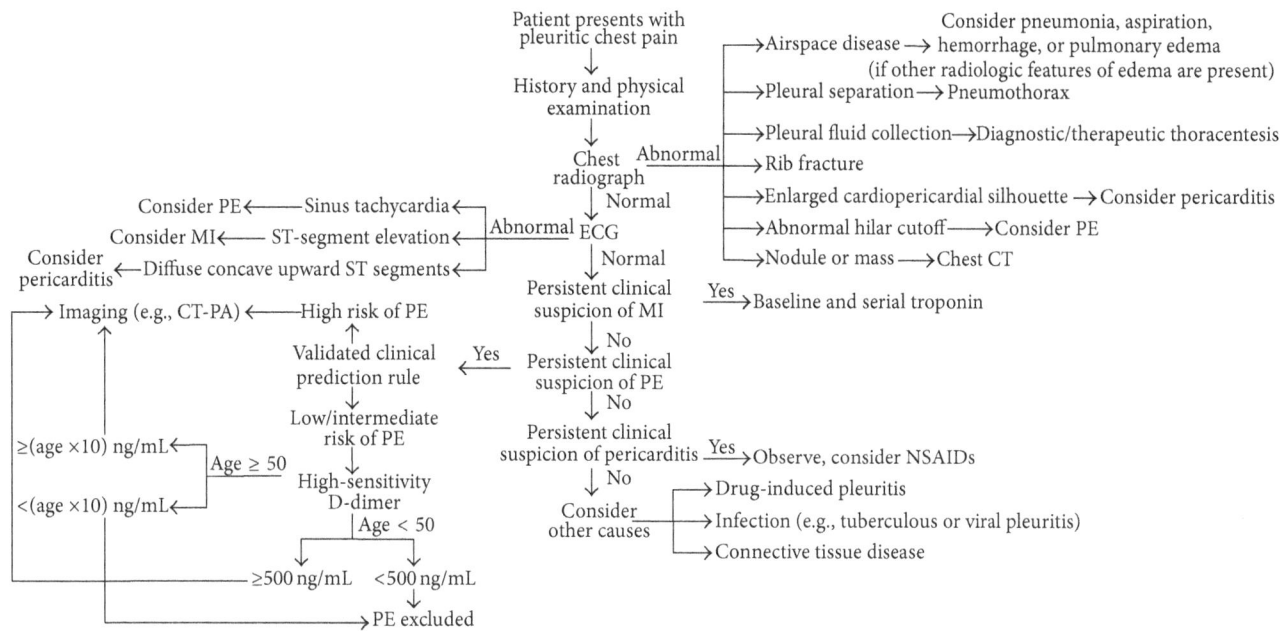

FIGURE 4: Diagnostic algorithm for pleuritic chest pain (modified from Kass et al. [18] and Cuker [21]).

of BML monitoring [23]. Surgical resection of the BML nodules, if feasible, should be considered for prophylaxis of complications observed by some authors [24]. Given the presence of estrogen and progesterone receptors [25], BML is thought to be hormonally responsive. Surgical removal of estrogen stimulation may be accomplished with bilateral oophorectomy. Alternatively, for unresectable lung nodules or patients who prefer nonsurgical management, hormonal therapeutic options that include tamoxifen, progesterone, aromatase inhibitors, luteinizing hormone-releasing hormone analogue, and estrogen receptor modulators should be considered [26, 27].

In conclusion, emergency physicians should be aware of BML and its range of clinical presentations. Although BML involving the lung is usually asymptomatic and found incidentally, it may be present with emergent symptoms. BML should be considered in women of reproductive age with current or previously diagnosed uterine smooth muscle tumor(s) who are found to have multiple pulmonary nodules in the absence of pertinent history, risk factors, or localizing findings suggestive of metastasis from other primary site.

## Abbreviations

ABG: Arterial blood gas
ALK-1: Anaplastic lymphoma kinase-1
Bcl-2: B-cell lymphoma-2
BMI: Body mass index
BML: Benign metastasizing leiomyoma
CD: Cluster of differentiation
CT: Computed tomography
CTPA: Computed tomography pulmonary angiogram
CXR: Chest X-ray
ECG: Electrocardiogram

FEU: Fibrinogen equivalent units
H&E: Hematoxylin and eosin
HMB-45: Human melanoma black-45
MI: Myocardial infarction
MIP: Maximum intensity projection
NSAID: Nonsteroidal anti-inflammatory drug
PA: Posterior-anterior
PE: Pulmonary embolus
SMA: Smooth muscle actin
VATS: Video-assisted thoracic surgery
WT-1: Wilms tumor-1.

## Consent

Written consent has been obtained from the patient and is available upon request.

## Conflict of Interests

The authors declare that there is no conflict of interests regarding the publication of this paper.

## References

[1] M. R. Nucci, R. Drapkin, P. D. Cin, C. D. M. Fletcher, and J. A. Fletcher, "Distinctive cytogenetic profile in benign metastasizing leiomyoma: pathogenetic implications," *The American Journal of Surgical Pathology*, vol. 31, no. 5, pp. 737–743, 2007.

[2] R. Maredia, B. J. Snyder, L. A. C. Harvey, and A. M. Schwartz, "Benign metastasizing leiomyoma in the lung," *Radiographics*, vol. 18, no. 3, pp. 779–782, 1998.

[3] S. Abramson, R. C. Gilkeson, J. D. Goldstein, P. K. Woodard, R. Eisenberg, and N. Abramson, "Benign metastasizing leiomyoma: clinical, imaging, and pathologic correlation," *American Journal of Roentgenology*, vol. 176, no. 6, pp. 1409–1413, 2001.

[4] Z. J. del Real-Romo, C. Montero-Cantú, O. Villegas-Cabello et al., "Incidental benign metastasizing leiomyoma in a patient with bone sarcoma: a case report," *Case Reports in Surgery*, vol. 2014, Article ID 439061, 4 pages, 2014.

[5] J. Wongsripuemtet, R. Ruangchira-Urai, E. J. Stern, J. P. Kanne, and N. Muangman, "Benign metastasizing leiomyoma," *Journal of Thoracic Imaging*, vol. 27, no. 2, pp. W41–W43, 2012.

[6] A. S. Rege, J. A. Snyder, and W. J. Scott, "Benign metastasizing leiomyoma: a rare cause of multiple pulmonary nodules," *Annals of Thoracic Surgery*, vol. 93, no. 6, pp. E149–E151, 2012.

[7] T. Uyama, Y. Monden, M. Harada, M. Sumitomo, and S. Kimura, "Pulmonary leiomyomatosis showing endobronchial extension and giant cyst formation," *Chest*, vol. 94, no. 3, pp. 644–646, 1988.

[8] E. Y. Ki, S. J. Hwang, K. H. Lee, J. S. Park, and S. Y. Hur, "Benign metastasizing leiomyoma of the lung," *World Journal of Surgical Oncology*, vol. 11, article 279, 2013.

[9] A. M. Ponea, C. P. Marak, H. Goraya, and A. K. Guddati, "Benign metastatic leiomyoma presenting as a hemothorax," *Case Reports in Oncological Medicine*, vol. 2013, Article ID 504589, 6 pages, 2013.

[10] H. Moon, S. J. Park, H. B. Lee et al., "Pulmonary benign metastasizing leiomyoma in a postmenopausal woman," *The American Journal of the Medical Sciences*, vol. 338, no. 1, pp. 72–74, 2009.

[11] S. D. Galvin, B. Wademan, J. Chu, and R. W. Bunton, "Benign metastasizing leiomyoma: a rare metastatic lesion in the right ventricle," *Annals of Thoracic Surgery*, vol. 89, no. 1, pp. 279–281, 2010.

[12] H. Wei, Y. Liu, H. Sun, F. Qian, and G. Li, "Benign pelvic metastatic leiomyoma: case report," *Clinical and Experimental Obstetrics and Gynecology*, vol. 40, no. 1, pp. 165–167, 2013.

[13] C.-Y. Jiang, W. Wang, and Z.-R. Yuan, "A rare pancreatic tumor in a 52-year-old chinese woman. Pancreatic benign metastasizing," *Gastroenterology*, vol. 144, no. 3, pp. 659–660, 2013.

[14] G. C. W. de Ruiter, B. W. Scheithauer, K. K. Amrami, and R. J. Spinner, "Benign metastasizing leiomyomatosis with massive brachial plexus involvement mimicking neurofibromatosis type 1," *Clinical Neuropathology*, vol. 25, no. 6, pp. 282–287, 2006.

[15] G. Alessi, M. Lemmerling, L. Vereecken, and L. de Waele, "Benign metastasizing leiomyoma to skull base and spine: a report of two cases," *Clinical Neurology and Neurosurgery*, vol. 105, no. 3, pp. 170–174, 2003.

[16] A. A. Loukeri, I. N. Pantazopoulos, R. Tringidou et al., "Benign metastasizing leiomyoma presenting as cavitating lung nodules," *Respiratory Care*, vol. 59, no. 7, pp. e94–e97, 2014.

[17] L. Tietze, K. Günther, A. Hörbe et al., "Benign metastasizing leiomyoma: a cytogenetically balanced but clonal disease," *Human Pathology*, vol. 31, no. 1, pp. 126–128, 2000.

[18] S. M. Kass, P. M. Williams, and B. V. Reamy, "Pleurisy," *American Family Physician*, vol. 75, no. 9, pp. 1357–1364, 2007.

[19] P. S. Wells, D. R. Anderson, M. Rodger et al., "Derivation of a simple clinical model to categorize patients probability of pulmonary embolism: increasing the models utility with the SimpliRED D-dimer," *Thrombosis and Haemostasis*, vol. 83, no. 3, pp. 416–420, 2000.

[20] M. Righini, J. Van Es, P. L. Den Exter et al., "Age-adjusted D-dimer cutoff levels to rule out pulmonary embolism: the ADJUST-PE study," *Journal of the American Medical Association*, vol. 311, no. 11, pp. 1117–1124, 2014.

[21] A. Cuker, "A D-dimer cutoff for excluding PE: one size does not fit all," *The Hematologist*, vol. 11, no. 5, p. 8, 2014.

[22] M. Naito, T. Kobayashi, M. Yoshida et al., "Solitary pulmonary nodule of benign metastasizing leiomyoma associated with primary lung cancer: a case report," *Journal of Medical Case Reports*, vol. 5, article 500, 2011.

[23] Y. Tsunoda, K. Tanaka, and M. Hagiwara, "A case of benign metastasizing leiomyoma of the lung complicated with primary lung cancer," *Japanese Journal of Lung Cancer*, vol. 49, no. 4, pp. 445–449, 2009.

[24] K. Hoetzenecker, H. J. Ankersmit, C. Aigner et al., "Consequences of a wait-and-see strategy for benign metastasizing leiomyomatosis of the lung," *Annals of Thoracic Surgery*, vol. 87, no. 2, pp. 613–614, 2009.

[25] G. Jautzke, E. Müller-Ruchholtz, and U. Thalmann, "Immunohistological detection of estrogen and progesterone receptors in multiple and well differentiated leiomyomatous lung tumors in women with uterine leiomyomas (so-called benign metastasizing leiomyomas): a report on 5 cases," *Pathology Research and Practice*, vol. 192, no. 3, pp. 215–223, 1996.

[26] J. A. Rivera, S. Christopoulos, D. Small, and M. Trifiro, "Hormonal manipulation of benign metastasizing leiomyomas: report of two cases and review of the literature," *Journal of Clinical Endocrinology and Metabolism*, vol. 89, no. 7, pp. 3183–3188, 2004.

[27] E. I. Lewis, R. J. Chason, A. H. DeCherney, A. Armstrong, J. Elkas, and A. M. Venkatesan, "Novel hormone treatment of benign metastasizing leiomyoma: an analysis of five cases and literature review," *Fertility and Sterility*, vol. 99, no. 7, pp. 2017–2024, 2013.

# Incidental Finding of Inferior Vena Cava Atresia Presenting with Deep Venous Thrombosis following Physical Exertion

**Shalini Koppisetty,**[1] **Alton G. Smith,**[1] **and Ravneet K. Dhillon**[2]

[1]*Department of Radiology, Beaumont Health System, Grosse Pointe, MI 48230, USA*
[2]*Emergency Medicine, Henry Ford Health System, West Bloomfield, MI 48322, USA*

Correspondence should be addressed to Shalini Koppisetty; shalini.koppisetty@beaumont.org

Academic Editor: Serdar Kula

Inferior vena cava atresia (IVCA) is a rare but well described vascular anomaly. It is a rare risk factor for deep venous thrombosis (DVT), found in approximately 5% of cases of unprovoked lower extremity (LE) DVT in patients <30 years of age. Affected population is in the early thirties, predominantly male, often with a history of major physical exertion and presents with extensive or bilateral DVTs. Patients with IVC anomalies usually develop compensatory circulation through the collateral veins with enlarged azygous/hemizygous veins. Despite the compensatory circulation, the venous drainage of the lower limbs is often insufficient leading to venous stasis and thrombosis. We describe a case of extensive and bilateral deep venous thrombosis following physical exertion in a thirty-six-year-old male patient with incidental finding of IVCA on imaging.

## 1. Introduction

Inferior vena cava atresia (IVCA) is an extremely rare vascular anomaly with an estimated prevalence of approximately 1% in general population [1]. It is also called IVC agenesis or aplasia. IVCA is found in approximately 5% of cases of unprovoked lower extremity (LE) deep venous thrombosis (DVT) in young adults, significantly occurring before the fourth decade of life [2].

## 2. Case Presentation

A previously healthy thirty-six-year-old male presented to the emergency department with acute onset of shortness of breath and diffuse bilateral lower extremity pain and swelling for two days. Patient was dancing for two hours in a party and the following day woke up with severe bilateral lower extremity and lumbar pain. The patient eventually developed shortness of breath and worsening pain in his legs and back. Past medical history and family history were insignificant.

*2.1. Hospital Course.* On arrival, the patient's vitals were as follows: blood pressure 130/100, pulse 88. Respiratory rate was 20, oxygen saturation 100% on room air. On physical examination there was bilateral lower extremity swelling, tenderness, tense skin, and blotchy purplish discoloration of both legs. Additional lab work including prothrombin time, basic metabolic profile, and complete blood picture was unremarkable. Venous Duplex scan of LE revealed extensive, bilateral DVT. Computer tomography (CT) scan of the chest was negative for pulmonary embolism.

*2.2. Bilateral Venous Duplex Ultrasound Lower Extremity.* Total occluding acute thrombosis of right external iliac vein, right and left common femoral vein, right and left femoral veins, right and left greater saphenous vein, right and left small saphenous vein, right and left popliteal vein, right and left gastrocnemius vein, left peroneal veins, right and left posterior tibial veins, and right and left soleal vein was observed.

*2.3. CT Scan of the Chest, Abdomen, and Pelvis with Contrast.* Approximately 5.7 × 4.1 cm right retroperitoneal mass at the level of L3 adjacent to the IVC, differential, would be large venous varix or lymph node (Figure 1). Atretic intrahepatic portion of the IVC with multiple collaterals is seen in

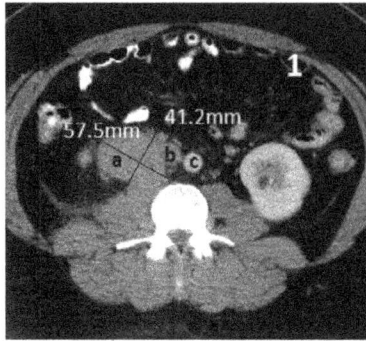

FIGURE 1: Abdomen CT axial view: (a) inferior vena cava (IVC) varix measuring 57.5 mm × 41.2 mm, (b) IVC, and (c) aorta.

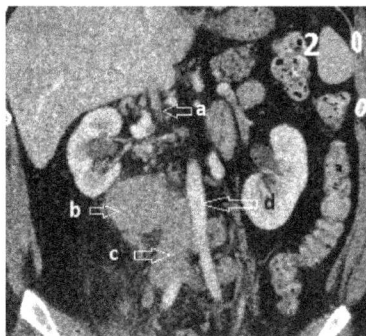

FIGURE 2: Abdomen CT coronal view: (a) atretic intrahepatic IVC, (b) IVC venous varix, (c) thrombosed IVC, and (d) aorta.

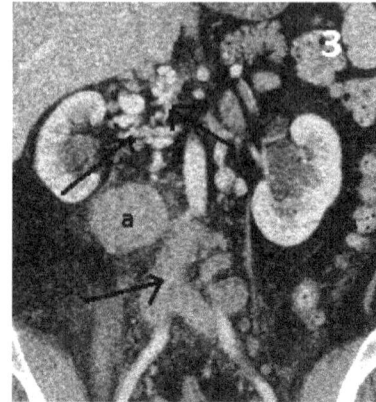

FIGURE 3: Abdomen CT coronal view: (a) IVC venous varix. Arrows pointing enlarged, multiple retroperitoneal/paralumbar collateral veins.

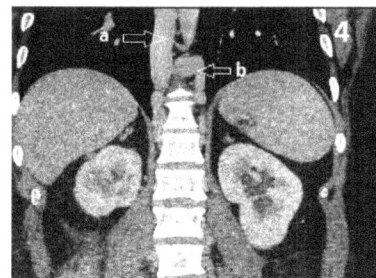

FIGURE 4: Abdomen CT coronal view: (a) enlarged azygous vein, (b) enlarged hemizygous vein.

the retroperitoneum as well as a dilated hemiazygous and azygous system and response to the atretic intrahepatic IVC (Figures 2, 3, and 4).

*2.4. Treatment.* Patient was transferred to surgical unit for pharmacomechanical catheter-directed thrombolysis (PCDT). Patient underwent a venogram, ultrasound guided venous puncture bilateral popliteal veins, sheath placement, and placement of bilateral Ekos infusion catheters. He received continuous thrombolysis with tissue plasminogen activator (tPA) and heparin infusions. Subsequent venogram showed moderate improvement in bilateral venous flow. Balloon angioplasty was performed on the bilateral common iliac veins with subsequent sluggish venous flow. Mechanical thrombectomy of left and right iliac veins was then performed using Trellis device with infusion of tPA on both sides. Serial fibrinogen levels were monitored during the procedure. Final venogram showed patency of the iliac veins and lower IVC with persistent but improved sluggish flow. Patient was discharged home on oral Xarelto (rivaroxaban) and compression stockings.

*2.5. Outcome and Follow-Up.* Magnetic resonance imaging (MRI) of the abdomen with and without contrast performed after 2 weeks confirmed the retroperitoneal mass most likely related to large thrombosed venous varix. The IVC was patent and of normal caliber at and above the level of the hepatic

veins. IVC above the level of the renal veins was occluded with multiple collaterals. The left renal vein was small in caliber but patent. There was a small amount of residual eccentric nonocclusive thrombus within the right external iliac vein. Patient was in regular follow-up for one year without any recurrent DVT.

*2.6. Diagnosis.* Diagnosis of the patient was as follows: (1) inferior vena cava atresia and (2) deep venous thrombosis, bilateral lower limbs.

## 3. Discussion

Inferior vena cava anomalies are rare and have an estimated prevalence of 0.07% to 8.7% in general population [2]. IVC atresia is a type of IVC anomaly and accounts for up to 5% of unprovoked DVTs in young patients aged 20–40 years. IVC atresia can be congenital or acquired and is thought to be due to embryonic dysgenesis or thrombosis during the intrauterine or perinatal period [2, 3]. During embryogenesis (6–8 weeks of gestation), the IVC is formed by the fusion of three sets of paired veins (posterior cardinal, subcardinal, and supracardinal veins) [4]. Failure of these paired veins to fuse into a unilateral right-sided venous structure results in anomaly of IVC. Patients with IVCA develop a robust collateral deep venous system with or without azygous and hemizygous continuation of the IVC. Lambert et al. propose that the collaterals are unable to cope with the demands of increasing blood flow, thereby generating venous stasis, ulceration, and recurrent DVT [5]. Most of the patients with IVCA are asymptomatic and detected incidentally during radiological procedures or abdominal surgery [6]. Common symptoms are lower extremity pain, swelling, ulcers, and sometimes nonspecific pain in the lower back and abdomen. Pulmonary embolism is not a frequent finding with IVCA, because the emboli get trapped in the azygous/hemizygous system preventing it from reaching the pulmonary circulation [5]. The characteristic findings of IVCA-DVT include occurrence before the fourth decade of life, male predominance, extensive or bilateral LE DVT, and history of major physical exertion [5, 7, 8]. The DVT most frequently involves the distal IVC, common, internal, and external iliac and femoral veins [8]. Data suggests that approximately one-third of patients with IVCA had associated hypercoagulability disorders [9]; hence screening is recommended for any coagulation abnormalities. IVC anomalies can cause diagnostic problems because of tumor like appearance of the enlarged azygous or collateral veins on imaging, which was indeed what happened in this case. Our patient had a nonspecific retroperitoneal mass at the level of L3 on CT scan of the abdomen, which was confirmed most likely as a venous varix of IVC on MRI. Although ultrasound and venography are excellent tools in identification of DVT, they can often miss the diagnosis of IVCA. CT or MRI studies are more effective in identifying IVC anomalies and are recommended if there is history of unprovoked DVT in younger patients. Review of the literature revealed that IVC anomalies may be associated with renal anomalies, with a handful of case reports reported in literature. Most of these cases had absent IVC with renal anomalies involving the right kidney (agenesis, hypoplasia, and aplasia). Gayer et al. reported the occurrence of congenital anomalies of the IVC and right renal aplasia in three patients detected on CT scan. The authors proposed that the association between absent IVC and right renal anomalies was not coincidental and may be due to abnormal embryogenesis [10]. Absent IVC can lead to impaired venous drainage of the right metanephros, resulting in right kidney abnormalities. The left metanephros drain via gonadal vein and lumbar perforators, leading to less common involvement of the left kidney. However there are few reported cases of absent IVC with left renal hypoplasia and atrophy [11–13]. Van Veen et al. suggested the term KILT syndrome, due to the occurrence of kidney and IVC abnormalities associated with leg thrombosis [11]. There are no standard guidelines for the treatment of IVCA-DVT and further research is required on optimal treatment strategies. Patients are initially treated with intravenous heparin followed by oral anticoagulation. Recently, Broholm et al. described the efficacy of catheter directed thrombolysis (CDT) for rapid thrombus removal in patients with IVCA with acute DVT, especially involving iliofemoral venous thrombosis [14]. Further the authors proposed that CDT provides immediate symptom relief and significantly decrease thrombus burden that may otherwise takes days to weeks to resolve with systemic anticoagulation alone [14]. In patients with extensive iliofemoral DVT, pharmacomechanical catheter directed thrombolysis (PCDT), which refers to the combination of mechanical thrombectomy and CDT, has been shown to significantly decrease the thrombus burden, incidence of recurrent DVT, and incidence of post thrombotic syndrome compared to systemic anticoagulation alone [15]. Observational studies demonstrated promising results with PCDT; however more research trials are necessary to look into long term efficacy [16–19]. Patients are strongly advised to wear elastic stocking support and leg elevation and also avoid risk factors such as excessive physical exertion, prolonged immobilization, smoking, and hormonal contraceptive use [5, 8]. Long term anticoagulation may be required if associated with hereditary thrombophilia and other risk factors due to risk of recurrent thrombosis.

## 4. Conclusion

It is essential for physicians to consider the possibility of IVC anomalies in a young adult presenting with unexplained, extensive, or bilateral LE DVT. The diagnosis can be challenging and requires detailed imaging studies with computed tomography and magnetic resonance imaging to identify IVC anomalies. Further diagnostic workup and management should be considered for any coagulation abnormalities and long term anticoagulation. Pharmacomechanical catheter-directed thrombolysis followed by systemic anticoagulation seems a promising therapy with significant reduction of thrombus burden.

## Conflict of Interests

The authors declare that there is no conflict of interests regarding the publication of this paper.

## References

[1] S. Eifert, J. L. Villavicencio, T.-C. Kao, B. M. Taute, and N. M. Rich, "Prevalence of deep venous anomalies in congenital vascular malformations of venous predominance," *Journal of Vascular Surgery*, vol. 31, no. 3, pp. 462–471, 2000.

[2] A. Obernosterer, M. Aschauer, W. Schnedl, and R. W. Lipp, "Anomalies of the inferior vena cava in patients with iliac venous thrombosis," *Annals of Internal Medicine*, vol. 136, no. 1, pp. 37–41, 2002.

[3] T. Ramanathan, T. M. D. Hughes, and A. J. Richardson, "Perinatal inferior vena cava thrombosis and absence of the infrarenal inferior vena cava," *Journal of Vascular Surgery*, vol. 33, no. 5, pp. 1097–1099, 2001.

[4] K. L. Moore and T. V. N. Persaud, *The Developing Human: Clinically Oriented Embryology*, Saunders, Philadelphia, Pa, USA, 6th edition, 1998.

[5] M. Lambert, P. Marboeuf, M. Midulla et al., "Inferior vena cava agenesis and deep vein thrombosis: 10 patients and review of the literature," *Vascular Medicine*, vol. 15, no. 6, pp. 451–459, 2010.

[6] N. L. Shah, C. J. Shanley, M. R. Prince, and T. W. Wakefield, "Deep venous thrombosis complicating a congenital absence of the inferior vena cava," *Surgery*, vol. 120, no. 5, pp. 891–896, 1996.

[7] K. Atmatzidis, B. Papaziogas, T. Pavlidis, G. Paraskevas, C. Mirelis, and T. Papaziogas, "Surgical images: soft tissue: reccurent deep vein thrombosis caused by hypoplasia of the inferior vena cava," *Canadian Journal of Surgery*, vol. 49, no. 4, article 285, 2006.

[8] S. Cizginer, S. Tatli, J. Girshman, J. A. Beckman, and S. G. Silverman, "Thrombosed interrupted inferior vena cava and retroaortic left renal vein mimicking retroperitoneal neoplasm," *Abdominal Imaging*, vol. 32, no. 3, pp. 403–406, 2007.

[9] D. B. O'Connor, N. O'Brien, T. Khani, and S. Sheehan, "Superficial and deep vein thrombosis associated with congenital absence of the infrahepatic inferior vena cava in a young male patient," *Annals of Vascular Surgery*, vol. 25, no. 5, pp. 697.el–697.e4, 2011.

[10] G. Gayer, R. Zissin, S. Strauss, and M. Hertz, "IVC anomalies and right renal aplasia detected on CT: a possible link?" *Abdominal Imaging*, vol. 28, no. 3, pp. 395–399, 2003.

[11] J. Van Veen, K. K. Hampton, and M. Makris, "Kilt syndrome?" *British Journal of Haematology*, vol. 118, no. 4, pp. 1199–1200, 2002.

[12] J. Iqbal and E. Nagaraju, "Congenital absence of inferior vena cava and thrombosis: a case report," *Journal of Medical Case Reports*, vol. 2, article 46, 2008.

[13] R. A. Lawless and D. A. Dangleben, "Caval agenesis with a hypoplastic left kidney in a patient with trauma on warfarin for deep vein thrombosis," *Vascular and Endovascular Surgery*, vol. 46, no. 1, pp. 75–76, 2012.

[14] R. Broholm, M. Jorgensen, S. Just, L. P. Jensen, and N. Bækgaard, "Acute iliofemoral venous thrombosis in patients with atresia of the inferior vena cava can be treated successfully with catheter-directed thrombolysis," *Journal of Vascular and Interventional Radiology*, vol. 22, no. 6, pp. 801–805, 2011.

[15] A. J. Comerota and M. H. Gravett, "Iliofemoral venous thrombosis," *Journal of Vascular Surgery*, vol. 46, no. 5, pp. 1065–1076, 2007.

[16] R. L. Bush, P. H. Lin, J. T. Bates, L. Mureebe, W. Zhou, and A. B. Lumsden, "Pharmacomechanical thrombectomy for treatment of symptomatic lower extremity deep venous thrombosis: safety and feasibility study," *Journal of Vascular Surgery*, vol. 40, no. 5, pp. 965–970, 2004.

[17] H. S. Kim, A. Patra, B. E. Paxton, J. Khan, and M. B. Streiff, "Adjunctive percutaneous mechanical thrombectomy for lower-extremity deep vein thrombosis: clinical and economic outcomes," *Journal of Vascular and Interventional Radiology*, vol. 17, no. 7, pp. 1099–1104, 2006.

[18] P. H. Lin, W. Zhou, A. Dardik et al., "Catheter-direct thrombolysis versus pharmacomechanical thrombectomy for treatment of symptomatic lower extremity deep venous thrombosis," *The American Journal of Surgery*, vol. 192, no. 6, pp. 782–788, 2006.

[19] S. Vedantham, T. M. Vesely, G. A. Sicard et al., "Pharmacomechanical thrombolysis and early stent placement for iliofemoral deep vein thrombosis," *Journal of Vascular and Interventional Radiology*, vol. 15, no. 6, pp. 565–574, 2004.

# Ovarian Hyperstimulation Syndrome, the Master of Disguise?

**Emily Charlotte Ironside and Andrew James Hotchen**

*Oxford University Hospitals, Headley Way, Headington, Oxford OX3 9DU, UK*

Correspondence should be addressed to Andrew James Hotchen; andy.hotchen@gmail.com

Academic Editor: Yuh-Feng Wang

The use of IVF has risen dramatically over the past 10 years and with this the complications of such treatments have also risen. One such complication is ovarian hyperstimulation syndrome with which patients can present acutely to hospital with shortness of breath. On admission, a series of blood tests are routinely performed, including the d-dimer. We present a case of a 41-year-old lady who had recently undergone IVF and presented with chest pain and dyspnoea. In the emergency department, a d-dimer returned as mildly elevated. Consequential admission onto MAU initiated several avoidable investigations for venous thromboembolism. Careful examination elicited a mild ascites and a thorough drug history gave recent low molecular weight heparin usage. Ultrasound scan of the abdomen subsequently confirmed the diagnosis of severe OHSS. The d-dimer should therefore be used to negate and not to substantiate a diagnosis of VTE. This case report aims to highlight the importance of OHSS as an uncommon cause of dyspnoea but whose prevalence is likely to increase in the forthcoming years. We discuss the complications of the misdiagnosis of OHSS, the physiology behind raised d-dimers, and the potential harm from incorrect treatment or inappropriate imaging.

## 1. Introduction

Ovarian hyperstimulation syndrome (OHSS) is a well-recognized iatrogenic complication of assisted conception techniques, including *in vitro* fertilization (IVF) [1]. Although the majority of presentations are mild, severe cases can result in systemic capillary leakage, causing life-threatening complications such as thromboembolic phenomena and multiple organ dysfunctions [2].

OHSS is common, occurring in mild forms in 33% of IVF cycles and in moderate or severe forms in 3% to 8% of IVF cycles [3]. Although it can occur in all age groups, it is less common in women over the age of 39 years [4]. In the last 10 years, in the United States, there has been a 50% increase in the number of IVF treatments in women over 41 years of age [5]. OHSS is particularly topical following a recent update of guidelines in the United Kingdom, which extends the age of those who can receive treatment to 42 years [6]. This recent increase in the usage of IVF will inevitably result in a rise in the number of cases of OHSS seen in the emergency department (ED). Ultimately, this will give the emergency physician an important role in expediting and optimizing treatment for these patients. On admission to the ED, a plethora of blood investigations are requested for those who present with acute shortness of breath including complete blood count, urea and electrolytes, troponin, and a d-dimer. The results of these investigations need to be interpreted with care as misinterpretation can lead to serious consequences for the patient and a delay in treatment.

We report a case of OHSS that was initially misdiagnosed in the ED, attributable to a mildly raised d-dimer, resulting in transfer to the inappropriate specialty and incorrect treatment being commenced. We discuss the potential complications for misdiagnosis of OHSS and the pathophysiology behind the raised d-dimer. This case report highlights an important message for the emergency physician and raises awareness of this increasingly common iatrogenic condition.

## 2. Case Report

A 41-year-old woman, undergoing her second cycle of IVF treatment, presented to the ED with acute chest pain. The chest pain was central, was worse on inspiration, and was not induced or exacerbated by exercise. The patient had associated dyspnea and observations revealed oxygen saturations to be 90% on air. Her thrombogenic risk factors

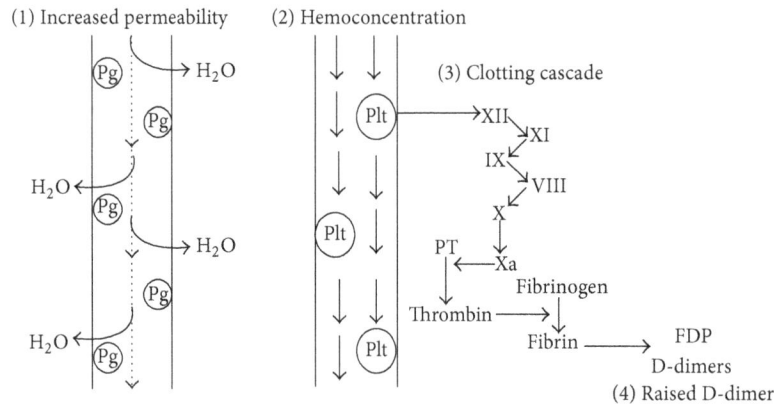

FIGURE 1: Schematic illustration of how OHSS causes a rise in d-dimers. Pg = prostaglandin; Plt = platelets; FDP = fibrin degradation productions; PT = prothrombin. (1) Dotted arrow represents normal blood flow. Prostaglandins are increased in OHSS which causes increased capillary permeability. This forces water out of the capillaries and into the tissues. (2) Loss of water causes hemoconcentration of the blood which is represented by thick arrows. Due to this, activation of platelets occurs. (3) Activation of platelets causes activation of the clotting cascade (simplified without the activated factors). (4) The final products of the coagulation cascade are fibrin degradation products which can be measured in the blood as d-dimers.

included reduced immobility due to back pain and recent IVF [7]. Past medical history included one failed cycle of IVF and a recent embryo implantation in her second IVF cycle. Examination revealed a woman in substantial pain, with associated tachypnea, tachycardia, and bilateral reduction in air entry to the lung bases.

The presence of thrombogenic risk factors and the clinical presentation gave the patient a modified Wells score of six, rendering pulmonary embolus a likely diagnosis [8]. Consequently, the patient was placed on high flow oxygen and routine bloods, a d-dimer, and a clotting profile were requested. The d-dimer returned as mildly raised (430 mg/L, upper limit of normal in our laboratory was 250 mg/L) and the patient was sent to the medical admissions unit (MAU) for further clerking and therapeutic thromboembolic treatment.

In the MAU, two important inconsistencies with the original assessment were established. Firstly, the chest pain appeared to be epigastric and was associated with new onset abdominal bloating. Secondly, a thorough drug history highlighted that the patient had been taking a low molecular weight heparin following her previous IVF failure. These findings significantly reduced the likelihood of a pulmonary embolus. Consequently, beta-human chorionic gonadotropin (beta-hCG) levels and abdominal ultrasound scan were requested. The beta-hCG returned as raised and the scan revealed bilateral ovarian enlargement, ascites, and a right-sided pleural effusion, uniting the symptoms and thus confirming the diagnosis of severe OHSS.

Subsequently, the patient was transferred to gynecology where she was closely monitored. During her stay, the ascites reduced, the shortness of breath improved and the following week, she was discharged home with no symptoms.

## 3. Discussion

This case has illustrated a diagnosis that is important in patients who are of reproductive age. We have reported a case

of severe OHSS which was mistaken for thromboembolic disease due to an inadequate history combined with a reliance on blood tests that could have potentially led to serious complications.

The complications of OHSS depend on the severity of the condition although a misdiagnosis and mistreatment can potentially become fatal. Complications from mild cases are usually self-limiting. In the more severe forms, fluid shifts can lead to dehydration resulting in acute kidney injury, multiple organ failure, and adult respiratory distress syndrome. Dehydration also increases the risk of thromboembolic phenomena and this occurs in 0.7% to 10% of OHSS patients [9]. Thromboembolic disease is therefore an important condition to rule out in any potential patient who has had assisted reproductive technologies (ART). This promotes the rationale behind the referral of our patient to the MAU with a suspected pulmonary embolus. However, it also highlights the importance of taking a thorough medication history, which revealed that the patient had recently been started on a low-molecular weight heparin in addition to thromboembolic stockings, two factors that reduce the risk of a thromboembolic disease.

In OHSS, the pathophysiology behind the raised d-dimer is thought to be due to an elevation of prostaglandins, which increase vascular permeability and result in extravasation of fluids into the third space. Extravasation leads to hemoconcentration, which in turn increases serum viscosity and slows blood flow. The hematological changes increase endothelial adherence of platelets and activate the coagulation cascade. In order to prevent the formation of thrombi, the body generates endogenous hormones to dissolve the fibrin clot. This ultimately increases fibrin degradation products which are measured as the d-dimer [10]. This whole process is illustrated in Figure 1.

This case imparts an important lesson regarding the interpretation of the investigations performed in the ED, especially the d-dimer. D-dimers are fibrin degradation products, which have a high sensitivity but low specificity. They can be elevated in a plethora of conditions including infection, inflammatory disease, malignancy, OHSS, and pregnancy [11]. In this case, the d-dimer was used to substantiate the diagnosis of a thromboembolic disease. Acting on a raised d-dimer is of particular significance as radiological investigations, which are often required for diagnoses of emboli, could be harmful to both the expectant mother and her fetus [12]. This supports the use of d-dimers only to rule out a pulmonary embolus and not to substantiate the history and clinical findings. The case also highlights that there is a relationship between thromboembolic disease and OHSS and that both conditions need to be considered when treated patients have undergone ART. This needs to be highlighted so that vital treatments are not omitted with potentially life threatening complications.

## 4. Why Should an Emergency Physician Be Aware of This?

Shortness of breath is a common presenting complaint to the ED. For this, it is important to consider multiple etiologies for abnormal blood results, especially d-dimers. D-dimer testing is useful only for negating and not substantiating a diagnosis of pulmonary embolism. This case report aims to highlight the importance of OHSS as an uncommon cause of dyspnea, but whose prevalence is likely to increase in the forthcoming years as a number of ART procedures are performed.

## Conflict of Interests

The authors declare no conflict of interests for this study.

## References

[1] R. Klemetti, T. Sevón, M. Gissler, and E. Hemminki, "Complications of IVF and ovulation induction," *Human Reproduction*, vol. 20, no. 12, pp. 3293–3300, 2005.

[2] J. A. Stewart, P. J. Hamilton, and A. P. Murdoch, "Thromboembolic disease associated with ovarian stimulation and assisted conception techniques," *Human Reproduction*, vol. 12, no. 10, pp. 2167–2173, 1997.

[3] A. Delvinge and S. Rozenberg, "Epidemiology and prevention of ovarian hyperstimulation syndrome (OHSS): a review," *Human Reproduction Update*, vol. 8, no. 6, pp. 559–577, 2002.

[4] L. F. J. M. M. Bancsi, F. J. M. Broekmans, M. J. C. Eijkemans, F. H. de Jong, J. D. F. Habbema, and E. R. Te Velde, "Predictors of poor ovarian response in in vitro fertilization: a prospective study comparing basal markers of ovarian reserve," *Fertility and Sterility*, vol. 77, no. 2, pp. 328–336, 2002.

[5] SartCors, "Clinical Summary Report," 2014, https://www.sart-corsonline.com/.

[6] NICE, *Fertility: Assessment and Treatment or People with Fertility Problems. Clinical Guidelines*, vol. 156, NICE, 2013.

[7] M. H. Aurousseau, M. M. Samama, A. Belhassen, F. Herve, and J. N. Hugues, "Risk of thromboembolism in relation to an in-vitro fertilization programme: three case reports," *Human Reproduction*, vol. 10, no. 1, pp. 94–97, 1995.

[8] P. S. Wells, J. S. Ginsberg, D. R. Anderson et al., "Use of a clinical model for safe management of patients with suspected pulmonary embolism," *Annals of Internal Medicine*, vol. 129, no. 12, pp. 997–1005, 1998.

[9] A. Delvigne and S. Rozenberg, "Review of clinical course and treatment of ovarian hyperstimulation syndrome (OHSS)," *Human Reproduction Update*, vol. 9, no. 1, pp. 77–96, 2003.

[10] M. M. Alper, L. P. Smith, and E. S. Sills, "Ovarian hyperstimulation syndrome: current views on pathophysiology, risk factors, prevention, and management," *Journal of Experimental and Clinical Assisted Reproduction*, vol. 6, article 3, 2009.

[11] G. Y. H. Lip and G. D. Lowe, "Fibrin D-dimer: a useful clinical marker of thrombogenesis?" *Clinical Science*, vol. 89, no. 3, pp. 205–214, 1995.

[12] M. Moradi, "Pulmonary thromboembolism in pregnancy: diagnostic imaging and related consideration," *Journal of Research in Medical Sciences*, vol. 18, no. 3, pp. 255–259, 2013.

# Acute Headache at Emergency Department: Reversible Cerebral Vasoconstriction Syndrome Complicated by Subarachnoid Haemorrhage and Cerebral Infarction

M. Yger,[1,2] C. Zavanone,[1,3] L. Abdennour,[4] W. Koubaa,[4] F. Clarençon,[2,5]
S. Dupont,[2,3,6] and Y. Samson[1,2]

[1]Unité Neurovasculaire, Hôpital de la Pitie-Salpetrière, APHP, 75013 Paris, France
[2]Université Pierre et Marie Curie, 75006 Paris, France
[3]Service de Rééducation Neurologique, Hôpital de la Pitie-Salpetrière, APHP, 75013 Paris, France
[4]Unité de Réanimation Neurologique, Hôpital de la Pitie-Salpetrière, APHP, 75013 Paris, France
[5]Neuroradiologie, Hôpital de la Pitie-Salpetrière, APHP, 75013 Paris, France
[6]Service d'Épilpeptologie, Hôpital de la Pitie-Salpetrière, APHP, 75013 Paris, France

Correspondence should be addressed to M. Yger; marionyger@gmail.com

Academic Editor: Kazuhito Imanaka

*Introduction.* Reversible cerebral vasoconstriction syndrome is becoming widely accepted as a rare cause of both ischemic and haemorrhagic stroke and should be evocated in case of thunderclap headaches associated with stroke. We present the case of a patient with ischemic stroke associated with cortical subarachnoid haemorrhage (cSAH) and reversible diffuse arteries narrowing, leading to the diagnosis of reversible vasoconstriction syndrome. *Case Report.* A 48-year-old woman came to the emergency department because of an unusual thunderclap headache. The computed tomography of the brain completed by CT-angiography was unremarkable. Eleven days later, she was readmitted because of a left hemianopsia. One day after her admission, she developed a sudden left hemiparesis. The brain MRI showed ischemic lesions in the right frontal and occipital lobe and diffuse cSAH. The angiography showed vasoconstriction of the right anterior cerebral artery and stenosis of both middle cerebral arteries. Nimodipine treatment was initiated and vasoconstriction completely regressed on day 16 after the first headache. *Conclusion.* Our case shows a severe reversible cerebral vasoconstriction syndrome where both haemorrhagic and ischemic complications were present at the same time. The history we reported shows that reversible cerebral vasoconstriction syndrome is still underrecognized, in particular in general emergency departments.

## 1. Introduction

Reversible cerebral vasoconstriction syndrome (RCVS) is characterised by acute and severe headaches, with or without other acute neurological symptoms, associated with diffuse segmental constrictions of cerebral arteries that resolve spontaneously within 3 months.

There is a clear female predominance of RCVS with sex ratio ranging from 2,6 : 1 to 10 : 1 [1, 2].

Three large series of RCVS in different countries have contributed to the consideration of this syndrome as a cause of stroke [1–3].

Because of reporting biases, the frequency of stroke in RCVS is uncertain, ranging from 3 [1] to 30% [3]. Haemorrhagic complications (intracerebral haemorrhage and cortical subarachnoid haemorrhage, cSAH) occur mainly in the week after the first headache, whereas ischemic events occur preferentially later (two weeks after the first headache). cSAH is also more frequent (12%) than ischemic events (6%) [4]. The physiopathology of RCVS seems to involve genetic features, endothelial dysfunction, and variation of the adrenergic cerebral tone [4]. This physiopathology is close to that of posterior reversible encephalopathy syndrome and, therefore, the two entities are assimilated by some authors.

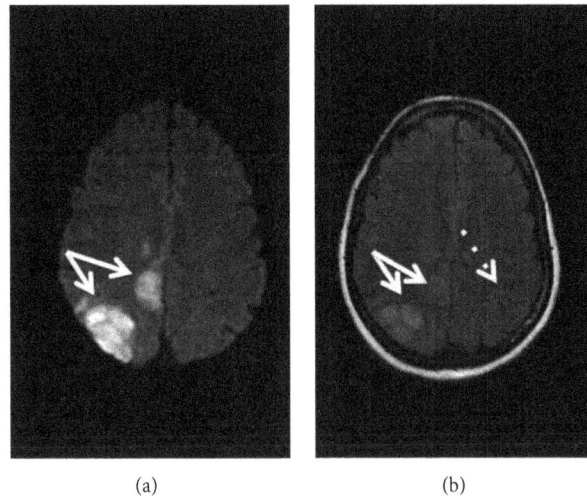

(a)                                      (b)

FIGURE 1: Diffusion-weighted imaging (a) and fluid-attenuated inversion recovery imaging (b) MRI of the patient, showing cytotoxic oedema in the right middle cerebral artery and anterior cerebral artery territories (plain arrows) and cSAH (discontinued arrow).

Since it remains poorly understood, the treatment of RCVS is uncertain and not consensual. We aim to expose, through a single but precise description of a case, our own experience of a complicated RCVS.

## 2. Case Report

A 48-year-old woman was admitted to the emergency department of a community hospital for an unusual thunderclap occipital headache associated with nausea, phonophobia, and photophobia, reaching peak intensity within one minute. Headache occurred during an emotional stress (while crying after having been informed of the death of a friend). She had never experienced such a brutal and painful headache. There was no prior history of headaches. Brain computed tomography (CT) and CT-angiography performed at the emergency department were unremarkable. On day four, the patient came back to the emergency department, because of the persistence of her headache. She was reassured and was rapidly discharged home without any further brain imaging. On day 11, she presented a sudden left hemianopsia and she was thus hospitalized. A brain magnetic resonance imaging (MRI) with diffusion-weighted imaging was performed the day of admission and showed hyperintense lesions in the right frontal lobe in the territory of anterior cerebral artery and in the right occipital lobe in the territory of posterior cerebral artery indicative of cytotoxic oedema. The same lesions were visible on fluid-attenuated inversion recovery imaging sequence. Images compatible with a cSAH were localised to the cortical sulcus in the right superior frontal lobe (Figure 1). Magnetic resonance angiography demonstrated diffuse severe arterial narrowing in the anterior and posterior circulations bilaterally. Injection of cervical vessels with gadolinium and fat saturation sequences excluded the presence of cervical dissections. On day 12, the patient experienced sudden weakness of the left upper and lower extremity and was immediately referred to our stroke unit. On admission, her blood pressure was 120/70 mmHg, her

pulse 64 beats per minute, and her temperature 36°C. The neurologic examination showed left hemiparesis predominant to the lower extremity, dysarthria, and spatial neglect. The National Institute of Health Stroke Score was 11. A second MRI was performed and showed an extension of ischemic lesions in frontal and occipital lobes and diffuse cSAH. Magnetic resonance angiography showed poor vascularisation of bilateral anterior and posterior circulations. A CT did not show recent cSAH and CT-angiography image showed vasoconstriction of the right anterior cerebral artery and stenosis of bilateral middle cerebral arteries, as well as vasoconstriction of the bilateral posterior cerebral arteries and vertebral arteries. A bedside transcranial Doppler ultrasonography revealed bilateral and asymmetrical elevated mean middle cerebral arteries velocities (right middle cerebral artery: 240 cm/s; left middle cerebral artery: 150 cm/s) and elevated mean anterior cerebral arteries velocities (right anterior cerebral artery: 102 cm/s; left anterior cerebral artery: 190 cm/s). Oral nimodipine (120 mg/day) and intravenous hydration were initiated and the patient was referred to the resuscitation department. Digital subtraction angiography performed on day 13 showed typical segmental vasoconstriction in the anterior and posterior circulation (Figure 2). There was neither sinus thrombosis nor arteriovenous malformation. A control of the digital subtraction angiography on day 16 showed complete regression of vasoconstriction. A MRI performed on day 24 did not evidence new ischemic lesions and showed a regression of vasospasm. The patient had no neurological residual impairments.

We diagnosed her as having RCVS complicated by cSAH and ischemic lesions, on the basis of reversibility of the vasoconstriction and brain imaging findings.

## 3. Discussion

Acute severe headache presenting to the emergency departments accounts for 1-2% of admissions [5]. Even if RCVS is one of the diagnoses to be evocated in the setting of

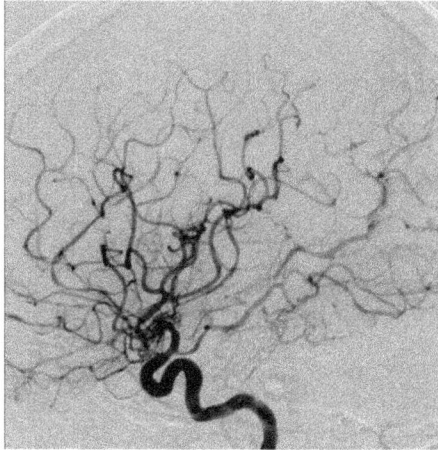

FIGURE 2: Digital subtraction angiography with injection of the right internal carotid artery showing narrowing of the arteries of both carotid and vertebrobasilar circulations.

nontraumatic headache and neurological emergency [6], the history that we report here demonstrates that this condition is still underrecognized, as suggested by numerous authors [2]. Despite a clinical and radiological presentation compatible with RCVS, the patient has been discharged from the emergency department without any advice or medication. The precipitating factor (emotional stress due to the death of a friend) may have led the emergency physicians to the wrong conclusion but could be a real source of adrenalin surge that might be related. We can suppose that an earlier diagnosis may have prevented severe complications. In front of a clinical presentation of RCVS, after having ruled out other differential diagnoses, advice should be given to the patient such as resting, avoiding any vasoconstrictive medication, and coming back in case of reoccurrence of a thunderclap headache or apparition of a new symptom.

Nimodipine is commonly used in RCVS without any proof of its efficiency on the outcome. Resting can also improve the outcome of RCVS, since thunderclap headaches occur especially during physical activity.

Even if haemorrhagic complications occur preferentially sooner than ischemic ones [4] the patient experienced a severe RCVS with both haemorrhagic and ischemic complications at the same time (day 12). She had no prior history of headache but she was aged 48 years, an age more frequently linked with haemorrhagic complications [4]. This case reminds physicians to be careful with any clinical presumption of RCVS, especially in a woman in the forties-fifties.

## Disclosure

M. Yger and C. Zavanone are co-first authors.

## Conflict of Interests

The authors declare no conflict of interests regarding the publication of this paper.

## References

[1] A. Ducros, M. Boukobza, R. Porcher, M. Sarov, D. Valade, and M.-G. Bousser, "The clinical and radiological spectrum of reversible cerebral vasoconstriction syndrome. A prospective series of 67 patients," *Brain*, vol. 130, no. 12, pp. 3091–3101, 2007.

[2] S.-P. Chen, J.-L. Fuh, and S.-J. Wang, "Reversible cerebral vasoconstriction syndrome: an under-recognized clinical emergency," *Therapeutic Advances in Neurological Disorders*, vol. 3, no. 3, pp. 161–171, 2010.

[3] A. B. Singhal, R. A. Hajj-Ali, M. A. Topcuoglu et al., "Reversible cerebral vasoconstriction syndromes: analysis of 139 cases," *Archives of Neurology*, vol. 68, no. 8, pp. 1005–1012, 2011.

[4] A. Ducros, "Reversible cerebral vasoconstriction syndrome," *The Lancet Neurology*, vol. 11, no. 10, pp. 906–917, 2012.

[5] T. N. Ward, M. Levin, and J. M. Phillips, "Evaluation and management of headache in the emergency department," *The Medical Clinics of North America*, vol. 85, no. 4, pp. 971–985, 2001.

[6] T. J. Schwedt, M. S. Matharu, and D. W. Dodick, "Thunderclap headache," *The Lancet Neurology*, vol. 5, no. 7, pp. 621–631, 2006.

# The Unexpected Pitter Patter: New-Onset Atrial Fibrillation in Pregnancy

**Sarah White, Janna Welch, and Lawrence H. Brown**

*Dell School of Medicine, University of Texas at Austin, USA*

Correspondence should be addressed to Janna Welch; drjannawelch@gmail.com

Academic Editor: Aristomenis K. Exadaktylos

*Background.* Atrial fibrillation is a relatively uncommon but dangerous complication of pregnancy. Emergency physicians must know how to treat both stable and unstable tachycardias in late pregnancy. In this case, a 40-year-old female with a cerclage due to incompetent cervix and previous preterm deliveries presents in new-onset atrial fibrillation. *Case Report.* A previously healthy 40-year-old African American G2 P1 female with a 23-week twin gestation complicated by an incompetent cervix requiring a cervical cerclage presented to the emergency department with intermittent palpitations and shortness of breath for the past two months. EMS noted the patient to have a tachydysrhythmia, atrial fibrillation with rapid ventricular response. She was placed on a diltiazem drip, which was titrated to 15 mg/hr without successful rate control. Her heart rate remained in the 130s and the rhythm continued to be atrial fibrillation with RVR. Digoxin was then added as a second agent, and discussions about the potential risks of cardioversion in pregnancy ensued. Fortunately, the patient converted to sinus rhythm before cardioversion became necessary. The digoxin was discontinued; the diltiazem was also discontinued after the patient subsequently developed hypotension. *"Why Should Emergency Physicians Be Aware of This?"* New-onset atrial fibrillation is rare in pregnancy but can increase the mortality and morbidity of the mother and fetus if not treated promptly.

## 1. Introduction

Atrial fibrillation is a relatively uncommon but dangerous complication of pregnancy. Emergency physicians must know how to treat both stable and unstable tachycardias in late pregnancy. In this case, a 40-year-old female with a cerclage due to incompetent cervix and previous preterm deliveries presents in new-onset atrial fibrillation.

## 2. Case Report

A previously healthy 40-year-old African American G2 P1 female with a 23-week twin gestation complicated by an incompetent cervix requiring a cervical cerclage presented to the emergency department with intermittent palpitations and shortness of breath for the past two months. The patient arrived via EMS complaining of persistent shortness of breath and palpitations for the past six hours. She was noted by EMS to have a tachydysrhythmia, atrial fibrillation with rapid ventricular response (RVR), and received two doses of diltiazem en route: 20 mg and then another 25 mg without rate control.

Upon arrival, the patient's shortness of breath had resolved but she continued to have palpitations. The patient denied dehydration, alcohol or caffeine use, lack of sleep, recent illness, or any other precipitating factors. Her past medical history was significant only for a previous preterm delivery at 20 weeks due to an incompetent cervix. She denied any cardiomyopathies, prior arrhythmias, or other structural heart diseases.

On physical exam, the patient was afebrile, normotensive, with a heart rate in the 130s–140s, and a respiratory rate of 25–42. Abnormal physical exam findings included bilateral crackles in the lung bases and an irregularly irregular heartbeat. Fetal heart tones were observed in both fetuses.

Initial work-up included an EKG, CBC, CMP, UA with microscopy, chest X-ray, cardiac enzymes, D-Dimer, BNP, and thyroid studies. On EKG, rate was 142 and rhythm was atrial fibrillation with rapid ventricular response. The chest radiograph revealed cardiac hypertrophy and right greater than left perihilar opacities suggestive of pulmonary edema. Laboratory examination revealed mild leukocytosis and mild elevation of D-Dimer, with the remainder of the results within normal limits.

The patient was placed on a diltiazem drip, which was titrated to 15 mg/hr without successful rate control. Her heart rate remained in the 130s and the rhythm continued to be atrial fibrillation with RVR. Digoxin was then added as a second agent, and discussions about the potential risks of cardioversion in pregnancy ensued. Fortunately, the patient converted to sinus rhythm before cardioversion became necessary. The digoxin was discontinued; the diltiazem was also discontinued after the patient subsequently developed hypotension.

The patient was admitted to hospital and was followed closely in an intermediate care unit by cardiology and OB/GYN. An ECHO was completed during her hospital admission that showed moderate left ventricular hypertrophy (LVH), and on further laboratory examination she appeared to likely have gestational diabetes. Due to her LVH, flecainide was not recommended, and due to her pregnancy it was decided that aspirin would be used for anticoagulation. The patient was discharged with follow-up with cardiology, high-risk obstetrics, and maternal fetal monitoring for the remainder of her pregnancy.

## 3. Discussion

There are many physiologic changes that occur during pregnancy, including increased demands on the cardiovascular system. Physiologic changes in the cardiovascular system include peripheral vasodilation resulting in decreased systemic vascular resistance, requiring increased cardiac output. This increase in cardiac output is accomplished by an increase in ventricular end-diastolic volume, wall mass, and contractility, which creates an increase in stroke volume and heart rate. Due to these alterations, pregnant women are placed at higher risk for developing comorbidities such as cardiac arrhythmias that range from benign to life threatening [4, 5].

While most cases of atrial fibrillation in pregnancy are the result of an underlying cardiac arrhythmia or structural abnormality, there is a very small percentage of women who develop new-onset "lone" atrial fibrillation during their pregnancy. While these cases are known in the OB/GYN literature, their presentation and management in the emergency department have not previously been described in emergency medicine literature.

In evaluating new-onset "lone" atrial fibrillation in the pregnant woman, it is important to discern the etiology of the abnormality. The initial work-up should attempt to rule out cardiac conduction and structural abnormalities, as well as extracardiac etiologies such as pulmonary embolus, hyperthyroidism, electrolyte disturbances, and pharmacologic effects. This assessment should include an EKG, echocardiogram, serum electrolytes, thyroid studies, and urine drug screen. The EKG should reveal the diagnosis of atrial fibrillation as well as any other conduction abnormalities once the rate is controlled, and an echocardiogram

will be able to evaluate any structural abnormalities that would predispose the patient to developing an arrhythmia. A thorough evaluation of medications as well as illicit drug use should be completed, as many pharmacologic agents are arrhythmogenic. If clinically indicated, an evaluation for pulmonary embolus should be completed using laboratory and radiologic evidence and therapy should be initiated [6].

Emergency department treatment is divided between pharmacologic and nonpharmacologic interventions for rate and rhythm control. The initial goal should be to control the rate; however, in order to maintain consistent blood-flow to the patient's end organs including the placenta, sinus rhythm should be restored as soon as possible. The European Society of Cardiology established guidelines in 2011 for management of cardiovascular diseases in pregnancy. Beta-blockers are the first choice for rate control of atrial fibrillation in pregnancy, followed by calcium-channel blockers. They recommend digoxin as well, with the caveat that digoxin blood concentrations are unreliable in pregnancy due to interference with immunoreactive serum components [7].

When choosing therapeutic interventions, adverse events to both mother and fetus must be taken into consideration, as many antiarrhythmic drugs are teratogenic. The FDA classifies the risk and benefits of medications during pregnancy as follows:

> A: controlled studies showed no risk in the fetus in any trimester of pregnancy.
>
> B: no evidence of risk in humans. The chance of fetal harm is remote.
>
> C: the risk cannot be ruled out. There are no well-controlled clinical studies, and animal studies show risk to the fetus. Fetal damage is likely if the drug is administered during pregnancy, but the potential benefits could exceed the potential risk.
>
> D: sure evidence of risk. However, the potential benefits of use of the drug may outweigh the potential risk.
>
> X: contraindicated in pregnancy. Studies in animals or humans showed certain evidence or risk of fetal abnormality and clearly outweigh any benefit to the patient [8].

Table 1 shows the FDA classification and safety profile for the pharmacologic agents used in the emergency department treatment of atrial fibrillation, modified from Oishi and Xing [9].

Emergency physicians frequently encounter patients with atrial fibrillation that does not respond to pharmacologic intervention, and cardioversion is a common emergency department intervention. Pregnant women with unresponsive, new-onset "lone" atrial fibrillation are rare, and emergency physicians are likely not as conversant with the risks and benefits of cardioversion in this patient group. In hemodynamically unstable patients, in patients who are not responding to pharmacologic therapy, or whenever the risk of ongoing atrial fibrillation is considered high for the mother or the fetus cardioversion up to 400 J can be performed safely

TABLE 1

| Drug | Rate versus rhythm control | Class of recommendation/level of evidence | FDA category | Dosage | Adverse effects |
| --- | --- | --- | --- | --- | --- |
| Beta-blockers | Rate | Class IIa/C | C | | Pregnancy: born small for gestational age, preterm birth, and perinatal mortality [1]. General: bradycardia, hypotension, AV block, bronchospasm |
| Esmolol | | | | Loading: 0.5 mg/kg over 1 min. Maintenance: 0.06–0.2 mg/k/min | |
| Metoprolol | | | | 2.5–5 mg bolus over 2 min, up to 3 doses | |
| Propranolol | | | | 0.15 mg/kg | |
| Nondihydropyridine calcium channel blockers | Rate | Class IIa/C | C | | Pregnancy: increased risk of neonatal seizures, jaundice, and hematologic disorders [2]. General: hypotension, heart failure |
| Diltiazem | | | | Loading: 0.25 mg/kg/dose over 2 min; may give a second dose at 0.35 mg/kg/dose. Maintenance: 5–15 mg/kg for <24 hr. | |
| Verapamil | | | | 0.075–0.15 mg/kg over 2 min | |
| Cardiac glycoside | | | | | |
| Digoxin | Rate | Class IIb/C | C | Loading: 0.25 mg IV every 2 h, up to 1.5 mg. Maintenance 0.125–0.375 mg daily IV or orally | Pregnancy: digitalis toxicity may cause fetal demise [3]. General: digitalis toxicity, heart block |
| Class I C antiarrhythmic agent | | | | | |
| Flecainide | Rhythm | Class IIb/C | C | | General: heart block, ventricular arrhythmias, and heart failure |
| Class III antiarrhythmic agent | | | | | |
| Ibutilide | Rhythm | Class IIb/C | C | 1 mg IV; may repeat dose if no response after 10 min | General: bradycardia, AV block, Torsades |
| Adjunctive therapies | | | | | |
| Magnesium | | NA | B | 2 g over 15 min | General: respiratory depression |

at all stages of pregnancy [6]. It is a Class I recommendation with a C level of evidence [9]. That is, risk to the fetus cannot be ruled out. While maternal cardioversion is unlikely to have significant effects on the fetus due to a high threshold for arrhythmogenesis and the minimal amount of current that reaches the uterus [10], continuous fetal monitoring should be utilized during the procedure, and cardioversion should be performed in a facility with the ability to perform an emergency C-section if needed. Previous reports note fetal arrhythmia developing as bradycardia or loss of variability after maternal cardioversion; both of which are indications for C-section [11].

In cases of atrial fibrillation occurring for longer than 48 hours, a transesophageal ECHO should be completed to evaluate atrial thrombus, and anticoagulation should be initiated prior to cardioversion [6, 8]. Vitamin K agonists, however, are teratogenic and therefore unfractionated or low molecular weight heparin should be used during the first trimester. During the third trimester, frequent laboratory testing is recommended to maintain appropriate levels of anticoagulation [8, 12].

3.1. "Why Should Emergency Physicians Be Aware of This?" New-onset atrial fibrillation is rare in pregnancy but can increase the mortality and morbidity of the mother and fetus if not treated promptly. In the case of an unstable patient, cardioversion should be completed as quickly as possible. In a stable patient, effort should be made to determine the etiology of the arrhythmia, and treatment should follow accordingly. In the emergency department pharmacological intervention should be targeted toward rate control with Beta-blockers, calcium-channel blockers, or digoxin. In the case of our patient, management with diltiazem and digoxin was within European Society of Cardiology guidelines. Strict adherence to guidelines would have included beta-blocker as a first line medication. Once the rate is controlled, the provider should attempt to restore sinus rhythm chemically or electrically. In this case, the patient may require anticoagulation prior to cardioversion, with unfractionated or low molecular weight heparin. A high-risk obstetrician for the remainder of their pregnancy should follow these patients, and continued monitoring and treatment of her arrhythmia should be performed in conjunction with a cardiologist.

## Conflict of Interests

The authors declare that there is no conflict of interests regarding the publication of this paper.

## References

[1] K. M. Petersen, E. Jimenez-Solem, J. T. Andersen et al., "$\beta$-Blocker treatment during pregnancy and adverse pregnancy outcomes: a nationwide population-based cohort study," *The British Medical Journal Open*, vol. 2, no. 4, Article ID e001185, 2012.

[2] R. L. Davis, D. Eastman, H. McPhillips et al., "Risks of congenital malformations and perinatal events among infants exposed to calcium channel and beta-blockers during pregnancy," *Pharmacoepidemiology and Drug Safety*, vol. 20, no. 2, pp. 138–145, 2011.

[3] H. L. Tan and K. I. Lie, "Treatment of tachyarrhythmias during pregnancy and lactation," *European Heart Journal*, vol. 22, no. 6, pp. 458–464, 2001.

[4] C. C. Burt and J. Durbridge, "Management of cardiac disease in pregnancy," *Continuing Education in Anaesthesia, Critical Care and Pain*, vol. 9, no. 2, pp. 44–47, 2009.

[5] J. A. Joglar and R. L. Page, "Management of arrhythmia syndromes during pregnancy," *Current Opinion in Cardiology*, vol. 29, no. 1, pp. 36–44, 2014.

[6] L. T. A. Dicarlo-Meacham and L. J. Dahlke, "Atrial fibrillation in pregnancy," *Obstetrics and Gynecology*, vol. 117, no. 2, pp. 489–492, 2011.

[7] V. Regitz-Zagrosek, C. Blomstrom Lundqvist, C. Borghi et al., "ESC Guidelines on the management of cardiovascular diseases during pregnancy," *European Heart Journal*, vol. 32, no. 24, pp. 3147–3197, 2011.

[8] A. Perez-Silva and J.-L. Merino, "Tachyarrhythmias in pregnancy," *ESC Council for Card Practice*, vol. 9, no. 31, 2011.

[9] M. L. Oishi and S. Xing, "Atrial fibrillation: management strategies in the emergency department," *Emergency Medicine Practice*, vol. 15, no. 2, pp. 1–28, 2013.

[10] R. A. DeSilva, T. B. Graboys, P. J. Podrid, and B. Lown, "Cardioversion and defibrillation," *American Heart Journal*, vol. 100, no. 6, part 1, pp. 881–895, 1980.

[11] E. J. Barnes, F. Eben, and D. Patterson, "Direct current cardioversion during pregnancy should be performed with facilities available for fetal monitoring and emergency caesarean section," *British Journal of Obstetrics and Gynaecology*, vol. 109, no. 12, pp. 1406–1407, 2002.

[12] S. M. Bates, I. A. Greer, I. Pabinger, S. Sofaer, and J. Hirsh, "Venous thromboembolism, thrombophilia, antithrombotic therapy, and pregnancy: American College of Chest Physicians evidence-based clinical practice guidelines (8th edition)," *Chest*, vol. 133, no. 6, pp. 844–886, 2008.

# 8

# A Case Report of Prilocaine-Induced Methemoglobinemia after Liposuction Procedure

**Birdal Yildirim,**[1] **Ulku Karagoz,**[2] **Ethem Acar,**[1] **Halil Beydilli,**[1] **Emine Nese Yeniceri,**[3] **Ozgur Tanriverdi,**[4] **Omer Dogan Alatas,**[2] **and Şükrü Kasap**[5]

[1]*Department of Emergency Medicine, Muğla Sıtkı Koçman University Medical Faculty, Orhaniye Mahallesi Haluk Ozsoy Caddesi, 48000 Mugla, Turkey*

[2]*Emergency Clinic, Muğla Sıtkı Koçman University Training and Investigation Hospital, Orhaniye Mahallesi Haluk Ozsoy Caddesi, 48000 Mugla, Turkey*

[3]*Department of Family Medicine, Muğla Sıtkı Koçman University Medical Faculty, Orhaniye Mahallesi Haluk Ozsoy Caddesi, 48000 Mugla, Turkey*

[4]*Department of Internal Medicine and Medical Oncology, Muğla Sıtkı Koçman University Medical Faculty, Orhaniye Mahallesi Haluk Ozsoy Caddesi, 48000 Mugla, Turkey*

[5]*Clinic of Plastic and Reconstructive Surgery, Muğla Sıtkı Koçman University Training and Investigation Hospital, Orhaniye Mahallesi Haluk Ozsoy Caddesi, 48000 Mugla, Turkey*

Correspondence should be addressed to Emine Nese Yeniceri; neseyeniceri@mu.edu.tr

Academic Editor: Chih Cheng Lai

Prilocaine-induced methemoglobinemia is a rarely seen condition. In this paper, a case is presented with methemoglobinemia developed secondary to prilocaine use in a liposuction procedure, and the importance of this rarely seen condition is emphasized. A 20-year-old female patient presented with complaints of prostration, lassitude, shivering, shortness of breath, and cyanosis. It was learned that the patient underwent nearly 1000 mg prilocaine infiltration 8 hours priorly during a liposuction procedure. At admission, her blood pressure (130/80 mmHg), pulse rate (140 bpm), body temperature (36°C), and respiratory rate (40/min) were recorded. The patient had marked acrocyanosis. The arterial blood gas methemoglobin level was measured as 40%. The patient received oxygen therapy with a mask and was administered vitamin C in normal saline (500 mg tid), N-acetylcysteine (300 mg tid), and 50 mg 10% methylene blue in the intensive care unit of the internal medicine department. Methemoglobin level dropped down to 2% after her treatment with methylene blue and she was clinically cured and discharged 2 days later. Emergency service physicians should remember to consider methemoglobinemia when making a differential diagnosis between dyspnea and cyanosis developing after prilocaine infiltration performed for liposuctions in the adult age group.

## 1. Introduction

Methemoglobinemia is defined as an increase in the blood methemoglobin level, and it is an important cause of cyanosis [1]. When ferrous ($Fe^{2+}$) hemoglobin oxidizes iron and transforms it into a ferric ($Fe^{3+}$) cation, methemoglobin forms. The methemoglobin level is held at low levels via the reductizing cytochrome b5 reductase enzyme (NADH-methemoglobin reductase) levels in erythrocytes [1]. Indeed, methemoglobin is not functional in contrast with oxygen-carrying hemoglobin, and conditions with increased blood methemoglobin levels convey clinical importance [2]. The most important clinical symptom of methemoglobinemia is cyanosis, and it should be considered in particular in cyanotic patients with normal cardiovascular and pulmonary functions [2]. In mild cases, clinical signs and symptoms may not be observed; however, severe cases may present with cyanosis, tachypnea, hypotension, tachycardia, and confusion. Advanced cases may be fatal [2].

The pathophysiology of methemoglobinemia involves an imbalance between oxidation and reduction [1, 2]. It may emerge as a hereditary or acquired condition [2]. The most important cause of acquired methemoglobinemia is exposure of healthy individuals to drugs or chemical substances [2]. Such chemicals as nitrite, nitrate, aniline, and benzene compounds and drugs like sulfonamides, dapsone, phenacetin, primaquine, and benzocaine make up the most important agents [2, 3]. Prilocaine, an amide compound that is frequently used as a local anesthetic, can also cause methemoglobinemia [3].

Based on a literature review, cases with prilocaine-induced methemoglobinemia are frequently seen in neonatal and early pediatric ages [4, 5]. Prilocaine-induced methemoglobinemia during liposuction is rarely seen. In this paper, in consideration of the rarity of this condition, a severe case of prilocaine-induced methemoglobinemia in a patient who underwent regional liposuction is presented.

## 2. Case Presentation

A 20-year-old female patient without any previous systemic disease applied to this emergency service with complaints of shivering, prostration, lassitude, fatigue, shortness of breath, and cyanosis of the lips. The general health state of the patient was deteriorated. An inspection of the patient revealed a tachypneic pulse and cyanotic lips. The patient's blood pressure (130/80 mm/Hg), respiratory rate (40/min), pulse rate (rhythmic, 140 bpm), body temperature (36°C), and oxygen saturation (SpO$_2$, 82%) were measured with normal pulmonary and cardiovascular examination findings. Her chest X-ray and electrocardiographic examination results were within normal limits. The whole blood cell count and blood biochemistry did not yield any abnormal results, which would explain the clinical health state and metabolic, hematological, infective, renal, and hepatic diseases of the patient. Similarly, no respiratory or cardiovascular abnormality that could account for her actual clinical health state was detected. With an arterial blood gas pH, 7.46, pCO$_2$, 31.1 mm Hg, pO$_2$, 83.3 mm Hg, HCO$_3$, 20 mEq/L, lactate, 3.6 mmol/L, and methemoglobin, 40%, the patient was considered to have methemoglobinemia. Despite the initiation of a saline infusion (100 mL/hr) and oxygen delivery with a mask at a rate of 10 mL/kg, her cyanosis persisted, and the patient was monitored in the intensive care unit of the department of internal medicine.

When the patient was stabilized, it was learned from her detailed anamnesis that she had undergone liposuction from her medial aspects of both femoral regions eight hours prior to the onset of her complaints. A total of 1000 mg prilocaine was used during the liposuction procedure, and 100–200 mg of the drug might be retained within the procedural site. Her treatment was continued with a vitamin C (3 × 500 mg) infusion in normal saline, N-acetylcysteine (3 × 300 mg), and 50 mg 10% methylene blue. Her methemoglobin level dropped to 2%, and her clinical findings improved. She was discharged two days after her admission into the intensive care unit.

## 3. Discussion

In this case report, in consideration of its rarity, an adult patient who consulted emergency services with clinical manifestations of severe methemoglobinemia which developed after the application of prilocaine during a regional liposuction is presented.

Methemoglobinemia can develop under the influence of hereditary and acquired factors [2]. Many drugs and chemical substances are known to induce acquired methemoglobinemia. The local anesthetic prilocaine is among these methemoglobinemia-inducing drugs [2, 6].

As a local anesthetic drug, the therapeutic dose of prilocaine has been reported as 1-2 mg/kg, and, in cases with methemoglobinemia emerging at its therapeutic doses, cyanosis cannot be observed [7]. The maximum safe dose of prilocaine is 8 mg/kg, while the daily maximum dose is 600 mg [8]. However, increasingly higher doses have been used during liposuction procedures [9]. It has been reported that, despite higher doses of prilocaine being used in the tumescent liposuction method, the risk of methemoglobinemia is lower, which indicates the safety of this liposuction method [9]. In a study of 25 cases in which patients had undergone liposuction with this technique, methemoglobinemia had not developed [10]. In the tumescent infiltrative liposuction technique, a substantial amount of local anesthetic infiltrated subcutaneously is removed from the body via the aspiration method [11]. The biological half-life of prilocaine is 55 minutes, and the time required for the development of methemoglobinemia is 20–60 minutes [8]. In this case, 1000 mg prilocaine was infiltrated and nearly 800–900 mg of the drug was aspirated. A total of 100–200 mg was aspirated by the body cavities. It is believed that, despite the use of lower than toxic doses of prilocaine, the prolongation of the procedure for 6–8 hours induced the development of methemoglobinemia.

Methemoglobinemia should be taken into consideration in the differential diagnosis of patients with normal circulatory and respiratory system findings who consult with cyanosis [2]. Under physiological conditions, methemoglobin constitutes 1% of Hb and does not exceed more than 2-3% of Hb [1]. However, a derangement of the balance between oxidation and reduction can increase the prilocaine concentration above physiologic levels [2]. Exposure to some oxidant substances can induce methemoglobinemia even in healthy individuals. However, in healthy individuals, the increased methemoglobin concentration is lowered to normal levels by means of the cytochrome b5 reductase enzyme found in red blood cells [1, 3, 6]. In some cases, the compensation mechanism does not function properly, and increasing levels of methemoglobin cannot transport O$_2$, which shifts the hemoglobin-oxygen dissociation curve to the left, thereby complicating the delivery of oxygen to the tissues [1, 3, 6].

Mild cases can be asymptomatic, but, in severe cases, cyanosis, tachypnea, tachycardia, hypotension, confusion, or even death may be observed [4]. In cases with methemoglobinemia, varying degrees of cyanosis can be detected which are associated with blood methemoglobin levels [3, 6].

When blood methemoglobin levels exceed 10%, peripheral cyanosis becomes apparent, and, in cases with methemoglobin levels of ≥35%, tissue hypoxia and diffuse cyanosis are seen. When methemoglobin levels approach 70%, the patient enters a coma and if untreated may die [1, 3, 6].

The patient who received prilocaine during a regional liposuction had a methemoglobin level of 40% at admission and presented clinically with fatigue, shivering, diffuse perioral and peripheral cyanosis, tachypnea, and tachycardia. The methemoglobinemia level of this patient and the clinical findings were compatible with the literature findings.

During the first months of life, a transient deficiency of cytochrome b5 reductase enzyme activity predisposes newborns and infants to methemoglobinemia [1]. However, since during the first 3 months of life the cytochrome b5 reductase activity is 50% of the level found in adults, even with therapeutic doses of prilocaine, methemoglobinemia can develop [7]. Therefore, many cases with methemoglobinemia can be found in the literature which have been encountered during surgical procedures performed on newborns with local anesthesia [4, 5, 12].

The first measure to be applied after the development of methemoglobinemia following an exposure to a chemical agent or drug is the prevention of exposure to this substance. Patients with levels of methemoglobin over 20% can improve spontaneously, and it must be remembered that, above this level, clinical manifestations can worsen [13]. As treatment alternatives, methylene blue, ascorbic acid, and riboflavin are recommended for these patients. The mortality risk is higher in cases with methemoglobin levels of ≥70%; hyperbaric oxygen therapy is recommended for these patients [14]. However, methylene blue is the first treatment alternative for all cases. Animal and *in vitro* human experiments have demonstrated that ascorbic acid decreases the methemoglobin levels through a nonenzymatic process [14]. Additionally, in previous *in vitro* studies, N-acetylcysteine has been reported to be an important alternative approach in the treatment of nitric oxide related methemoglobinemia [15, 16]. However, N-acetylcysteine was shown to have no effect on human volunteers in a study conducted by Tanen et al. [17]. Similarly, in a study carried out by Dötsch et al. [18], effects of treatment with methylene blue, riboflavin, and N-acetylcysteine were compared in patients with methemoglobinemia but N-acetylcysteine and low-dose riboflavin were found not to change methemoglobin formation. Therefore, N-acetylcysteine has not yet found a place in clinical practice as treatment for methemoglobinemia [18, 19]. However, it should be kept in mind that methylene blue is contraindicated in patients with glucose-6-phosphate dehydrogenase deficiency whose methemoglobinemia, paradoxically, may worsen [19].

Since this patient's level of methemoglobinemia was 40%, systemic toxic symptoms were in the foreground, and intravenous infusion of methylene blue at a rate of 1-2 mg/kg/5 min was initiated when the antioxidant therapy failed to elicit an adequate response.

In conclusion, methemoglobinemia should be considered in patients with incompatible oxygen saturation and $pO_2$ results who developed cyanosis following minimally invasive surgical interventions. With perfect history taking and appropriate differential diagnoses, methemoglobinemia treatment can be improved without giving rise to the deterioration of the clinical picture.

## Conflict of Interests

The authors declare that there is no conflict of interests regarding the publication of this paper.

## References

[1] G. R. Honig, "Hemoglobin disorder," in *Nelson Textbook of Pediatrics*, R. E. Behrman, R. M. Kleigman, and H. B. Jenson, Eds., pp. 1478–1488, Saunders, Philadelphia, Pa, USA, 2000.

[2] E. Türkmen, G. Kocabay, A. S. Yavuz et al., "A case of methemoglobinemia induced by the administration of prilocaine prior to an epilation procedure," *Journal of 1st Faculty of Medicine*, vol. 68, pp. 19–21, 2005.

[3] M. D. Coleman and N. A. Coleman, "Drug induced methemoglobinemia," *Drug Safety*, vol. 14, no. 6, pp. 394–405, 1996.

[4] D. Benini, L. Vivo, and V. Fanos, "Acquired methemoglobinemia: a case report," *La Pediatria Medica e Chirurgica*, vol. 20, no. 6, pp. 411–413, 1998.

[5] B. T. Çelik and N. Çelik, "Methemoglobinemia due to prilocaine: a case report," *Van Tıp Dergisi*, vol. 21, no. 1, pp. 44–45, 2014.

[6] D. Svecová and D. Böhmer, "Congenital and acquired methemoglobinemia and its therapy," *Casopis Lékaru Ceských*, vol. 137, pp. 168–170, 1998.

[7] S. G. Aygencel, E. Akinci, and G. Pamukcu, "Prilocaine induced methemoglobinemia," *Saudi Medical Journal*, vol. 27, no. 1, pp. 111–113, 2006.

[8] E. Lunenfeld and G. C. Kane, "Methemoglobinemia: sudden dyspnea and oxyhemoglobin desaturation after esophagoduodenoscopy," *Respiratory Care*, vol. 49, no. 8, pp. 940–942, 2004.

[9] W. Hanke, S. E. Cox, N. Kuznets, and W. P. Coleman III, "Tumescent liposuction report performance measurement initiative: national survey results," *Dermatologic Surgery*, vol. 30, no. 7, pp. 967–978, 2004.

[10] N. Lindenblatt, L. Belusa, B. Tiefenbach, W. Schareck, and R. R. Olbrisch, "Prilocaine plasma levels and methemoglobinemia in patients undergoing tumescent liposuction involving less than 2,000 ml," *Aesthetic Plastic Surgery*, vol. 28, no. 6, pp. 435–440, 2004.

[11] O. Lapid, "Syringe-delivered tumescent anesthesia made easier," *Aesthetic Plastic Surgery*, vol. 35, no. 4, pp. 601–602, 2011.

[12] T. Yılmaz, S. Ayşe, G. Serdal, and Ö. Ünsal, "Sünnet öncesi uygulanan lokal prilokaine bağlı methemoglobinemi olgusu," *Dicle Tıp Dergisi*, vol. 3, no. 1, pp. 53–55, 2009.

[13] Y. F. Su, L. H. Lu, T. H. Hsu, S. L. Chang, and R. T. Lin, "Successful treatment of methemoglobinemia in an elderly couple with severe cyanosis: two case reports," *Journal of Medical Case Reports*, vol. 6, article 290, 2012.

[14] R. B. Abu-Laban, P. J. Zed, R. A. Purssell, and K. G. Evans, "Severe methemoglobinemia from topical anesthetic spray: case report, discussion and qualitative systematic review," *Canadian Journal of Emergency Medicine*, vol. 3, no. 1, pp. 51–56, 2001.

[15] R. O. Wright, B. Magnani, M. W. Shannon, and A. D. Woolf, "N-acetylcysteine reduces methemoglobin in vitro," *Annals of Emergency Medicine*, vol. 28, no. 5, pp. 499–503, 1996.

[16] R. O. Wright, A. D. Woolf, M. W. Shannon, and B. Magnani, "N-acetylcysteine reduces methemoglobin in an in-vitro model of glucose-6-phosphate dehydrogenase deficiency," *Academic Emergency Medicine*, vol. 5, no. 3, pp. 225–229, 1998.

[17] D. A. Tanen, F. LoVecchio, and S. C. Curry, "Failure of intravenous N-acetylcysteine to reduce methemoglobin produced by sodium nitrite in human volunteers: a randomized controlled trial," *Annals of Emergency Medicine*, vol. 35, no. 4, pp. 369–373, 2000.

[18] J. Dötsch, S. Demirakça, M. Kratz, R. Repp, I. Knerr, and W. Rascher, "Comparison of methylene blue, riboflavin, and N-acetylcysteine for the reduction of nitric oxide-induced methemoglobinemia," *Critical Care Medicine*, vol. 28, no. 4, pp. 958–961, 2000.

[19] S. M. Bradberry, "Occupational methaemoglobinaemia: mechanisms of production, features, diagnosis and management including the use of methylene blue," *Toxicological Reviews*, vol. 22, no. 1, pp. 13–27, 2003.

# 9

# Damage Control Surgery for Hepatocellular Cancer Rupture in an Elderly Patient: Survival and Quality of Life

**Konstantinos Bouliaris, Grigorios Christodoulidis, Dimitrios Symeonidis, Alexandros Diamantis, and Konstantinos Tepetes**

*Surgical Department, University Hospital of Larissa, Mezurlo, 4110 Larissa, Greece*

Correspondence should be addressed to Konstantinos Bouliaris; kwstisbool@yahoo.com

Academic Editor: Aristomenis K. Exadaktylos

Spontaneous rupture of hepatocellular carcinoma (HCC) is a rare emergency condition with high mortality rate. Successful management depends on patients' hemodynamic condition upon presentation and comorbidities, correct diagnosis, HCC status, liver function, and future liver remnant, as well as available sources. There is still a debate in the literature concerning the best approach in this devastating complication. Nevertheless, the primary goal should be a definitive bleeding arrest. In most cases, patients with spontaneous rupture of HCC present with hemodynamic instability, due to hemoperitoneum, necessitating an emergency treatment modality. In such cases, transcatheter arterial embolization (TAE) should be the treatment of choice. Emergency liver resection is an option when TAE fails or in cases with preserved liver function and limited tumors. Otherwise, damage control strategies, as in liver trauma, are a reasonable alternative. We report a case of an elderly patient with hemoperitoneum and hypovolemic shock from spontaneous rupture of undiagnosed HCC, who was treated successfully by emergency surgery and damage control approach.

## 1. Introduction

Hepatocellular carcinoma (HCC) is an aggressive tumor that often occurs in the setting of chronic liver disease and cirrhosis and it is typically diagnosed late in its course. It is the sixth most common malignancy in the world and the third commonest cause of death from cancer [1]. One of the most life-threatening conditions associated with HCC is spontaneous rupture which occurs in 3–26% of all HCC cases [2, 3]. Thirty-day mortality can be very high ranging from 32 to 75% [4]. This poor outcome can be attributed to incorrect diagnosis, concomitant impaired liver function, advanced HCC status, inappropriate treatment, and patient's general condition and comorbidities upon presentation. In most cases, patients with spontaneous rupture of HCC present with hemodynamic instability, due to hemoperitoneum, necessitating an emergency treatment modality. Therapeutic options include transcatheter arterial embolization (TAE), surgical ligation of the hepatic artery, perihepatic packing, oversewing of the bleeding surface, and hepatectomy. Efforts for hemostasis in such patients should be directed by the available sources and the hemodynamic status. Thus, when TAE is not available, surgery with or without hepatectomy should be the first choice. Herein, we present a case of a successful two-stage surgical treatment of a ruptured HCC in an elderly patient who presented with hypovolemic shock.

## 2. Case Presentation

A 87-year-old male patient was transferred to the emergency department after an episode of sudden upper abdominal pain and vomiting. On arrival, the patient was pale, tachycardic with a heart rate of 103 beats per minute, and tachypnoeic with a blood pressure of 110/60 mmHg. Physical examination revealed guarding of the right upper quadrant with tenderness. Laboratory examination revealed a hemoglobin level of 10.2 g/dL, normal platelets count, prolonged INR = 1.41, normal liver enzymes, and slightly elevated $\gamma$GT = 70 U/I (normal values < 50). Past medical history included coronary artery disease with coronary artery bypass surgery

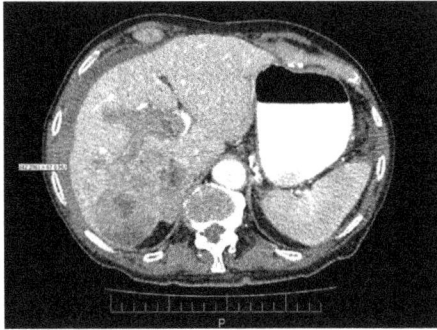

FIGURE 1: Abdomen CT showing a 7.5 cm mass occupying the right lobe of the liver, thrombosis of the right portal vein, and hemoperitoneum (HU = 67).

and carotid artery stenting. However, electrocardiogram and cardiac enzymes were within normal values. Abdominal ultrasound showed a hepatic lesion with free intraperitoneal fluid. A contrast enhanced abdominal CT was ordered which demonstrated a heterogenous mass of 7.5 cm diameter occupying the right lobe of the liver, thrombosis of the right portal vein, and free quantity of blood in the peritoneal cavity (Figure 1). These findings indicated a spontaneous rupture of a possible HCC since there was no past history of HCC disease. During the examination, the patient became hemodynamically unstable, with loss of consciousness. He was intubated and transferred to the operating room for an emergency exploratory laparotomy since TAE was not feasible at that time. During surgery, there was a notable amount of fresh and clotted blood in the abdomen and a large hepatic ruptured mass was detected, located in the right hepatic lobe. Although a right hepatectomy was technically feasible, this was not performed due to critical patient's situation. Under these circumstances, it was decided to perform damage control surgery with enucleation of the tumor, ligation of the hepatic artery, and perihepatic packing. Patient's condition did not permit us to check intraoperatively the patency of the main portal vein, but the CT had shown that the left portal vein was patent and there was also a collateral circulation due to cirrhosis. The haemorrhage was successfully controlled and the patient was transferred to the intensive care unit (ICU) for further supportive treatment. Forty-eight hours later, a second laparotomy was performed to remove the packing and apply RF ablation to the tumor's bed. After 4 days in the ICU, the patient was transferred to surgical ward and he was discharged on the 18th postoperative day. The histopathological examination showed HCC, while serological tests were positive for hepatitis B virus infection. One year after the operation, he is still alive, in good condition living at his village.

## 3. Discussion

Hepatocellular cancer is a hypervascular tumor with a high tendency for vascular invasion. However, the mechanism of spontaneous rupture is still not exactly known. Possible causes are rapid growth and necrosis, erosion of a vessel,

increased intratumoral pressure caused from the occlusion of hepatic veins by tumor thrombi or invasion, and coagulopathy [5]. Spontaneous rupture is the third most common cause of death due to HCC, after neoplastic progression and liver failure, and it is more frequent in males [6]. An important condition for intraperitoneal bleeding is tumor's location with tumors at the edge of the liver being at greater risk compared with intraparenchymal HCC. Typical symptoms of spontaneous rupture are epigastric pain of sudden onset with or without clinical signs of shock and peritoneal irritation. Diagnosis of ruptured HCC can be difficult especially when there is no history of HCC, cirrhosis, or HBV infection and the patient is in hemodynamic instability [5, 6]. Abdominal CT scans are useful in demonstrating the presence of hemoperitoneum and liver tumor with the additional advantage of showing tumor characteristics, the amount of ascites, related vascular abnormalities, patency of portal vein, and the likelihood of metastasis [4]. The primary aim of management in such cases should be the restoration and support of intravascular volume and attempts for hemostasis and preservation of liver parenchyma as much as possible [5, 6]. It is known that bleeding and hemodynamic instability are factors which strongly influence the prognosis [7–9]. Thus, the therapeutic choice must take into account the hemodynamic conditions, functional status of the liver, and stage of the cancer [6]. TAE has been increasingly used for hemostasis in ruptured HCC especially when there is hepatic insufficiency or liver cirrhosis [6, 10–12]. Even if TAE is associated with rebleeding, liver abscess, and a mortality rate of around 30%, this technique remains the best method to achieve hemostasis without surgery with a success rate up to 99% in cases of ruptured HCC [11, 13–15]. Moreover, when feasible, super selective TAE has the advantage of preserving liver function and can be used either as a definitive treatment or as a bridge to liver resection. When TAE fails or is not available, surgical hemostasis is the only alternative. Surgical hemostasis can be achieved by various techniques, including perihepatic packing, suture plication of bleeding tumor, hepatic artery ligation, and liver resection. Although open surgical procedures achieve a high rate of hemostasis and better survival outcome than TAE [16], they are associated with a high in-hospital mortality rate especially following emergency liver resections due to the damage of the residual hepatic function, leading to postoperative liver failure [4]. Furthermore, the presence of hemorrhagic shock renders the liver function poorer than usual. Therefore, emergency one-stage liver resection is feasible in patients with adequate liver function and limited tumors [5]. When patient's condition is too critical for emergency liver resection, a damage control strategy should be selected, as in liver trauma cases. In our patient, a combination of enucleation of the tumor, perihepatic packing, and hepatic artery ligation (HAL) was performed due the hemodynamic instability and his comorbidities associated with his age. In ruptured HCC, HAL has a hemostatic success rate of 68% to 100% and can either be selective or at the level of the hepatic artery, but its use is limited due to its high in-hospital mortality rate of 50% to 77% [17–19]. Packing of a bleeding tumor achieves hemostasis by tamponade effect and it is effective especially for oozing tumors. The duration of pack should be 24 to 48 hours. Packing for longer time increases the rate of intra-abdominal infection and sepsis according to clinical evidence from perihepatic packing in liver trauma cases [20, 21]. Perihepatic packing is a reliable method in hemodynamically unstable patients who require a fast damage control laparotomy providing early resuscitation and stabilization.

In summary, the management of spontaneous rupture of HCC is always a troublesome situation for emergency physicians and surgeons. The treatment of this devastating emergency should be closely scrutinized, with stabilization of vital signs and maintenance of hepatic perfusion as soon as possible. Nevertheless, the primary goal should be a definitive bleeding arrest. Although there is no consensus on the most effective treatment, the therapeutic choice must take into account the hemodynamic conditions, functional status of the liver, and stage of the cancer. In general, TAE should be the method of choice as it is less invasive and very efficacious technique and can be done with regional anesthesia. However, for patients with stable vital signs, noncirrhotic liver, and limited tumors, as shown in the abdominal CT scan, immediate hepatectomy can also be considered [4]. For unstable patients with poor liver function or questionable posthepatectomy functional residual volumes, TAE is very effective in achieving immediate hemostasis [4, 6]. Whether TAE is to be followed by staged hepatectomy depends on the recovery of liver function and thorough investigation of the tumor characteristics [4]. In cases of unstable patients and TAE failure, surgical hemostasis should be performed. Liver resection maybe attempted in cases with small tumors, adequate FLR (future liver remnant), and well preserved liver function but with a high rate of mortality. Otherwise, damage control strategies, as in liver trauma, are a reasonable alternative.

## Conflict of Interests

The authors declare that there is no conflict of interests regarding the publication of this paper.

## References

[1] P. Ferenci, M. Fried, D. Labrecque et al., "Hepatocellular carcinoma (HCC): a global perspective," Journal of Clinical Gastroenterology, vol. 44, no. 4, pp. 239–245, 2010.

[2] M.-F. Chen, T.-L. Hwang, L.-B. Jeng, Y.-Y. Jan, and C.-S. Wang, "Clinical experience with hepatic resection for ruptured hepatocellular carcinoma," Hepato-Gastroenterology, vol. 42, no. 2, pp. 166–168, 1995.

[3] V. Vergara, A. Muratore, H. Bouzari et al., "Spontaneous rupture of hepatocelluar carcinoma: surgical resection and long-term survival," European Journal of Surgical Oncology, vol. 26, no. 8, pp. 770–772, 2000.

[4] K.-C. Hsueh, H.-L. Fan, T.-W. Chen et al., "Management of spontaneously ruptured hepatocellular carcinoma and hemoperitoneum manifested as acute abdomen in the emergency room," World Journal of Surgery, vol. 36, no. 11, pp. 2670–2676, 2012.

[5] E. C. H. Lai and W. Y. Lau, "Spontaneous rupture of hepatocellular carcinoma: a systematic review," Archives of Surgery, vol. 141, no. 2, pp. 191–198, 2006.

[6] N. Bassi, E. Caratozzolo, L. Bonariol et al., "Management of ruptured hepatocellular carcinoma: implications for therapy," World Journal of Gastroenterology, vol. 16, no. 10, pp. 1221–1225, 2010.

[7] C.-L. Liu, S.-T. Fan, C.-M. Lo et al., "Management of spontaneous rupture of hepatocellular carcinoma: single-center experience," Journal of Clinical Oncology, vol. 19, no. 17, pp. 3725–3732, 2001.

[8] F. L.-S. Tan, Y.-M. Tan, A. Y.-F. Chung, P. C. Cheow, P. K.-H. Chow, and L. L. Ooi, "Factors affecting early mortality in spontaneous rupture of hepatocellular carcinoma," ANZ Journal of Surgery, vol. 76, no. 6, pp. 448–452, 2006.

[9] H. Kirikoshi, S. Saito, M. Yoneda et al., "Outcomes and factors influencing survival in cirrhotic cases with spontaneous rupture of hepatocellular carcinoma: a multicenter study," BMC Gastroenterology, vol. 9, article 29, 2009.

[10] L. Castells, M. Moreiras, S. Quiroga et al., "Hemoperitoneum as a first manifestation of hepatocellular carcinoma in Western patients with liver cirrhosis: effectiveness of emergency treatment with transcatheter arterial embolization," Digestive Diseases and Sciences, vol. 46, no. 3, pp. 555–562, 2001.

[11] A. Tanaka, R. Takeda, S. Mukaihara et al., "Treatment of ruptured hepatocellular carcinoma," International Journal of Clinical Oncology, vol. 6, no. 6, pp. 291–295, 2001.

[12] R. Shimada, H. Imamura, M. Makuuchi et al., "Staged hepatectomy after emergency transcatheter arterial embolization for ruptured hepatocellular carcinoma," Surgery, vol. 124, no. 3, pp. 526–535, 1998.

[13] W.-H. Li, E. C.-Y. Cheuk, P. C.-H. Kowk, and M.-T. Cheung, "Survival after transarterial embolization for spontaneous ruptured hepatocellular carcinoma," Journal of Hepato-Biliary-Pancreatic Surgery, vol. 16, no. 4, pp. 508–512, 2009.

[14] C.-T. Kung, B.-M. Liu, S.-H. Ng et al., "Transcatheter arterial embolization in the emergency department for hemodynamic instability due to ruptured hepatocellular carcinoma: analysis of 167 cases," American Journal of Roentgenology, vol. 191, no. 6, pp. W231–W239, 2008.

[15] C.-N. Yeh, W.-C. Lee, L.-B. Jeng, M.-F. Chen, and M.-C. Yu, "Spontaneous tumour rupture and prognosis in patients with hepatocellular carcinoma," British Journal of Surgery, vol. 89, no. 9, pp. 1125–1129, 2002.

[16] Y.-J. Jin, J.-W. Lee, S.-W. Park et al., "Survival outcome of patients with spontaneously ruptured hepatocellular carcinoma treated surgically or by transarterial embolization," World Journal of Gastroenterology, vol. 19, no. 28, pp. 4537–4544, 2013.

[17] G. B. Ong, E. P. Chu, F. Y. Yu, and T. C. Lee, "Spontaneous rupture of hepatocellular carcinoma," The British Journal of Surgery, vol. 52, pp. 123–129, 1965.

[18] O. Chearanai, U. Plengvanit, C. Asavanich, D. Damrongsak, K. Sindhvananda, and S. Boonyapisit, "Spontaneous rupture of primary hepatoma: report of 63 cases with particular reference to the pathogenesis and rationale treatment by hepatic artery ligation," Cancer, vol. 51, no. 8, pp. 1532–1536, 1983.

[19] E. C. S. Lai, K. M. Wu, T. K. Choi, S. T. Fan, and J. Wong, "Spontaneous ruptured hepatocellular carcinoma: an appraisal of surgical treatment," Annals of Surgery, vol. 210, no. 1, pp. 24–28, 1989.

[20] J. Saifi, J. B. Fortune, L. Graca, and D. M. Shah, "Benefits of intra-abdominal pack placement for the management of nonmechanical hemorrhage," *Archives of Surgery*, vol. 125, no. 1, pp. 119–122, 1990.

[21] J. A. Abikhaled, T. S. Granchi, M. J. Wall, A. Hirshberg, and K. L. Mattox, "Prolonged abdominal packing for trauma is associated with increased morbidity and mortality," *American Surgeon*, vol. 63, no. 12, pp. 1109–1113, 1997.

# 10

# Phencyclidine Induced Oculogyric Crisis Responding Well to Conventional Treatment

**Hassan Tahir and Vistasp Daruwalla**

*Department of Internal Medicine, Temple University/Conemaugh Memorial Hospital, 1086 Franklin Street, Johnstown, PA 15905, USA*

Correspondence should be addressed to Hassan Tahir; htahir@conemaugh.org

Academic Editor: Oludayo A. Sowande

*Background.* Oculogyric crisis is a form of acute dystonic reaction characterized by involuntary upward deviation of eye ball. Its causes are broad with antipsychotics and antiemetics as the most common causes. *Case Presentation.* A 25-year-old man with the past medical history of marijuana use presented to ED with involuntary upward deviation of eye 1 day after using phencyclidine (PCP) for the first time. He did not have any other symptoms and was hemodynamically stable. All laboratory investigations were normal except urine drug screen which was positive for PCP. Patient was treated with IV diphenhydramine which improved his symptoms. *Conclusion.* Illicit drug abuse is a growing problem in our society with increasingly more patients presenting to ED with its complications. The differential diagnosis of acute dystonic reactions should be extended to include illicit drugs as the potential cause of reversible acute dystonias especially in high risk patients.

## 1. Introduction

Dystonia is a movement disorder characterized by sustained or intermittent muscle contractions causing abnormal, often repetitive, movements, postures, or both. Dystonic movements are typically patterned, twisting, and may be tremulous. Dystonia is often initiated or worsened by voluntary action and associated with overflow muscle activation [1]. Drug induced acute dystonia (DID) is one of the commonest forms of secondary dystonia, along with tardive dystonia. This complication occurs in wide frequency range, depending on the specific drugs prescribed, indications, and studied populations [2]. Clinical presentation commonly includes craniocervical distribution with blepharospasm, buccolingual, mandibular, face and neck dystonia, and oculogyric crisis with contracture of the extraocular muscles leading to conjugate eyes deviation, usually with a predominance of the superior rectus muscle and consequent upward eye deviation [3]. Drug abuse is a rising problem in our society with increasing number of drug abusers being brought to the emergency department because of its complications. Hallucinogens are a class of illicit drugs that cause profound distortion in person's sense of reality. Phencyclidine (PCP), also known as angel dust, is the most dangerous of all hallucinogens due to its effect on behaviour. Unfortunately, there has been a recent increase in the number of emergency visits involving PCP [4]. Rare manifestations and complications of PCP are increasingly seen due to the rising burden of its use [5]. We report a case of 25-year-old man who developed acute oculogyric crisis after using PCP for the first time.

## 2. Case Presentation

A 25-year-old man presented to emergency department with involuntary sustained upward deviation of eyes for one day. According to the patient, he had been using marijuana almost once in a week for the last 5 years but this time he wanted to try a different drug. One day ago, he smoked angel dust with tobacco and also snorted it a little. This was the first time he was using PCP and as per the patient he used very small quantity. After that he felt dizzy and slept whole night. When patient woke up in the morning, he had both of his eyes involuntary deviated in upward direction. His girlfriend immediately brought him to ED for further evaluation. The patient denied any fever, headache, light headedness, slurred speech, weakness, diplopia, and auditory or visual hallucinations. Patient did not have any major medical illness other than marijuana use. He denied any family history of seizures, stroke, or cancer. Patient was not on any medication and also denied any accidental use of antiemetics or antipsychotics recently.

He was hemodynamically stable at the time of his admission. On neurological examination, he was well oriented in time, place, and space. Pupils were equal and reactive to light. Sustained conjugate upward deviation of eyes was noted. The patient was able to bring his eyes back to normal position with forceful effort but eyes used to deviate back to upward position within few seconds. Visual field, visual acuity, and ocular movements testing could not be done due to his upward deviation of eyes. Intraocular pressure was normal and fundoscopy showed normal retina and fundus. Cranial nerve functions were intact, power was 5/5 in all extremities, and there was no sensory loss. The rest of the physical examination was unremarkable. All laboratory data including complete blood count, serum electrolytes, and renal and liver function tests were within normal limits. Urine drug screen was done which came back positive for phencyclidine (PCP). Based on the onset of oculogyric crisis after taking PCP and positive urine drug screen, the diagnosis of PCP induced oculogyric crisis was made. Patient was seen by a neurologist for the evaluation of oculogyric crisis who recommended against any neurological imaging as the case was typical of dystonia and the patient did not have any headache, neck stiffness, seizure, or focal neurological deficits suggestive of intracranial pathology. Decision was made to give IV Benadryl and check response first.

Patient was given 50 mg of diphenhydramine (Benadryl) intravenously once. After 30 minutes, patient's eyes reverted back to normal position. Repeat neurological examination showed equal and reactive pupil. Eye movements were normal in all directions with normal visual acuity and no visual field defect. There was no motor or sensory deficit and his gait was normal. Patient was discharged on 25 mg of Benadryl TID for the next 2 days and also counselled about cessation of illicit drugs. Patient did not have any acute dystonia on follow-up.

## 3. Discussion

Acute dystonia is a movement disorder characterized by intermittent or sustained involuntary muscle contractions involving face, pelvis, trunk, neck, or rarely larynx [6]. Oculogyric crisis is a type of acute dystonia characterized by spasmodic movement of eyeball, usually upward, and each spasm lasts from seconds to hours. Oculogyric crisis is not usually life threatening but it can be very distressing to the patient and family. The causes of acute dystonic reaction are broad with drugs being the most common cause. Rarely, brain stem lesions, encephalitis, and trauma can also cause acute dystonias [7]. Cocaine and ecstasy have also been reported to cause acute dystonic reaction [8]. Although the main mechanism of acute dystonic reactions is still unclear, it is believed that central dopamine blockage with resulting increase in striatal acetylcholine may be the underlying mechanism [9]. Differential diagnosis of oculogyric crisis

also includes epilepsy, encephalitis, tetanus, hypocalcemia, brainstem lesions, cystic glioma, and Wilson's disease [10, 11], so it is important to rule out these conditions before making a diagnosis of oculogyric crisis due to drugs. Thorough history, physical examination, and baseline laboratory investigations can help to rule out important differential diagnoses.

Acute dystonic reactions are treated by anticholinergic medications like benztropine, promethazine, or diphenhydramine. Antihistamines like promethazine and diphenhydramine can be successfully used for treating acute dystonias due to their additional anticholinergic effects. Patient is given 2 mg of benztropine or 50 mg of diphenhydramine and watched for improvement of dystonia over the next 15 minutes. This step is both therapeutic and diagnostic. Medication should be preferably given via IV route and in majority of cases, symptoms resolve in 10 mins [12]. In some cases, more than one dosing is necessary for complete resolution of dystonia. In refractory cases or in the presence of contraindications to anticholinergics, diazepam can be used to treat dystonias with variable success [12]. Patient should be followed up for at least 2-3 days, as dystonia caused by long acting drugs may cause relapse of dystonia.

PCP or "angel dust" is a common hallucinogen that is sold illegally in many different forms and is usually smoked with marijuana or tobacco [4]. Depending on route and dose, its effects can last approximately 4–6 hours. PCP, like other hallucinogens, can distort the patient's perception of reality and produces feeling of detachment from environment and self. Delusions, hallucinations, and paranoia mimicking schizophrenia are possible. In extreme cases, seizures and coma can occur [13]. Unlike other hallucinogens, PCP is notorious for causing mood disturbances which can lead to very violent behaviour, thus making it the most dangerous hallucinogen [13]. Long term use can cause dementia, anxiety, and depression. PCP acts on glutamate receptors of brain where it acts as NMDA receptor antagonist and produces its effect. Glutamate receptor has a role in modulating learning, memory, and mood [14].

Our patient came with oculogyric crisis after using PCP for the first time. Interestingly, patient developed acute dystonic reaction after using only small quantities of PCP thus exhibiting idiosyncratic drug response. Patient did not have any hallucinations, delusions, or behaviour problems. CT scan of the head was not done because he did not have any headache, neck stiffness, seizure, or focal neurological deficit. IV Benadryl was given and patient response to it was used as a diagnostic test for acute dystonia. Acute dystonia resolved with Benadryl and patient did not have any symptoms on follow-up next day, after 6 weeks, and then 3 months, so the decision about not doing neurological imaging was considered appropriate. Urine drug screen was positive for PCP but the rest of laboratory investigations were within normal limits. Patient was not on any antipsychotic or antiemetic medication. Patient was given 50 mg of diphenhydramine to which he responded well. The fact that his symptoms were relieved by anticholinergics indicates that pathogenesis of PCP induced oculogyric crisis might be similar to acute dystonias caused by antipsychotics. The exact mechanism is still unclear.

## 4. Conclusion

Acute dystonias including oculogyric crisis have been well known to be caused by antipsychotics and antiemetics. Illicit drugs can very rarely cause similar movement disorders. Due to increasing number of patients with drug abuse being brought to the emergency department, it is imperative to include illicit drugs including PCP in the differential diagnosis of acute dystonias. The management is the same as for dystonias caused by antipsychotics, that is, anticholinergics and reassurance. Our case report highlights the fact that oculogyric crises caused by drugs may be reversible and prognosis may be good.

## Abbreviations

PCP: Phencyclidine
DID: Drug induced acute dystonia
NMDA: N-Methyl-D-aspartate.

## Conflict of Interests

The authors confirm that they have no competing interests.

## References

[1] A. Albanese, K. Bhatia, S. B. Bressman et al., "Phenomenology and classification of dystonia: a consensus update," *Movement Disorders*, vol. 28, no. 7, pp. 863–873, 2013.

[2] D. E. Casey, "Neuroleptic-induced acute dystonia," in *Drug-Induced Movement Disorders*, A. E. Lang, Ed., pp. 21–41, Futura Publishing, Mount Kisco, NY, USA, 1992.

[3] B. J. Robottom, S. A. Factor, and W. J. Weiner, "Movement disorders emergencies part 2: hyperkinetic disorders," *Archives of Neurology*, vol. 68, no. 6, pp. 719–724, 2011.

[4] U.S. Department of Justice and Drug Enforcement Administration, "PCP: the threat remains," *Microgram Bulletin*, vol. 36, no. 8, pp. 181–190, 2003.

[5] National Institute on Drug Abuse, "Research report series: hallucinogens and dissociative drugs," NIH Publication Number 01-4209, National Institute of Health, Washington, DC, USA, 2001.

[6] R. P. Munhoz, M. Moscovich, P. D. Araujo, and H. A. G. Teive, "Movement disorders emergencies: a review," *Arquivos de Neuro-Psiquiatria*, vol. 70, no. 6, pp. 453–461, 2012.

[7] G. T. Schumock and E. Martinez, "Acute oculogyric crisis after administration of prochlorperazine," *Southern Medical Journal*, vol. 84, no. 3, pp. 407–408, 1991.

[8] P. N. van Harten, H. W. Hoek, and R. S. Kahn, "Fortnightly review: acute dystonia induced by drug treatment," *British Medical Journal*, vol. 319, no. 7210, pp. 623–626, 1999.

[9] P. J. Blanchet, "Antipsychotic drug-induced movement disorders," *Canadian Journal of Neurological Sciences*, vol. 30, no. 1, pp. S101–S107, 2003.

[10] M. S. Lee, Y. D. Kim, and C. H. Lyoo, "Oculogyric crisis as an initial manifestation of Wilson's disease," *Neurology*, vol. 52, no. 8, pp. 1714–1715, 1999.

[11] M. T. Stechison, "Cystic glioma with positional oculogyric crisis," *Journal of Neurosurgery*, vol. 71, no. 6, pp. 955–956, 1989.

[12] A. S. Lee, "Treatment of drug-induced dystonic reactions," *Journal of the American College of Emergency Physicians*, vol. 8, no. 11, pp. 453–457, 1979.

[13] T. Bey and A. Patel, "Phencyclidine intoxication and adverse effects: a clinical and pharmacological review of an illicit drug," *California Journal of Emergency Medicine*, vol. 8, no. 1, pp. 9–14, 2007.

[14] W. E. Fantegrossi, K. S. Murnane, and C. J. Reissig, "The behavioral pharmacology of hallucinogens," *Biochemical Pharmacology*, vol. 75, no. 1, pp. 17–33, 2008.

# 11

# Food Particle Aspiration Associated with Hemorrhagic Shock: A Diagnostic Dilemma

**Basheer Tashtoush,[1] Jonathan Schroeder,[1] Roya Memarpour,[1] Eduardo Oliveira,[1] Michael Medina,[2] Anas Hadeh,[1] Jose Ramirez,[1] and Laurence Smolley[1]**

[1]*Department of Pulmonary and Critical Care Medicine, Cleveland Clinic Florida, Weston, FL, USA*
[2]*Department of Otolaryngology, Cleveland Clinic Florida, Weston, FL, USA*

Correspondence should be addressed to Basheer Tashtoush; tashtob@ccf.org

Academic Editor: Ritesh Agarwal

The hemodynamic compromise caused by a large aspirated food particle in the airway can become the focus of medical attention and a distraction from rare but fatal Heimlich maneuver related injuries after an incident of food aspiration. We herein present a case of an 84-year-old man who was brought to the emergency department after an episode of choking at a restaurant followed by several failed Heimlich maneuver attempts. Despite relieving the airway obstruction by extracting a large piece of steak from the airway, the patient remained hypotensive and required continued hemodynamic support. Repeated laboratory tests within 24 hrs of aspiration showed a significant decline in the hemoglobin level. A computed tomography (CT) scan of the abdomen and pelvis showed a lacerated liver with a large subcapsular hematoma draining into the pelvis. *Conclusion.* Hepatic rupture is a rare complication of Heimlich maneuver; this paper represents the second case report in the literature. It emphasizes the necessity of early identification and surveillance of fatal Heimlich maneuver complications in a high risk population.

## 1. Case Presentation

An 84-year-old Caucasian man was brought to the emergency department (ED) after an episode of choking at a restaurant. Reports from the emergency medical services (EMS) personnel, who responded to the scene, indicated that the patient had developed signs of choking when a bystander performed several unsuccessful attempts of Heimlich maneuver (HM). Upon EMS arrival, the patient was found to be unresponsive, apneic, and pulseless. Cardiopulmonary resuscitation (CPR) was performed with return of spontaneous circulation after two minutes of CPR. He was intubated in the field by EMS personnel, who reported difficulty during intubation, as an obstructing foreign body prevented proper advancement of the ET tube (size 7) into the trachea.

Upon arrival to the ED, the patient was found to be hypotensive, requiring immediate fluid resuscitation, vasopressors, and continued mechanical ventilation. He had signs of a persistent large food particle in the main airway as evidenced on the Flow/Time monitor, which showed auto-PEEP with a notched expiratory flow curve, an elevated peak pressure of 53 cm $H_2O$, and plateau pressure of 26 cm $H_2O$ (Figure 1).

Chest X-ray (Figure 2) showed inflated lungs with a right upper lobe opacity. Empiric antimicrobial treatment for aspiration pneumonia was initiated. A flexible bronchoscopy procedure to extract the food particle was attempted on admission but was unsuccessful, as the forceps could not properly grasp the meat particle without biting through it.

Over the following 12 hours, the patient developed severe refractory shock with multiorgan failure, despite adequate oxygenation. Laboratory test results (Table 1) revealed severe lactic acidosis, acute renal failure, and elevated liver enzymes.

After 24 hours of his initial presentation, the patient was transferred to our facility for rigid bronchoscopy and further management.

Upon arrival, the patient was found to be in severe shock, with a blood pressure of 60/49 mmHg, a heart rate of

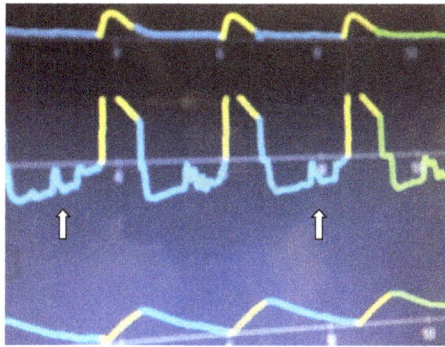

FIGURE 1: Flow/Time curve on the mechanical ventilator showing auto-PEEP with a notched expiratory flow curve appearing as an "inverted square root sign" (arrows); this represents a complete occlusion of the airway during expiration when the point of equalization of pressures reaches the level of airway obstruction.

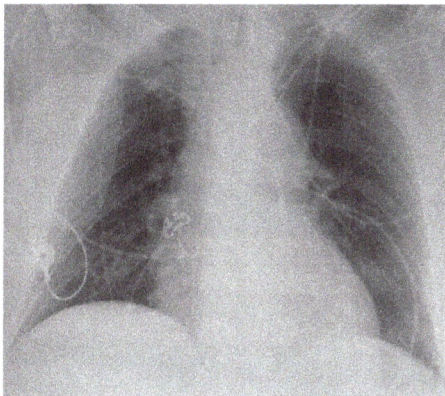

FIGURE 2: Chest X-ray. Inflated lungs with right upper lobe opacity and a high endotracheal tube position caused by a foreign body in the central airway.

150 bpm, and severe lactic acidosis, on maximum dose of IV norepinephrine and vasopressin.

Rigid bronchoscopy was performed immediately, where the patient was taken to the operating room and placed in neck extended, supine position. A 12 mm external diameter rigid bronchoscope was utilized during the procedure to visualize the trachea and mainstem bronchi while being ventilated via an external side port. A large piece of meat was seen lodged in the distal trachea and extended into the right mainstem bronchus, which was successfully extracted with a grasping crocodile-jaw forceps (Figure 3).

Despite relieving the airway obstruction, the patient remained hypotensive and required continued hemodynamic support after the procedure. Repeated laboratory tests drawn upon arrival to our facility showed a significant decline in the hemoglobin level (~3 gm/dL) compared to 24 hours earlier (Table 1). With no obvious external bleed, an intra-abdominal or retroperitoneal hemorrhage was suspected, and immediate transfusion of packed RBCs with fresh frozen plasma was initiated. A CT scan of the abdomen and pelvis (Figure 4) revealed a lacerated liver with a large subcapsular hematoma draining into the pelvis. In the absence of any rib fractures or

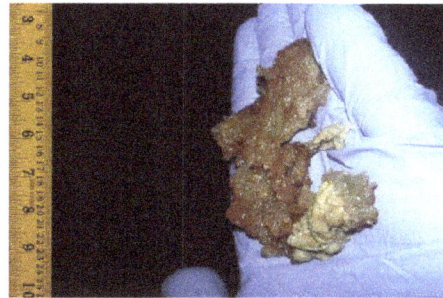

FIGURE 3: A large piece of steak removed from the trachea with rigid bronchoscopy, approximately 10 cm long.

TABLE 1: Laboratory test results on admission and repeated tests 24 hours later.

| Laboratory tests on arrival to ED | Laboratory tests 24 hrs after aspiration |
|---|---|
| Arterial blood gas analysis (ABG) | |
| PH: 7.21 | PH: 7.38 |
| $PCO_2$: 28 mmHg | $PCO_2$: 32 mmHg |
| $PO_2$: 423 mmHg | $PO_2$: 134 mmHg |
| $HCO_3$: 11.2 mmol/L | $HCO_3$: 19.3 mmol/L |
| Lactate: 12.9 mmol/L | Lactate: 14.34 |
| $FiO_2$: 100% | $FiO_2$: 60% |
| Serum chemistry tests | |
| Glucose: 120 mg/dL | Glucose: 174 mg/dL |
| K: 3.6 mmol/L | K: 4.9 mmol/L |
| Na: 143 mmol/L | Na: 148 mmol/L |
| Cl: 117 mmol/L | Cl: 105 mmol/L |
| $HCO_3$: 12 mmol/L | $HCO_3$: 22 mmol/L |
| Ca: 7.7 mg/dL | Ca: 8.2 mg/dL |
| Mg: 2.0 mg/dL | Mg: 2.2 mg/dL |
| BUN: 31 mg/dL | BUN: 36 mmol/L |
| Creatinine: 2.0 mg/dL | Creatinine: 2.1 mg/dL |
| ALB: 2.5 gm/dL | ALB: 2.5 gm/dL |
| TPROT: 4 gm/dL | TPROT: 3.8 gm/dL |
| ALKPHOS: 103 U/L | ALKPHOS: 156 U/L |
| ALT: 426 U/L | ALT: 3947 U/L |
| AST: 2307 U/L | AST: >7000 U/L |
| TBILI: 0.9 mg/dL | TBILI: 1.7 mg/dL |
| Complete blood count | |
| WBC: 12.56 k/$\mu$L | WBC: 13.09 k/$\mu$L |
| HB: 8.1 g/dL | HB: 5.3 g/L |
| HCT: 25% | HCT: 16.8% |
| PLT: 133 k/$\mu$L | PLT: 155 k/$\mu$L |
| Coagulation profile | |
| APTT: 31.0 sec | APTT: 31.8 sec |
| INR: 1.5 | INR: 1.6 |

prolonged CPR, the laceration was attributed to the repeated HM (abdominal thrusts) performed.

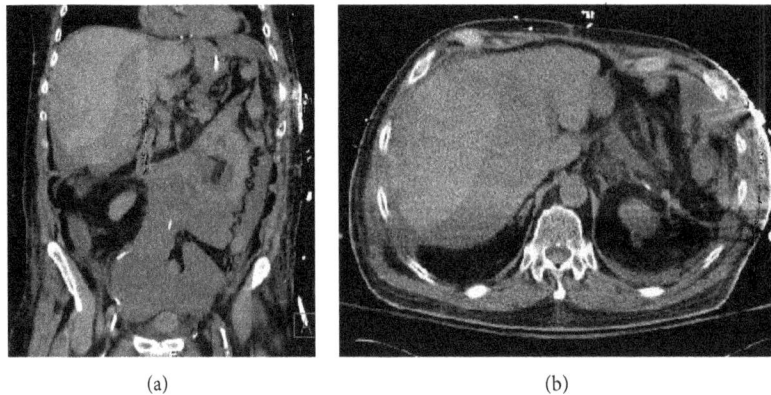

(a)                                                                                                     (b)

FIGURE 4: CT abdomen and pelvis. (a) Coronal view and (b) axial view, showing a liver laceration with a large subcapsular hematoma and hemoperitoneum.

Upon further inquiry, family members who witnessed the bystander performing the HM stated that more than ten abdominal thrusts were performed while the patient was in a seated position, as he was unable to stand.

The liver laceration was managed conservatively with transfusion of blood products and close monitoring. Over the following two days, the patient was weaned off vasopressors, and extubated on day three of admission to our facility. Liver enzymes trended down over the course of hospitalization, and the patient was discharged to a rehab facility three weeks later for extended nursing care and physical therapy.

## 2. Discussion

The Heimlich maneuver (HM) was first publicized by Heimlich in 1975 [1]. A year later, the National Research Council reported that 500 lives were saved by the HM [2]. Since that time, vigorous promotion of this technique has saved the lives of many choking victims and became widely accepted as the universal method for relieving foreign body upper airway obstruction [3]. However, several rare but life threatening complications have been reported from properly and improperly performed HM.

Complications such as rib and vertebral fractures, retinal detachment [4], diaphragmatic rupture [5], ruptured aortic valve [6], acute thrombosis of abdominal aortic aneurysm [7–10], aortic stent-graft displacement [11], mesenteric laceration [12], and many other fatal traumatic injuries of the gastrointestinal tract have also been reported [13–18].

Hepatic rupture is an extremely rare complication of HM with only one previously reported case in literature in 2007 by Palleiro et al. [19].

Our patient's family members stated that a Good Samaritan performed the maneuver more than ten times while the patient was in a seated position. This may have contributed to the hepatic injury, as the correct application of HM in a seated victim has not been well described, and abdominal thrusts may have been directly applied to the liver.

Common features shared with the case reported by Palleiro et al. include patients age, both in their 80s, and meat aspiration occurred in both cases. However, there was

no precise description of how the HM was performed in the previously reported case.

Even when performed correctly, the maneuver can be associated with rare complications. Rib fractures and gastric and esophageal perforations are among the most frequently reported [20, 21].

In this case, the large piece of meat in the airway performed as a ball valve, demonstrating auto-PEEP on the Flow/Time curve of the mechanical ventilator monitor (Figure 1), with a notched expiratory flow curve giving the "inverted square root sign," where the particle completely but transiently occludes the expiratory airflow towards the end of expiration when the point of equalization of pressures reaches the level of obstruction. After this transient flow cessation, expiratory airflow resumes as the point of equalization of pressures passes the level of obstruction.

Auto-PEEP can cause significant hemodynamic compromise and circulatory collapse, as the increased intrathoracic pressure associated with auto-PEEP reduces venous return (preload) and increases pulmonary vascular resistance, precipitating right ventricular strain and failure. In addition, auto-PEEP can augment left ventricular afterload due to increased negative intrapleural pressure generated by the patient when he/she triggers the ventilator. All these phenomena can severely reduce the cardiac output and precipitate shock [22, 23].

Urgent rigid bronchoscopy in a hemodynamically unstable patient with central airway obstruction is critical. In this patient the delay in performing rigid bronchoscopy occurred due to the flexible bronchoscopy attempt and the lack of resources for rigid bronchoscopy at the referring facility, in addition to the patient's hemodynamic instability, which delayed the decision to transfer the patient.

Because of the major airway obstruction in our patient, the auto-PEEP was thought to be the primary cause of the persistent hypotension and circulatory failure. However, when the obstruction was removed, the persistent shock and the decline in the hemoglobin level indicated that a concealed source of hemorrhage was overlooked.

Given the potential for critical abdominal organ injuries in association with the HM, there appears to be an emerging necessity to establish surveillance guidelines for internal organ injuries when evaluating high risk patients who undergo HM, for example, children, the elderly, and patients with impaired consciousness.

## 3. Conclusion

Hepatic rupture is a rare complication of Heimlich maneuver; this paper represents the second case report in the literature. It emphasizes the necessity of early identification and surveillance of fatal Heimlich maneuver complications in a high risk population.

## Conflict of Interests

The authors declare that there is no conflict of interests regarding the publication of this paper.

## References

[1] H. J. Heimlich, "A life-saving maneuver to prevent food-choking," *Journal of the American Medical Association*, vol. 234, no. 4, pp. 398–401, 1975.

[2] The National Safety Council, 2009, http://www.nsc.org/research/odds.aspx.

[3] H. J. Heimlich and E. A. Patrick, "The Heimlich maneuver. Best technique for saving any choking victim's life," *Postgraduate Medicine*, vol. 87, no. 6, pp. 38–48, 1990.

[4] J. A. Fink and R. L. Klein, "Complications of the Heimlich maneuver," *Journal of Pediatric Surgery*, vol. 24, no. 5, pp. 486–487, 1989.

[5] V. Ujjin, S. Ratanasit, and T. Nagendran, "Diaphragmatic hernia as a complication of the Heimlich maneuver," *International Surgery*, vol. 69, no. 2, pp. 175–176, 1984.

[6] J. H. Chapman, F. J. Menapace, and R. R. Howell, "Ruptured aortic valve cusp: a complication of the Heimlich maneuver," *Annals of Emergency Medicine*, vol. 12, no. 7, pp. 446–448, 1983.

[7] R. L. Kirshner and R. M. Green, "Acute thrombosis of abdominal aortic aneurysm subsequent to Heimlich maneuver: a case report," *Journal of Vascular Surgery*, vol. 2, pp. 594–596, 1985.

[8] E. F. Roehm, M. W. Twiest, and R. C. Williams Jr., "Abdominal aortic thrombosis in association with an attempted Heimlich maneuver," *Journal of the American Medical Association*, vol. 249, no. 9, pp. 1186–1187, 1983.

[9] L. Mack, T. L. Forbes, and K. A. Harris, "Acute aortic thrombosis following incorrect application of the Heimlich maneuver," *Annals of Vascular Surgery*, vol. 16, no. 1, pp. 130–133, 2002.

[10] J. Ayerdi, S. K. Gupta, L. N. Sampson, and N. Deshmukh, "Acute abdominal aortic thrombosis following the Heimlich maneuver," *Cardiovascular Surgery*, vol. 10, no. 2, pp. 154–156, 2002.

[11] P. H. Lin, R. L. Bush, and A. B. Lumsden, "Proximal aortic stent-graft displacement with type I endoleak due to Heimlich maneuver," *Journal of Vascular Surgery*, vol. 38, no. 2, pp. 380–382, 2003.

[12] V. Valero, "Mesenteric laceration complicating a Heimlich maneuver," *Annals of Emergency Medicine*, vol. 15, no. 1, pp. 105–106, 1986.

[13] M. J. Meredith and R. Liebowitz, "Rupture of the esophagus caused by the Heimlich maneuver," *Annals of Emergency Medicine*, vol. 15, no. 1, pp. 106–107, 1986.

[14] D. E. Haynes, B. E. Haynes, and Y. V. Yong, "Esophageal rupture complicating Heimlich maneuver," *American Journal of Emergency Medicine*, vol. 2, no. 6, pp. 507–509, 1984.

[15] M. Bintz and T. H. Cogbill, "Gastric rupture after the Heimlich maneuver," *The Journal of Trauma-Injury Infection & Critical Care*, vol. 40, no. 1, pp. 159–160, 1996.

[16] R. M. Razaboni, C. E. M. Brathwaite, and W. A. Dwyer Jr., "Ruptured jejunum following Heimlich maneuver," *Journal of Emergency Medicine*, vol. 4, no. 2, pp. 95–98, 1986.

[17] S. N. Feeney, W. Pegoli, and M. L. Gestring, "Pancreatic transection as a complication of the Heimlich maneuver: case report and literature review," *Journal of Trauma*, vol. 62, no. 1, pp. 252–254, 2007.

[18] G. Cecchetto, G. Viel, A. Cecchetto, S. Kusstatscher, and M. Montisci, "Fatal splenic rupture following Heimlich maneuver: case report and literature review," *The American Journal of Forensic Medicine and Pathology*, vol. 32, no. 2, pp. 169–171, 2011.

[19] M. M. O. Palleiro, C. B. López, M. C. F. Pretel, and J. S. Fernández, "Hepatic rupture after Heimlich maneuver," *Annals of Emergency Medicine*, vol. 49, no. 6, pp. 825–826, 2007.

[20] N. M. Fearing and P. B. Harrison, "Complications of the Heimlich maneuver: case report and literature review," *Journal of Trauma—Injury, Infection and Critical Care*, vol. 53, no. 5, pp. 978–979, 2002.

[21] D. A. Wolf, "Heimlich trauma: a violent maneuver," *American Journal of Forensic Medicine and Pathology*, vol. 22, no. 1, pp. 65–67, 2001.

[22] P. E. Pepe and J. J. Marini, "Occult positive end-expiratory pressure in mechanically ventilated patients with airflow obstruction: the auto-PEEP effect," *The American Review of Respiratory Disease*, vol. 126, no. 1, pp. 166–170, 1982.

[23] R. Brandolese, C. Broseghini, G. Polese et al., "Effects of intrinsic PEEP on pulmonary gas exchange in mechanically-ventilated patients," *European Respiratory Journal*, vol. 6, no. 3, pp. 358–363, 1993.

# 12

# Isolated Proximal Tibiofibular Dislocation during Soccer

**Casey Chiu and Johnathan Michael Sheele**

*Department of Emergency Medicine, University Hospitals Case Medical Center and Case Western Reserve University, Cleveland, OH 44106, USA*

Correspondence should be addressed to Casey Chiu; crishly@gmail.com and Johnathan Michael Sheele; jsheele@gmail.com

Academic Editor: Ching H. Loh

Proximal tibiofibular dislocations are rarely encountered in the Emergency Department (ED). We present a case involving a man presenting to the ED with left knee pain after making a sharp left turn on the soccer field. His physical exam was only remarkable for tenderness over the lateral fibular head. His X-rays showed subtle abnormalities of the tibiofibular joint. The dislocation was reduced and the patient was discharged from the ED with orthopedic follow-up.

## 1. Introduction

Isolated dislocation of the proximal tibiofibular joint is an uncommon injury but has been associated with multiple different sports injuries including parachuting, ballet, and rugby as well as motor vehicle accidents [1, 2]. Anterolateral dislocations are the most common tibiofibular joint dislocation and are seen in 85% of cases [3]. The mechanism leading to a tibiofibular joint dislocation usually involves a sudden internal rotation and plantar flexion of the foot and an external rotation of the leg with flexion of the knee or a fall on a flexed adducted leg [3].

The proximal tibiofibular joint is a synovial joint between the oval facet of the head of the fibula and the facet of the lateral tibial condyle. The anterior and posterior tibiofibular ligaments and the joint capsule provide stabilization for the joint [1]. The clinical signs of a tibiofibular joint dislocation include swelling and tenderness around the tibiofibular joint and the proximal fibula. Patients can present with a sensation that the knee feels "out of joint [1]."

Plain radiographs are helpful for diagnosing tibiofibular joint dislocations. The X-rays may show a laterally displaced fibular head and a widened interosseous space. If the diagnosis is uncertain, then X-rays of the unaffected contralateral tibiofibular joint can be helpful in making the diagnosis [1].

## 2. Case Presentation

A 21-year-old male soccer player with no history of prior knee injuries presents to the ED via private vehicle complaining of left proximal leg pain and difficulty ambulating. The patient comes to the ED directly from the soccer field where he states he was running and then made an abrupt cut to the left causing his ankle to roll. He then heard a crack from his knee and immediately felt pain along the lateral side of his proximal leg and proceeded to fall. The patient denied any pain while flexing or extending his knee. The patient states that he may have adducted his left leg while in a flexed position when he cut to the left. The patient complained of his left knee feeling "tight." The patient had no other injuries or complaints and the rest of his physical exam was unremarkable.

On examination, the patient appeared in no distress and his vital signs were stable. The patient had 5/5 strength with dorsiflexion and plantarflexion. Both knee joints were stable with Lachman, posterior drawer, varus stress, and valgus stress test. Just by visual inspection, the left fibular head appeared more pronounced when compared to the contralateral side. The patient also complained of severe tenderness upon palpation over the fibular head with varus stress of the left knee. There was no crepitus to flexion or

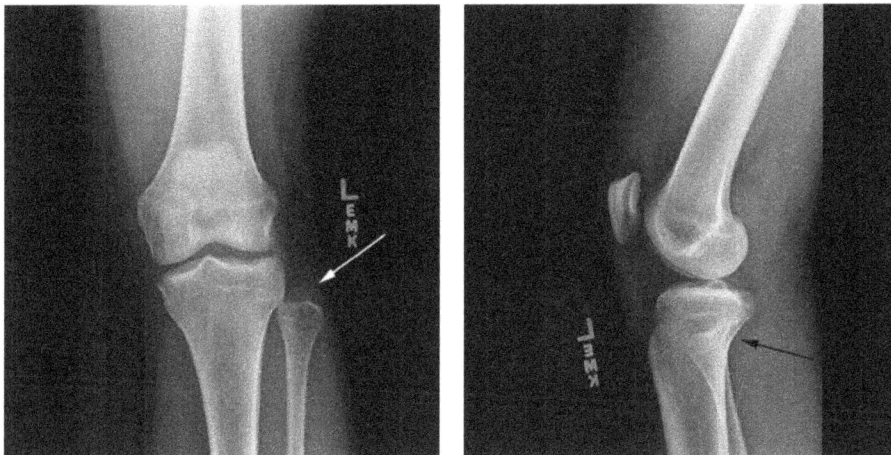

FIGURE 1: AP and lateral X-ray views of the left knee showing Type II anterolateral tibiofibular dislocation.

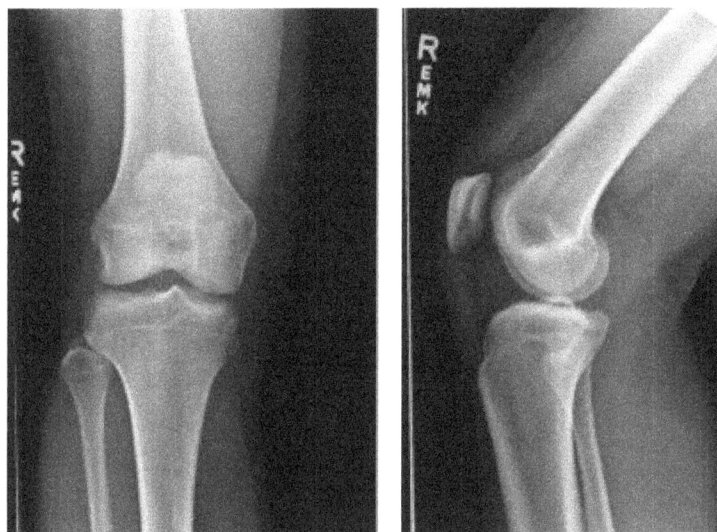

FIGURE 2: AP and lateral X-ray views of the right "unaffected" knee.

extension of the left knee. Anterior-posterior (AP) and lateral view X-rays of the left knee are shown in Figure 1. Figure 2 shows the contralateral AP and lateral X-ray views of the unaffected right knee. The AP view of the affected left knee shows that the fibular head was situated with a more lateral prominence and with less tibia-fibula overlap compared to the right knee. On the lateral views, the left fibular head is very slightly more anterior compared to the contralateral knee. The constellation of history, physical examination, and X-ray finding suggested that the patient had a proximal anterolateral fibular head dislocation. Closed reduction of the left fibular head dislocation was performed by orthopedics. Immediately after joint relocation the patient stated that the left knee pain had improved and the "tightness" had resolved. Figure 3 shows post-X-ray reduction films of the left knee and normal anatomical alignment of the left tibiofibular joint. The patient was placed in a knee immobilizer, given crutches, and referred to orthopedics.

## 3. Discussion

A tibiofibular dislocation is a clinical diagnosis that can often be misdiagnosed as a meniscal injury. If untreated, the patient may experience chronic pain, abnormal gait, and reduced sports performance [4]. A high index of suspicion for a tibiofibular joint dislocation needs to be maintained in all patients who present with lateral knee pain and an inability to bear weight.

There are four types of tibiofibular joint dislocations [2]. Type I is a subluxation of the proximal tibiofibular joint [2]. Type II, the most common type of dislocation, is an anterior dislocation that involves the anterior and posterior tibiofibular ligaments [2]. Type III dislocation involves a posteromedial dislocation that can rarely injure the peroneal nerve [2]. Type IV dislocation involves a superior dislocation and is associated with a tibial shaft fracture or ankle injury [2].

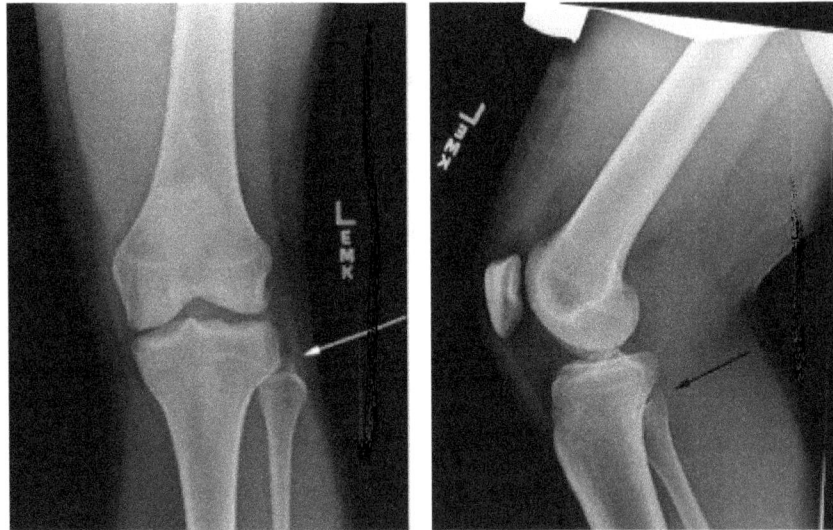

FIGURE 3: AP and lateral X-ray views of the left knee after reduction of the tibiofibular dislocation.

The physical examination for a tibiofibular joint dislocation may only show subtle findings such as a prominent fibular head that can be accentuated by knee flexion with an anterior dislocation [5]. The patient with a tibiofibular joint dislocation often presents with lateral knee pain, a normal range of motion of the affected knee, and no joint effusion [6, 7]. Patients with chronic tibiofibular joint dislocations may have a "popping" sensation in the knee and will often complain of maximal tenderness over the fibular head.

Obtaining X-rays of the AP and lateral views of the unaffected knee for comparison to the painful knee may suggest an abnormality at the tibiofibular joint. Alternatively a computed tomography (CT scan) or magnetic resonance imaging (MRI) can be used to make the diagnosis [8].

Tibiofibular joint dislocations need to be reduced, usually with the knee in flexion, and a "pop" may be heard or felt as the joint is reduced [7]. Patients are then instructed to remain non-weight-bearing until appropriate follow-up with orthopedics [2]. Peroneal nerve injury can occur in up to 5% of tibiofibular dislocations and patients may be more prone to degenerative joint disease in the future [5].

Our patient dislocated his tibiofibular joint after a twisting motion of his left knee. He presented to the ED with a prominent and painful fibular head. The patient had appropriate range of motion and normal laxity of the knee. Reduction of the dislocated joint was accomplished by direct manipulation. In summary, we report a rare case of a tibiofibular joint dislocation and we review the diagnosis and management of the condition. Suspicion for tibiofibular dislocation is needed for persons presenting to the ED with lateral knee pain after a fall and a twisting of the knee.

## Conflict of Interests

The authors declare that there is no conflict of interests regarding the publication of this paper.

## References

[1] J. A. Marx, R. S. Hockberger, R. M. Walls, and P. Rosen, "Knee and lower leg," in *Rosen's Emergency Medicine: Concepts and Clinical Practice*, vol. 1, pp. 720–722, Saunders/Elsevier, Philadelphia, Pa, USA, 8th edition, 2014.

[2] M. I. Iosifidis, I. Giannoulis, A. Tsarouhas, and S. Traios, "Isolated acute dislocation of the proximal tibiofibular joint," *Orthopedics*, vol. 31, no. 6, p. 605, 2008.

[3] Y. Goldstein, A. Gold, O. Chechik, and M. Drexler, "Dislocation of the proximal tibiofibular joint: a rare sports-related injury," *Israel Medical Association Journal*, vol. 13, no. 1, pp. 62–63, 2011.

[4] O. D. Crothers and J. T. Johnson, "Isolated acute dislocation of the proximal tibiofibular joint. Case report," *The Journal of Bone & Joint Surgery—American Volume*, vol. 55, no. 1, pp. 181–183, 1973.

[5] R. R. Simon, S. C. Sherman, G. Q. Sharieff, and R. R. Simon, "Knee," in *Emergency Orthopedics*, McGraw-Hill Medical, New York, NY, USA, 2011.

[6] L. A. Veerappa and C. Gopalakrishna, "Traumatic proximal tibiofibular dislocation with neurovascular injury," *Indian Journal of Orthopaedics*, vol. 46, no. 5, pp. 585–588, 2012.

[7] L. Camarda, A. Abruzzese, and M. D'Arienzo, "Proximal tibiofibular joint reconstruction with autogenous semitendinosus tendon graft," *Techniques in Orthopaedics*, vol. 28, no. 3, pp. 269–272, 2013.

[8] J. Horan and G. Quin, "Proximal tibiofibular dislocation," *Emergency Medicine Journal*, vol. 23, no. 5, article e33, 2006.

# 13

# Temporoparietal Headache as the Initial Presenting Symptom of a Massive Aortic Dissection

**Manan Parikh,**[1] **Abhinav Agrawal,**[1] **Braghadheeswar Thyagarajan,**[1]
**Sayee Sundar Alagusundaramoorthy,**[1] **and James Martin**[2]

[1]*Department of Internal Medicine, Monmouth Medical Center, Long Branch, NJ 07740, USA*
[2]*Department of Emergency Medicine, Monmouth Medical Center, Long Branch, NJ 07740, USA*

Correspondence should be addressed to Manan Parikh; manan_cnv@yahoo.com

Academic Editor: Kazuhito Imanaka

Aortic dissection is a life-threatening medical emergency often presenting with severe chest pain and acute hemodynamic compromise. The presentation of aortic dissection can sometimes be different thus leading to a challenge in prompt diagnosis and treatment as demonstrated by the following presentation and discussion. We present a case of a 71-year-old male who presented to the emergency department with complaints of left sided temporoparietal headache and was eventually diagnosed with a thoracic aortic dissection involving the ascending aorta and descending aorta, with an intramural hematoma in the descending aorta. This case illustrates the importance of keeping in mind aortic dissection as a differential diagnosis in patients with acute onset headaches in which any intracranial source of headache is not found.

## 1. Introduction

Aortic dissection is a relatively uncommon, though catastrophic, illness often presenting with severe chest pain and acute hemodynamic compromise. The presentation of aortic dissection can sometimes be different thus leading to a challenge in prompt diagnosis and treatment as demonstrated by the following presentation and discussion.

## 2. Case Presentation

This is a case of 71-year-old Caucasian male with past medical history significant for choroideremia who presented to the emergency department (ED) with complaints of left sided temporoparietal headache upon waking up on the day of admission.

Patient in his thirties had progressive vision loss and was diagnosed as choroideremia with the deletion of REP 1. He became completely blind by the age of 50. The other significant past medical history includes ablation for supraventricular tachycardia around 20 years ago, coronary artery disease with percutaneous coronary intervention in the left anterior descending artery around 10 years ago, hypertension, and hyperlipidemia. His social history is significant for no history of smoking, alcohol consumption, and drug abuse. His family history is significant for choroideremia in his brother (complete blindness) and carrier state in his sister (asymptomatic). His medications included aspirin, clopidogrel, losartan, and pravastatin.

On the day of admission, the patient woke up with a severe left sided temporoparietal headache with no numbness or weakness. Concerning this symptom, the patient contacted his primary care physician who advised the patient to go to the emergency department. His initial vitals in the ED were significant for blood pressure of 107/49 mm of hg and a heart rate of 38 beats per minute. The lab work was unremarkable with negative troponins; an ECG (Figure 1) that was done was significant for sinus bradycardia with some T wave abnormalities in lead V3 to V6 and the initial chest X-ray (Figure 2) was significant for prominence of the thoracic aorta. His physical examination was unremarkable except for his vision where the patient was able to perceive only shadows and otherwise he was completely blind. He had no focal neurological

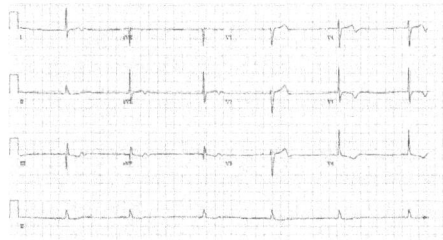

FIGURE 1: EKG showing sinus bradycardia with nonspecific ST-T wave abnormalities.

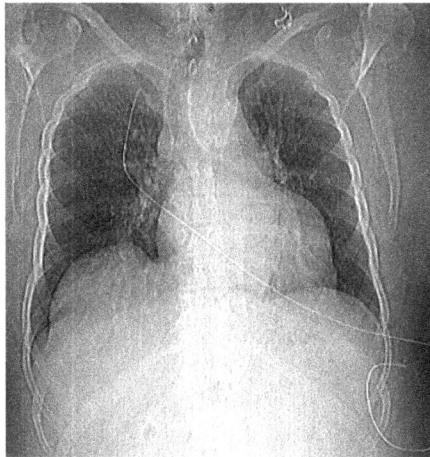

FIGURE 2: Chest X-ray showing prominence of thoracic aorta, no acute pulmonary disease.

deficits. The differential at this time due to his symptoms and physical exam was possibly a pulmonary embolism versus any intracranial hemorrhage versus acute coronary syndrome. The repeat blood pressure bilaterally showed 134/61 mm of hg on the right arm and 123/53 mm of hg on the left arm with a heart rate of around 49 beats per minute.

Concerning the persistent nature of the headache and prominent thoracic aorta on the X-ray, a CT head without contrast was done which was unremarkable and a CT of the chest with contrast (Figures 3(a)–3(d)) was also done which was significant for a thoracic aortic dissection involving the ascending aorta and descending aorta, with an intramural hematoma in the descending aorta. The dissection extended superiorly to the brachiocephalic/left common carotid trunk. Concerning the life-threatening emergency of the situation it was decided that the patient needed surgical intervention. His vitals continued to be unchanged with no worsening of symptoms. Patient was emergently transferred to a tertiary care center. The patient underwent an ascending aortic replacement and hemiarch replacement as well as a suspension of the aortic valve. Patient was subsequently discharged with a stable follow-up course.

## 3. Discussion

Aortic dissection is an uncommon medical emergency with incidence of around 3 per 100,000 person-years [1].

Despite the current advancements in cardiothoracic surgery it remains a lethal event with extremely variable case fatality rate. Surgical mortality rate has been noted to be ranging from 15 to 30% for acute aortic dissection in some reviews [2]. Dissection is a dynamic process that can rapidly evolve and progress to hemodynamic compromise; therefore urgency in diagnosis remains essential. Over 90% of cases classically present with one or more of the following findings: (1) abrupt onset sharp chest or abdominal pain, (2) chest radiograph suggestive of aortic or mediastinal widening, and (3) a variation in pulse or blood pressure [3]. Despite the chest pain being the most common complaint, diagnosis of aortic dissection is often missed in absence of any type of pain in about 6% cases [4]. Common extra cardiac manifestations are neurological deficits in about 18–30% cases as well as syncope in about 13% but rare cases of dissection presenting as gastrointestinal hemorrhage, pleural effusion, intestinal ischemia, or fever of unknown origin have also been previously described [5–10]. Of the neurological manifestations stroke, spinal cord ischemia, and hypoxic encephalopathy as well as ischemic neuropathy are commonly described. But only isolated cases of vertigo, uniocular blindness, or headache have been described as the presenting manifestation of aortic dissection [11].

On extensive review of medical literature we only found a handful of cases of aortic dissection presenting as headache. A literature search using the key words "aortic dissection" and "headache" was performed using Ovid, MEDLINE, and PubMed. Singh et al. [12] have reported a case of patient presenting bifrontal headache that subsequently became hemodynamically unstable and was found to have Stanford type A aortic dissection. Ko and Park [13] have reported a case where a patient that presented with bifrontal headache on further evaluation was found to have common carotid artery dissection along with aortic dissection. Our case demonstrates a similar but unique scenario where patient presented with frontal headache and remained hemodynamically stable prior to his diagnosis of the condition and was subsequently found to have an aortic dissection. Headaches can be seen in patients with primary carotid artery dissection [14]. Headache in these situations can be due to distension of the carotid artery, thus in turn stimulating pain receptors [15]. It has also been suggested that ischemia due to reduced blood flow resulting from an aortic dissection may stimulate the depolarizing sensory fibers in the pericarotid cavernous sinus plexus and lead to headache [12]. The aortic dissection extended to the left brachiocephalic trunk along with the left common carotid trunk, which might explain the cause of left sided temporoparietal headache in this patient.

Upon suspicion, the diagnosis of aortic dissection is made with CT scan with angiography or echocardiography or via magnetic resonance imaging. Based on the imaging studies patients are further classified. The DeBakey classification has three types: type I dissections originate in the ascending aorta and extend to at least the aortic arch; type II dissections involve the ascending aorta only; and type III dissections begin in the descending aorta, usually just distal to the left subclavian artery. The Stanford classification has two types: type A dissections involve the ascending aorta, and type B

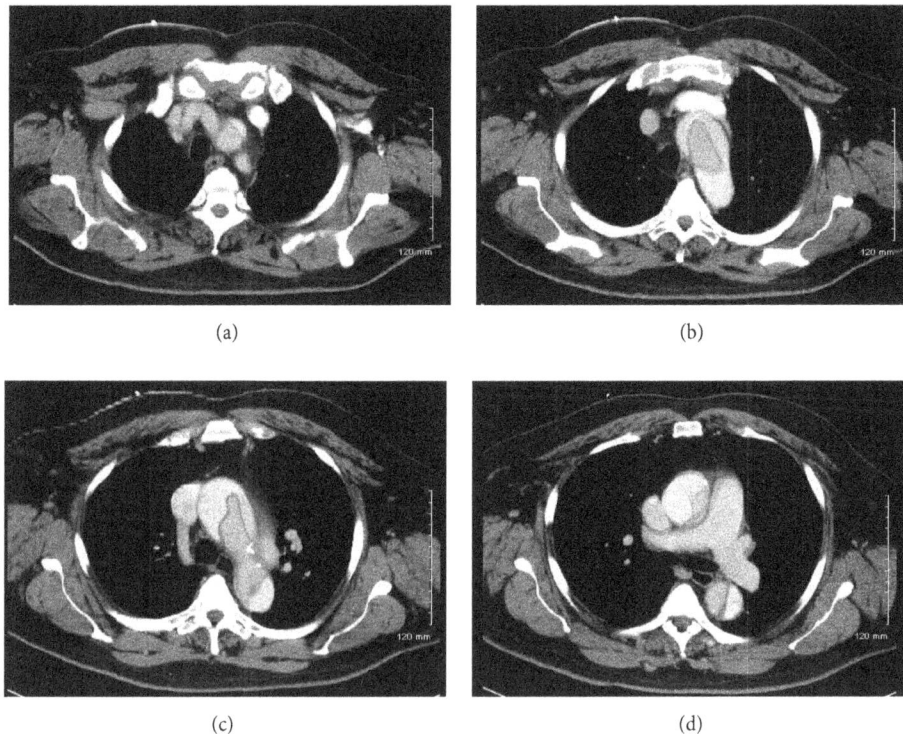

FIGURE 3: CT scan with contrast showing a thoracic aortic dissection involving the ascending aorta and descending aorta, with an intramural hematoma in the descending aorta. (a)–(d) show coronal sections at different levels.

dissections are those that do not involve the ascending aorta. Every dissection involving the ascending aorta (type A or I or II) has to be operated. Regarding the dissection involving the descending aorta (type B or III), the treatment is most often conservative around the world but many advanced centers have adopted endovascular treatment for cases with specific scenarios like untreatable pains, malperfusion, and pseudocoarctation with arterial hypertension in the upper body part [16–19].

## 4. Conclusion

Our case presents a unique scenario where a severe headache led to the patient's presentation to the emergency room that prompted further evaluation into his symptoms and led to the diagnosis of aortic dissection. The classical teaching professes that the classic chest pain syndrome radiating to the back should raise the suspicion regarding a dissecting aortic aneurysm. This case illustrates the importance of keeping in mind aortic dissection as a differential in patients with acute onset headaches in whom any intracranial source of headache is not found.

## Conflict of Interests

The authors declare that there is no conflict of interests regarding the publication of this paper.

## Acknowledgments

The authors acknowledge Department of Emergency Medicine at Monmouth Medical Center and Department of Cardiology at Monmouth Medical Center.

## References

[1] P. G. Hagan, C. A. Nienaber, E. M. Isselbacher et al., "The international registry of acute aortic dissection (IRAD): new insights into an old disease," *Journal of the American Medical Association*, vol. 283, no. 7, pp. 897–903, 2000.

[2] V. Rampoldi, S. Trimarchi, K. A. Eagle et al., "Simple risk models to predict surgical mortality in acute type A aortic dissection: the International Registry of Acute Aortic Dissection score," *Annals of Thoracic Surgery*, vol. 83, no. 1, pp. 55–61, 2007.

[3] Y. Von Kodolitsch, A. G. Schwartz, and C. A. Nienaber, "Clinical prediction of acute aortic dissection," *Archives of Internal Medicine*, vol. 160, no. 19, pp. 2977–2982, 2000.

[4] S. W. Park, S. Hutchison, R. H. Mehta et al., "Association of painless acute aortic dissection with increased mortality," *Mayo Clinic Proceedings*, vol. 79, no. 10, pp. 1252–1257, 2004.

[5] G. Gandelman, N. Barzilay, M. Krupsky, and P. Resnitzky, "Left pleural hemorrhagic effusion: a presenting sign of thoracic aortic dissecting aneurysm," *Chest*, vol. 106, no. 2, pp. 636–638, 1994.

[6] K. C. Edwards and B. T. Katzen, "Superior mesenteric artery syndrome due to a large dissecting abdominal aortic aneurysm," *The American Journal of Gastroenterology*, vol. 79, pp. 72–74, 1984.

[7] B. K. Nallamothu, R. H. Mehta, S. Saint et al., "Syncope in acute aortic dissection: diagnostic, prognostic, and clinical implications," *American Journal of Medicine*, vol. 113, no. 6, pp. 468–471, 2002.

[8] J. Alvarez Sabín, J. Vázquez, A. Sala, A. Ortega, and A. Codina Puiggrós, "Neurologic manifestations of dissecting aneurysms of the aorta," *Medicina Clinica*, vol. 92, no. 12, pp. 447–449, 1989.

[9] J. L. Prendes, "Neurovascular syndromes of aortic dissection," *American Family Physician*, vol. 23, no. 6, pp. 175–179, 1981.

[10] C. Veyssier-Belot, A. Cohen, D. Rougemont, C. Levy, P. Amarenco, and M.-G. Bousser, "Cerebral infarction due to painless thoracic aortic and common carotid artery dissections," *Stroke*, vol. 24, no. 12, pp. 2111–2113, 1993.

[11] C. Gaul, W. Dietrich, and F. J. Erbguth, "Neurological symptoms in aortic dissection: a challenge for neurologists," *Cerebrovascular Diseases*, vol. 26, no. 1, pp. 1–8, 2008.

[12] S. Singh, J. Y. Huang, K. Sin, and R. A. Charles, "Headache: an unusual presentation of aortic dissection," *European Journal of Emergency Medicine*, vol. 14, no. 1, pp. 47–49, 2007.

[13] J.-I. Ko and T. Park, "Headache: a rare manifestation of Debakey type I aortic dissection," *The American Journal of Emergency Medicine*, vol. 32, no. 3, pp. 291.e5–291.e6, 2014.

[14] M. Sturzenegger, "Spontaneous internal carotid artery dissection: early diagnosis and management in 44 patients," *Journal of Neurology*, vol. 242, no. 4, pp. 231–238, 1995.

[15] V. Biousse, J. D'Anglejan-Chatillon, H. Massiou, and M.-G. Bousser, "Head pain in non-traumatic carotid artery dissection: a series of 65 patients," *Cephalalgia*, vol. 14, no. 1, pp. 33–36, 1994.

[16] R. M. Doroghazi, E. E. Slater, R. W. DeSanctis, M. J. Buckley, W. G. Austen, and S. Rosenthal, "Long-term survival of patients with treated aortic dissection," *Journal of the American College of Cardiology*, vol. 3, no. 4, pp. 1026–1034, 1984.

[17] E. S. Crawford, "The diagnosis and management of aortic dissection," *Journal of the American Medical Association*, vol. 264, no. 19, article 2537, 1990.

[18] R. Erbel, F. Alfonso, C. Boileau et al., "Diagnosis and management of aortic dissection," *European Heart Journal*, vol. 22, no. 18, pp. 1642–1681, 2001.

[19] S. D. Xu, F. J. Huang, J. F. Yang et al., "Endovascular repair of acute type B aortic dissection: early and mid-term results," *Journal of Vascular Surgery*, vol. 43, no. 6, pp. 1090–1095, 2006.

# 14

# Disabling Orthostatic Headache after Penetrating Stonemason Pencil Injury to the Sacral Region

Carlo Brembilla,[1] Luigi Andrea Lanterna,[1] Paolo Gritti,[2] Emanuele Costi,[1] Gianluigi Dorelli,[1] Elena Moretti,[1] and Claudio Bernucci[1]

[1]Department of Neurosurgery, Pope John XXIII Hospital, OMS Square No. 1, 24100 Bergamo, Italy
[2]Department of Anesthesia and Intensive Care, Pope John XXIII Hospital, OMS Square No. 1, 24100 Bergamo, Italy

Correspondence should be addressed to Carlo Brembilla; carlinobrembo@hotmail.com

Academic Editor: Aristomenis K. Exadaktylos

Penetrating injuries to the spine, although less common than motor vehicle accidents and falls, are important causes of injury to the spinal cord. They are essentially of two varieties: gunshot or stab wounds. Gunshot injuries to the spine are more commonly described. Stab wounds are usually inflicted by knife or other sharp objects. Rarer objects causing incidental spinal injuries include glass fragments, wood pieces, chopsticks, nailguns, and injection needles. Just few cases of penetrating vertebral injuries caused by pencil are described. The current case concerns a 42-year-old man with an accidental penetrating stonemason pencil injury into the vertebral canal without neurological deficit. After the self-removal of the foreign object the patient complained of a disabling orthostatic headache. The early identification and treatment of the intracranial hypotension due to the posttraumatic cerebrospinal fluid (CSF) sacral fistulae were mandatory to avoid further neurological complications. In the current literature acute pattern of intracranial hypotension immediately after a penetrating injury of the vertebral column has never been reported.

## 1. Introduction

Penetrating injury is the third most frequent cause of spinal injuries in adults, only surpassed by traffic accidents and falls [1]. Gunshot wounds and knife stabbings account for the majority of penetrating spinal injuries [2, 3]. Other rare objects usually cause incidental penetrating spinal injury [4–6].

The current case concerns a 42-year-old man with an accidental penetrating stonemason pencil injury to the sacral region. The man was referred to the attention of Pope John XXIII Hospital Emergency Department in Bergamo with a disabling orthostatic headache.

## 2. Case Report

A 42-year-old man was referred to the attention of Pope John XXIII Hospital Emergency Department in Bergamo after falling while working. The man, a stonemason, fell walking backwards in the dockyard. A stonemason pencil (Figure 1(a)) carried in his work pouch stabbed him in the lumbosacral region. After the falling, the man removed from himself the foreign body. Immediately he complained of severe lumbosacral pain. After few minutes there appeared a disabling orthostatic headache that forced the man into supine position.

On admission the inspection revealed a wound in the lumbosacral region (Figure 1(b)), slightly to the right of the midline, with serohematic fluid attributable to cerebrospinal fluid (CSF) leakage. Physical examination revealed severe contracture of the lumbosacral muscles. At the neurological examination no deficit was detected on lower limbs. Bowel and bladder function were intact. The patient could not stand on his feet because of the orthostatic headache. The lumbosacral pain score on a visual analog scale (VAS) of 0–100, with 0 representing no pain and 100 representing severe pain, was 70; the headache, in standing position, was quantified 80. A complete blood count showed mild normocytic anemia and moderate leukocytosis. A lumbosacral CT scan showed a multifragmented fracture of the S1 lamina,

(a)

(b)

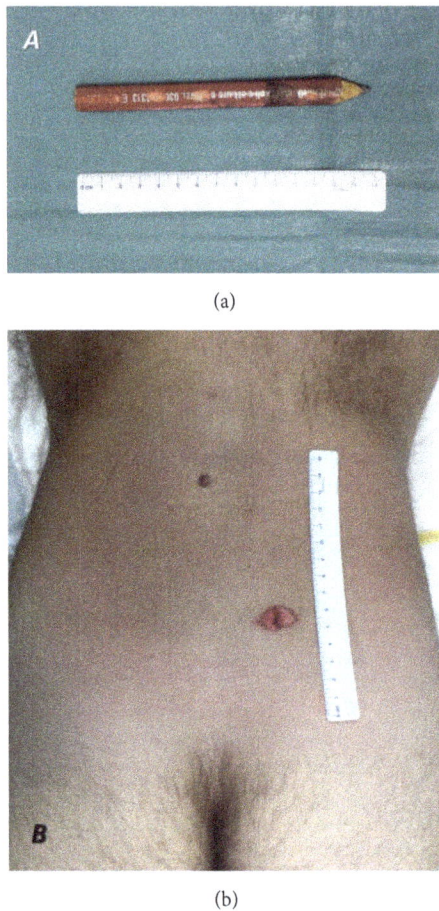

FIGURE 1: The wound caused by the penetrating object in the lumbosacral region (b), slightly to the right of the midline at the level of S1, and the penetrating object: a stonemason pencil (a).

with air bubbles in the epidural space (Figures 2(a), 2(b), and 2(c)). A lumbosacral RMI confirmed the presence of the S1 lamina fracture and the contusion of the lumbosacral muscles along the foreign object trajectory (Figure 2(d)). The neuroradiological exams also showed incidentally L5-S1 isthmic spondylolisthesis. In order to investigate the headache, a cranial CT scan showed diffused pneumocephalus (Figure 3), without dislocation of the cerebellar tonsils. In light of the patient's history as well as findings on physical examination and imaging studies, a diagnosis of intracranial hypotension due to posttraumatic CSF lumbosacral fistulae was made.

The patient underwent a surgical intervention. A linear skin incision on the midline at S1 level was made to expose the multifragmented fracture of the S1 lamina. After the removal of the bone fragments, the exposition of the vertebral canal was completed with a minimal laminectomy of S1. The dura mater was lacerated for about 1.5 centimeters (Figure 4(a)). No residual part of the pencil was detected into the dural sac. A watertight closure of the dural sac was achieved (Figure 4(b)). The entry point of the foreign body, after a surgical toilette, and the surgical incision were both closed in layers.

After surgery no neurological deficit appeared. The patient walked on postoperative day 3 with an elastic lower back support. A 7-day course of antibiotic was given for prophylaxis: amoxicillin-clavulanate 850 mg/125 mg (Augmentin) three times daily. A postoperative cranial CT scan showed an improvement of the pneumocephalus. After one month the patient reported no pain and episodes of fever. A new cranial CT scan showed the resolution of the pneumocephalus. After 3 months still no fever episodes and pain were reported.

## 3. Discussion

In adults, penetrating injuries constitute the third most frequent cause of spinal cord injuries [1]. Surpassed only by traffic accidents and falls, they account for four to seven cases per million persons per year [2]. Penetrating injuries are essentially of two varieties: gunshot or stab wounds. Gunshot injuries to the spine are more commonly described and are associated with a higher incidence of neurological damage [1–3]. Stab wounds are usually inflicted by knife or other sharp, knife-like objects. Commonly, the wound is inflicted from behind during an assault, and it results in an incomplete spinal cord injury [7].

Rarer objects causing accidental spinal injuries include glass fragments, wood pieces, chopsticks, nailguns, and injection needles [4–6]. In the current literature just few cases of penetrating vertebral injuries caused by pencil are described [8]. Between these only two cases regard the penetration of a pencil into the spinal canal, both being in pediatric patients. In 2006 Piqueras et al. [9] reported the case of a 10-year-old boy who sustained an injury to the cauda equina as a result of the accidental penetration during a fall of a wooden pencil into the spinal canal at the L5-S1 level. After neuroimaging evaluation, the foreign body was removed and the wound was repaired. As a precaution, the child was treated with antibiotics. After a follow-up period of 1 year, the boy's neurological deficits had completely resolved. Still in 2006 Ramaswamy et al. [10] reported the case of a 12-year-old boy that suffered a penetrating injury from a pencil contained in his coat pocket during a rough tumble with his friends. The pencil penetrated the posterior wall of his chest on the left side, extended through the dorsal paraspinal soft tissues into the neuroforaminal canal on the left at T12-L1 level, and across the midline reached the right neuroforaminal canal. The penetrating injury gave a complete spinal cord damage. After neuroimaging evaluation, the child underwent a surgical operation to decompress the spinal canal and remove the foreign object. In the postoperative time the patient did not improve the neurological deficit.

The initial principles in the management of penetrating intraspinal injuries should include a meticulous neurologic examination and the administration of prophylactic antibiotic agents. Particular attention should be paid and priority given to eventually life-threatening visceral and vascular injuries [1–11].

Radiograph and CT of the spine are essential to demonstrate bony injuries, retained foreign bodies, and signs of

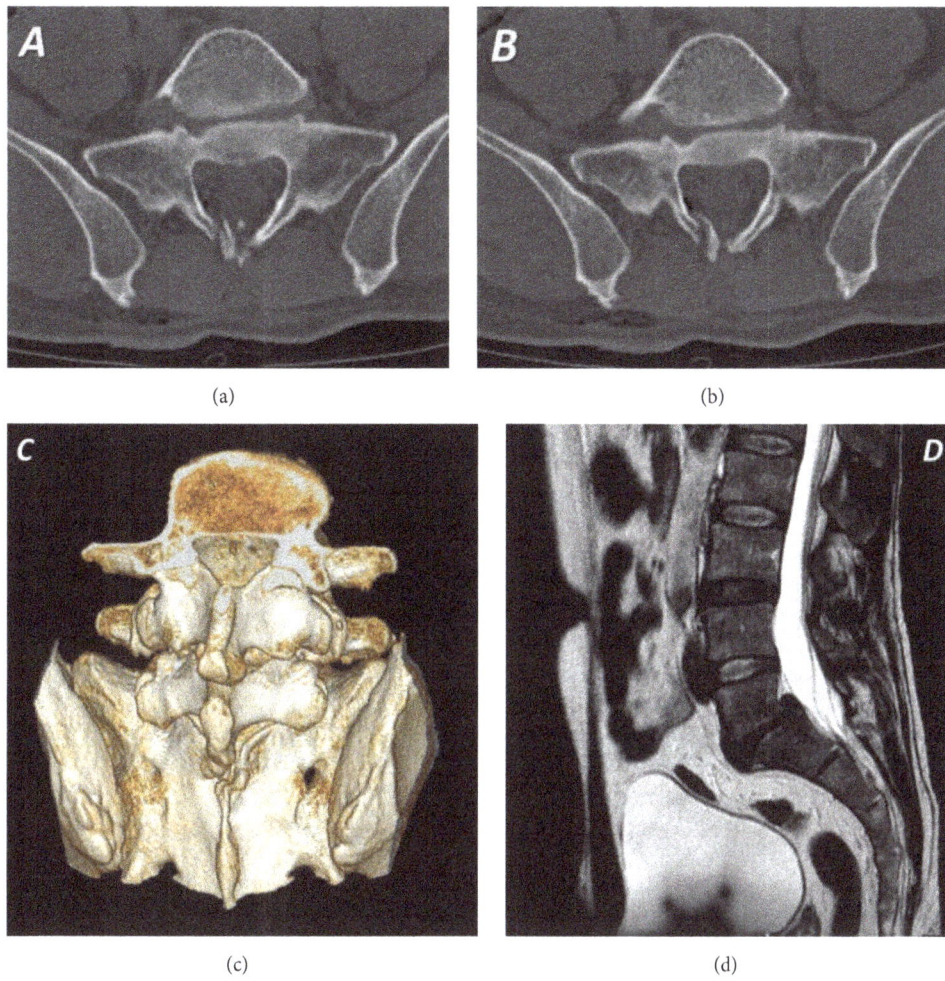

(a)

(b)

(c)

(d)

FIGURE 2: Lumbosacral CT scan ((a), (b), (c)) and RMI (d) showing a multifragmented fracture of the S1 lamina, with air bubbles in the epidural space.

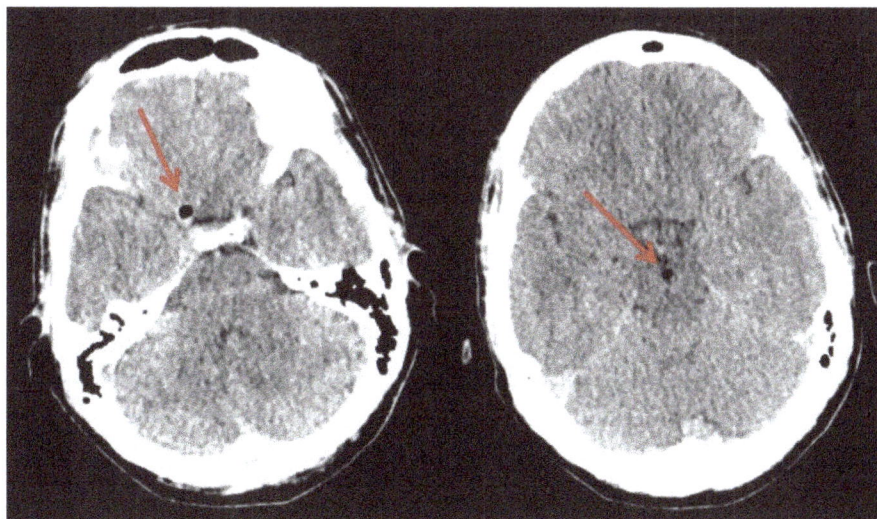

FIGURE 3: Cranial CT scan showing pneumocephalus.

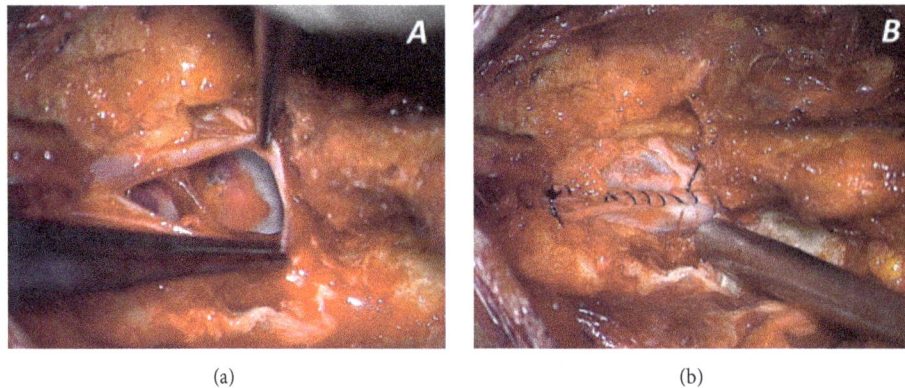

(a)                                                               (b)

FIGURE 4: Intraoperative pictures from the high resolution microscope. (a) The dural laceration, with sacral roots contused, and the impact point of the penetrating object in the anterior part of the dural sac, at the level of the posterior wall of S1 vertebral body; in the middle of the contusion some little graphite pigments from the pencil tip can be seen. (b) The watertight closure of the dural sac.

spinal instability [12]. Radiologic investigation of the vessel anatomy should be performed if the trajectory of the blade predicts damage to any important artery. In most cases, the foreign body is metal, plastic, or glass, all of which are usually easily detected on conventional radiograph [12]. However, wooden foreign bodies are difficult to detect with plain radiograph; therefore, their diagnosis is often missed or delayed. A CT scan is usually performed in cases where entry of the foreign bodies is suspected. But a wooden foreign body is known to initially be recognized as a hypodense image on the CT scan and consequently diagnosed as air. Therefore, MRI is advised to be used in adjunction with CT. MRI scan can be very useful to demonstrate and localize the foreign body and also to exclude any intra- or extradural hematoma or contusion in the cord or cauda equine [13].

The objective of the surgical treatment is to decompress the spinal cord, remove the foreign body, prevent cerebrospinal fluid leakage, and eventually stabilize the vertebral column [14–16]. Some authors emphasize surgery for removal of the retained object to avoid progressive neurological deterioration, especially if wood is involved, as wood in particular can be irritant to tissue. In 1993 Sawar et al. [17] reported a case in which penetrating injury to the midthoracic spine was caused by a piece of wood in a patient involved in a road traffic accident. The patient underwent a surgical intervention 3 years after the injury for indurated and fluctuant swelling over the penetrating injury. The wound had healed completely after the removing of a wood piece from the spinal canal and the toilette of the granulation tissue around. In 2000 Lunawat and Taneja [18] reported the case of 18-year-old boy who presented with weakness in his lower limbs and had an upper motor neuron lesion at the D12-L1 level. At laminectomy two stone-like objects were found which proved to be bundles of tiny pieces of wood. They are thought to have entered the cord through an abdominal penetrating injury sustained six years previously.

The current case concerns 42-year-old man with an accidental penetrating stonemason pencil injury into the vertebral canal without neurological deficit. After the removal of the foreign object the subsequent posttraumatic CSF fistulae

gave an acute clinical pattern of intracranial hypotension. An early identification and treatment of the intracranial hypotension was mandatory to avoid further neurological complications. In the current literature acute pattern of intracranial hypotension due to posttraumatic CSF fistulae by penetrating object into the spinal canal has never been reported.

## Conflict of Interests

The authors declare no conflict of interests.

## References

[1] G. I. Jallo, "Neurosurgical management of penetrating spinal injury," *Surgical Neurology*, vol. 47, no. 4, pp. 328–330, 1997.

[2] R. E. Burney, R. F. Maio, F. Maynard, and R. Karunas, "Incidence, characteristics, and outcome of spinal cord injury at trauma centers in North America," *Archives of Surgery*, vol. 128, no. 5, pp. 596–599, 1993.

[3] G. S. Sidhu, A. Ghag, V. Prokuski, A. R. Vaccaro, and K. E. Radcliff, "Civilian gunshot injuries of the spinal cord: a systematic review of the current literature," *Clinical Orthopaedics and Related Research*, vol. 471, no. 12, pp. 3945–3955, 2013.

[4] S. Gul, A. Dusak, M. Songur, M. Kalayci, and B. Acikgoz, "Penetrating spinal injury with a wooden fragment: a case report and review of the literature," *Spine*, vol. 35, no. 25, pp. E1534–E1536, 2010.

[5] D. J. Opel, D. A. Lundin, K. L. Stevenson, and E. J. Klein, "Glass foreign body in the spinal canal of a child: case report and review of the literature," *Pediatric Emergency Care*, vol. 20, no. 7, pp. 468–472, 2004.

[6] S. Yamaguchi, K. Eguchi, M. Takeda, T. Hidaka, P. Shrestha, and K. Kurisu, "Penetrating injury of the upper cervical spine by a chopstick—case report," *Neurologia Medico-Chirurgica*, vol. 47, no. 7, pp. 328–330, 2007.

[7] G. Rubin, D. Tallman, L. Sagan, and M. Melgar, "An unusual stab wound of the cervical spinal cord: a case report," *Spine*, vol. 26, no. 4, pp. 444–447, 2001.

[8] H. S. Meltzer, P. J. Kim, B. M. Ozgur, and M. L. Levy, "Vertebral body granuloma of the cervical region after pencil injury," *Neurosurgery*, vol. 54, no. 6, pp. 1527–1529, 2004.

[9] C. Piqueras, J. F. Martínez-Lage, M. J. Almagro, J. R. de San Pedro, P. T. Tortosa, and A. Herrera, "Cauda equina-penetrating injury in a child: case report," *Journal of Neurosurgery*, vol. 104, no. 4, supplement, pp. 279–281, 2006.

[10] R. Ramaswamy, G. Dow, and S. Bassi, "Pencil is mightier than the sword!," *Pediatric Neurosurgery*, vol. 42, no. 3, pp. 168–170, 2006.

[11] J. H. Kahn, "The management of stab wounds to the back," *Journal of Emergency Medicine*, vol. 17, no. 3, pp. 497–502, 1999.

[12] T. N. Pham, E. Heinberg, J. Cuschieri et al., "The evolution of the diagnostic work-up for stab wounds to the back and flank," *Injury*, vol. 40, no. 1, pp. 48–53, 2009.

[13] H. Imokawa, T. Tazawa, N. Sugiura, D. Oyake, and K. Yosino, "Penetrating neck injuries involving wooden foreign bodies: the role of MRI and the misinterpretation of CT images," *Auris Nasus Larynx*, vol. 30, supplement, pp. S145–S147, 2003.

[14] G. T. Tindall et al., "Penetrating spinalsurgery," in *The Practice of Neurosurgery*, part 5, section 3, p. 114, Lippincott Williams & Wilkins, London, UK, 1997.

[15] J. S. Harrop, G. E. Hunt Jr., and A. R. Vaccaro, "Conus medullaris and cauda equina syndrome as a result of traumatic injuries: management principles," *Neurosurgical Focus*, vol. 16, no. 6, p. E4, 2004.

[16] R. K. Osenbach and A. H. Menezes, "Pediatric spinal cord and vertebral column injury," *Neurosurgery*, vol. 30, no. 3, pp. 385–390, 1992.

[17] O. Sawar, C. Inman, and D. C. Jaffray, "We could not see the wood for the tree," *Injury*, vol. 24, no. 7, pp. 491–493, 1993.

[18] S. K. Lunawat and D. K. Taneja, "A foreign body in the spinal canal. A case report," *The Journal of Bone and Joint Surgery—British Volume*, vol. 82, no. 2, pp. 267–268, 2000.

# 15

# Death after Sexual Intercourse

**Christian T. Braun,[1] Meret E. Ricklin,[1] Andreina Pauli,[2] Daniel Ott,[2] Aristomenis K. Exadaktylos,[1] and Carmen A. Pfortmueller[1,3]**

[1]*Department of Emergency Medicine, Inselspital, University Hospital Bern, Freiburgstrasse 10, 3010 Bern, Switzerland*
[2]*University Institute of Diagnostic, Interventional and Pediatric Radiology, Inselspital, University Hospital Bern, Freiburgstrasse 10, 3010 Bern, Switzerland*
[3]*Department of General Anesthesiology, Intensive Care and Pain Management, Medical University of Vienna, Waehringerguertel 18-22, 1090 Vienna, Austria*

Correspondence should be addressed to Carmen A. Pfortmueller; cpfortmueller@gmail.com

Academic Editor: Henry David

Sexuality is an essential aspect of quality of life. Nevertheless, sexual intercourse is physically challenging and leads to distinct changes in blood pressure, heart, and respiratory rate that may lead to vital complications. We present a case report of a 22-year-old female suffering from subarachnoid hemorrhage after sexual intercourse. The patient was immediately transported to hospital by emergency medical services and, after diagnosis, transferred to a tertiary hospital with neurosurgical expertise but died within 24 hours. After postcoital headaches, subarachnoid hemorrhage is the second most common cause of neurological complications of sexual intercourse and therefore patients admitted to an emergency department with headache after sexual intercourse should always be carefully evaluated by cerebral imaging.

## 1. Introduction

Sexuality is an essential aspect of quality of life [1–3]. Nevertheless, sexual intercourse is physically challenging and leads to distinct changes in blood pressure, heart, and respiratory rate [3, 4]; for an overview see Table 1.

The complications of sexual intercourse are apparently rare relative to the frequency of coitus in the general population [3, 5, 6]. The true incidence is not known, as patients may not report the sexual circumstances of their health problems to health care professionals [5, 6]. Nevertheless, it has been reported that sexual intercourse may lead to severe injury [3, 4].

## 2. Case Presentation

We present a case of a 22-year-old female admitted unconscious to the emergency department by emergency medical services. The medical history revealed that the woman suffered from a seizure followed by unconsciousness while having sexual intercourse. The patient had never had a seizure before and had no prior history of headaches, migraine, head trauma, substance abuse, or intoxication. The patient had previously been in excellent health and with physical fitness appropriate to her age. Her only regular medication was an oral anticontraceptive.

On admission to the emergency department (ED) of a secondary care hospital, the clinical findings were as follows: unconsciousness with a Glasgow Coma Scale (GCS) of 3 and unilaterally (left) light reactive pupil; no seizure was observed. The patient was breathing spontaneously through a nasal cannula, with a normal respiratory rate and 4l oxygen saturation. Blood pressure, heart rate, and temperature were normal. After immediate airway management, computed tomography (CT) of the head was performed. She was found to have an extensive subarachnoid hemorrhage (Fisher grade 4), with breach in the fourth ventricle; see Figure 1. Clinical examination and laboratory analysis did not reveal any further pathologic features. The patient was urgently transferred by helicopter to our tertiary hospital for neurosurgical intervention.

TABLE 1: Overview on stages of the sexual cycle [3, 13].

| Stage | Explanation | Body's response |
| --- | --- | --- |
| 1 | Excitement (initial state of arousal) | Increases in muscular tone, heart rate, and blood pressure |
| 2 | Plateau (full arousal immediately preceding orgasm) | Further increases in muscular tone, heart rate, and blood pressure and increased relative vascular resistance |
| 3 | Orgasm | Associated with muscle spasms, massive elevation of heart rate, blood pressure, and respiratory rate |
| 4 | Resolution | Normalization of physical function |

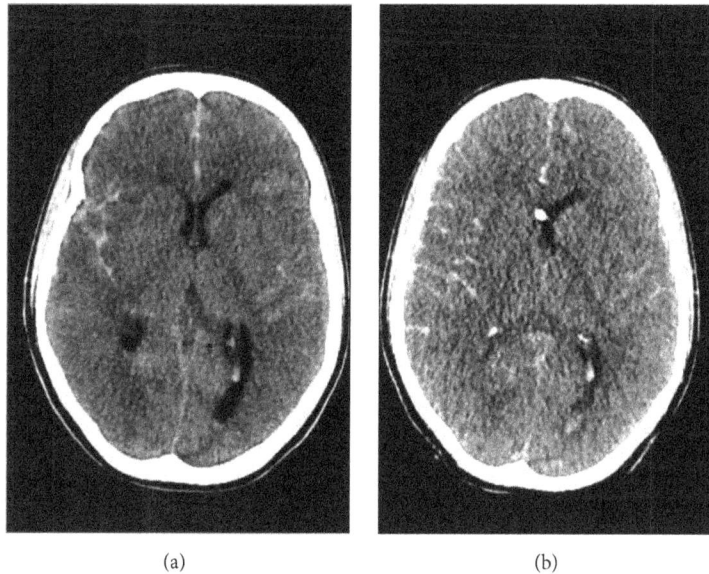

(a)                                      (b)

FIGURE 1: (a) First computed tomography of the head (01:25 am) and (b) follow-up computed tomography of the head (02:30 am).

On admission to our emergency department (ED), clinical examination showed bilaterally wide pupils with bilaterally absent pupillary reflexes, irregularities in the pupillary margin, and absent brain stem reflexes; for a timeline of changes in neurological findings see Table 2. A ventricle drainage was immediately placed and showed an opening pressure of 86 mmHg. Thus, conservative measurements to lower intracerebral pressure were started (head up placement, hyperventilation, intravenous mannitol, maximal sedation, and muscle relaxation) and computed tomography with angiography was performed. This showed an extensive and progressive subarachnoid hemorrhage (now Fisher grade 4) with diminished perfusion during the arterial phase, collapsed ventricles, cerebral herniation, pan-cerebrally diminished perfusion, and a potential aneurysm at the carotid artery cross; see Figure 2. Despite maximal conservative therapy (see above) a decline in cerebral pressure could not be achieved.

After careful consideration by all specialists involved and with the consent of the patient's relatives, it was decided that further neurosurgery would not be performed, as the brain stem reflexes were extinct and the intracerebral pressure had remained at 80 mmHg for more than one hour despite maximal conservative therapy. The patient was transferred to the intensive care unit for organ saving therapy and died 48 hours after admission.

## 3. Discussion

Our case features sexual intercourse as a trigger of an acute intracerebral hemorrhage in a young female. Several studies have shown that sexual intercourse may provoke intracerebral hemorrhage, especially subarachnoid hemorrhage [3, 4]. It has been reported that 14.5% of all subarachnoid hemorrhages are precipitated by sexual activity [7, 8]. Our patients most likely had a preexisting vascular aneurysm as a precipitating lesion for subarachnoid bleeding, as the second computed tomography showed. It has been reported that the acute elevation in blood pressure during sexual intercourse increases the vessels' wall tension and the subsequent risk of its rupture by 15-fold [4, 9]. Nevertheless, this connection has only been seen in the few existing observational studies on this topic; further scientific evaluation of the cohesion between sexual intercourse and cerebral aneurysm rupture should be performed.

Although the published literature is sparse on the topic of sexual intercourse-related subarachnoid hemorrhage, several studies have found a male predominance [7, 9–11]. This is

TABLE 2: Timeline of neurological findings.

|  | 00:35 | 00:55 | 01:25 | 02:30 | 08:00 |
|---|---|---|---|---|---|
| Event | Sexual intercourse | Ambulance arrived | Arrival at secondary care hospital | Arrival at tertiary care hospital | Neurological re-evaluation on ICU |
| Pupils | Normal | Miotic bilaterally light reactive pupils | Unilaterally light reactive pupil (left), right pupil wide and nonreactive | Bilaterally wide pupils with absent pupillary reflexes bilaterally, irregularities to pupillary margin | Bilaterally wide pupils with absent pupillary reflexes bilaterally, irregularities to pupillary margin |
| Brainstem reflexes | Present | Present | Unclear | Lack of brainstem reflexes | Lack of brainstem reflexes |
| CT | — | — | Figure 1 | Figures 1 and 2 | — |
| Intracerebral pressure | — | — | — | 86 mmHg | 90 mmHg |
| Other findings | Generalized seizure, comatose |  |  | Lack of corneal reflexes | Lack of corneal reflexes |

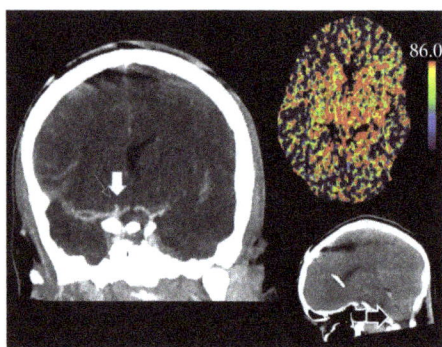

FIGURE 2: Second computed tomography of the head (02:30 am) shows an aneurysm at the right carotid T cross, pan-cerebral diminished perfusion, and developing tonsillar herniation.

striking for two reasons: firstly it is known that the incidence of cerebral aneurysms is higher in females [12] and secondly as women may experience multiple and longer orgasms than men, it would be expected that wall tension in cerebral vessels would be elevated for longer than in males [9].

Patients with sexually triggered subarachnoid hemorrhage most often present with severe headache [3, 4]. Headaches are the most common symptoms and pathology of patients presenting with sexual intercourse-related problems to the emergency department [3], amounting to almost 50% of the total [14]. The explosive character of coital headache makes it difficult to differentiate from more severe disease [6]; therefore, subarachnoid hemorrhage and arterial dissection should always be excluded by radiological image study [6, 15, 16]. The pathophysiology of orgasmic headache is not yet completely understood [15, 16]; arterial vasospasm secondary to impaired myogenic cerebral autoregulation may play a role [8, 17, 18].

In contrast to the overall frequency of headaches in sexual intercourse-related admissions to the emergency department, our patient suffered a seizure followed by unconsciousness. Her seizure was certainly due to the massive

subarachnoid hemorrhage. Nonetheless, in rare cases, epileptic seizures are induced by sexual orgasm [19]. They are predominant in females and their origin is thought to be in the right hemisphere [19, 20].

Unfortunately the patient featured in our case report died. Death due to sexual intercourse is rare [3, 4]. In two large autopsy studies with 5559 patients, the rate of death due to sexual intercourse was estimated to be about 0.6% [10, 21]. Male gender and extramarital sexual activity as well as excessive alcohol consumption and large meals are a risk factor for death related to intercourse [1, 22, 23].

## 4. Conclusion

In conclusion, sexual intercourse might be a precipitating factor for subarachnoid hemorrhage with a potentially fatal outcome, as this case report shows. Nonetheless, further studies are needed to prove a direct relationship between the sexual intercourse and cerebral aneurysm rupture. After excluding intracerebral pathologies such as subarachnoid hemorrhage or intracranial bleeding by cerebral computed tomography, further differential diagnosis should involve seizures triggered by postcoital headaches and sexual intercourse.

## Conflict of Interests

The authors declare that there is no conflict of interests regarding the publication of this paper.

## References

[1] X. Chen, Q. Zhang, and X. Tan, "Cardiovascular effects of sexual activity," *The Indian Journal of Medical Research*, vol. 130, no. 6, pp. 681–688, 2009.

[2] Y. Drory, "Sexual activity and cardiovascular risk," *European Heart Journal Supplements*, vol. 4, pp. H13–H18, 2002.

[3] C. A. Pfortmueller, J. N. Koetter, H. Zimmermann, and A. K. Exadaktylos, "Sexual activity-related emergency department admissions: eleven years of experience at a Swiss university

hospital," *Emergency Medicine Journal*, vol. 30, no. 10, pp. 846–850, 2013.

[4] C. A. Pfortmueller, A. C. Schankath, P. Mordasini et al., "Radiological findings of sexual intercourse related emergency department admissions: a first overview," *PLoS ONE*, vol. 9, no. 8, Article ID e104170, 2014.

[5] N. Eke, "Urological complications of coitus," *BJU International*, vol. 89, no. 3, pp. 273–277, 2002.

[6] A. Banerjee, "Coital emergencies," *Postgraduate Medical Journal*, vol. 72, no. 853, pp. 653–656, 1996.

[7] F. Portunato, M. C. Landolfa, M. Botto, A. Bonsignore, F. De Stefano, and F. Ventura, "Fatal subarachnoid hemorrhage during sexual activity: a case report," *The American Journal of Forensic Medicine and Pathology*, vol. 33, no. 1, pp. 90–92, 2012.

[8] M. M. Valença, L. P. A. A. Valença, C. A. Bordini et al., "Cerebral vasospasm and headache during sexual intercourse and masturbatory orgasms," *Headache*, vol. 44, no. 3, pp. 244–248, 2004.

[9] M. R. Reynolds, J. T. Willie, G. J. Zipfel, and R. G. Dacey, "Sexual intercourse and cerebral aneurysmal rupture: potential mechanisms and precipitants," *Journal of Neurosurgery*, vol. 114, no. 4, pp. 969–977, 2011.

[10] M. R. C. Parzeller and H. Bratzke, "Sudden cardiovascular death during sexual intercourse: results of a legal medicine autopsy study," *Zeitschrift für Kardiologie*, vol. 88, pp. 44–48, 1999.

[11] J. Lee, B. Singh, F. G. Kravets, A. Trocchia, W. C. Waltzer, and S. A. Khan, "Sexually acquired vascular injuries of the penis: a review," *The Journal of Trauma—Injury, Infection and Critical Care*, vol. 49, no. 2, pp. 351–358, 2000.

[12] T. A. R. Dinning and M. A. Falconer, "Sudden or unexpected natural death due to ruptured intracranial aneurysm; survey of 250 forensic cases," *The Lancet*, vol. 262, no. 6790, pp. 799–801, 1953.

[13] M. Pines, "Human sexual response: discussion of the work of Masters and Johnson," *Revue de Médecine Psychosomatique et de Psychologie Médicale*, vol. 11, no. 4, pp. 459–471, 1969.

[14] K. Kriz, "Coitus as a factor in the pathogenesis of neurologic complications," *Ceskoslovenska Neurologie*, vol. 33, no. 3, pp. 162–167, 1970.

[15] C.-M. Hu, Y.-J. Lin, Y.-K. Fan, S.-P. Chen, and T.-H. Lai, "Isolated thunderclap headache during sex: orgasmic headache or reversible cerebral vasoconstriction syndrome?" *Journal of Clinical Neuroscience*, vol. 17, no. 10, pp. 1349–1351, 2010.

[16] A. J. Larner, "Transient acute neurologic sequelae of sexual activity: headache and amnesia," *The Journal of Sexual Medicine*, vol. 5, no. 2, pp. 284–288, 2008.

[17] J. G. Heckmann, M. J. Hilz, M. Muck-Weymann, and B. Neundorfer, "Benign exertional headache/benign sexual headache: a disorder of myogenic cerebrovascular autoregulation?" *Headache*, vol. 37, no. 9, pp. 597–598, 1997.

[18] D. Schlegel and B. Cucchiara, "Orgasmic headache with transient basilar artery vasospasm," *Headache*, vol. 44, no. 7, pp. 710–712, 2004.

[19] C. Ozkara, S. Ozdemir, A. Yilmaz, M. Uzan, N. Yeni, and M. Ozmen, "Orgasm-induced seizures: a study of six patients," *Epilepsia*, vol. 47, no. 12, pp. 2193–2197, 2006.

[20] A. Sengupta, A. Mahmoud, S. Z. Tun, and P. Goulding, "Orgasm-induced seizures: male studied with ictal electroencephalography," *Seizure*, vol. 19, no. 5, pp. 306–309, 2010.

[21] W. U. T. Krauland, *Herzinfarkt und Sexualität aus der Sicht des Rechtsmediziners*, Sexualmedizin, 1976.

[22] G. Gorge, S. Flüchter, M. Kirstein, and T. Kunz, "Sex, erectile dysfunction, and the heart: a growing problem," *Herz*, vol. 28, no. 4, pp. 284–290, 2003.

[23] G. N. Levine, E. E. Steinke, F. G. Bakaeen et al., "Sexual activity and cardiovascular disease: a scientific statement from the American Heart Association," *Circulation*, vol. 125, pp. 1058–1072, 2012.

# 16

# Subcutaneous Emphysema, Pneumomediastinum, and Pneumorrhachis after Cocaine Inhalation

**Tuğba Atmaca Temrel,[1] Alp Şener,[1] Ferhat İçme,[1] Gül Pamukçu Günaydın,[1] Şervan Gökhan,[2] Yavuz Otal,[1] Gülhan Kurtoğlu Çelik,[1] and Ayhan Özhasenekler[2]**

[1]*Department of Emergency Medicine, Ankara Atatürk Training and Research Hospital, Üniversiteler Mahallesi Bilkent Caddesi No. 1, Çankaya, 06800 Ankara, Turkey*
[2]*Department of Emergency Medicine, Faculty of Medicine, Yildirim Beyazit University, Üniversiteler Mahallesi Bilkent Caddesi No. 1, Çankaya, 06800 Ankara, Turkey*

Correspondence should be addressed to Gül Pamukçu Günaydın; gulpamukcu@gmail.com

Academic Editor: Ching H. Loh

*Introduction.* The most prominent complications of cocaine use are adverse effects in the cardiovascular and central nervous systems. Free air in the mediastinum and subcutaneous tissue may be observed less frequently, whereas free air in the spinal canal (pneumorrhachis) is a very rare complication of cocaine abuse. In this report we present a case of pneumorrhachis that developed after cocaine use. *Case.* A 28-year-old male patient was admitted to the emergency department with shortness of breath, chest pain, and swelling in the neck and face which started four hours after he had sniffed cocaine. On physical examination, subcutaneous crepitations were felt with palpation of the jaw, neck, and upper chest area. Diffuse subcutaneous emphysema, pneumomediastinum, and pneumorrhachis were detected in the computed tomography imaging. The patient was treated conservatively and discharged uneventfully. *Discussion.* Complications such as pneumothorax, pneumomediastinum, and pneumoperitoneum that are associated with cocaine use may be seen due to increased intrathoracic pressure. The air then may flow into the spinal canal resulting in pneumorrhachis. Emergency physicians should know the possible complications of cocaine use and be prepared for rare complications such as pneumorrhachis.

## 1. Introduction

Cocaine leads to the most emergency department visits in the USA due to illicit drug use and it is the most frequently abused substance in Europe after cannabis [1]. Cocaine can be consumed in several ways such as smoking (crack) or sniffing or in an intravenous way. The mortality and morbidity associated with cocaine abuse usually occur due to acute cardiovascular or neurological complications [1].

The complications associated with inhaled cocaine use such as pneumothorax, pneumomediastinum, pneumopericardium, pneumoperitoneum, and pneumorrhachis are thought to occur due to barotrauma caused by increased intrathoracic pressure. Increased intrathoracic pressure is a result of either deep inhalation followed by the prolonged valsalva maneuver that is done by the individuals in order

to augment absorption and enhance the desired effect of the drug or cough caused by the sniffed substance [2, 3].

In this paper we presented a case of subcutaneous emphysema, pneumomediastinum, and pneumorrhachis that developed after cocaine use.

## 2. Case

A 28-year-old male patient was admitted to the emergency department with shortness of breath, chest pain, and swelling in the neck and face which developed four hours after he had sniffed cocaine. The patient had a history of cocaine addiction; there was no history of other diseases, drugs, trauma, recent surgery, or air travel. The vital signs were blood pressure of 150/80 mmHg, pulse of 150 beats/min, body temperature of 37.8°C, and SpO2 of 96%. On his

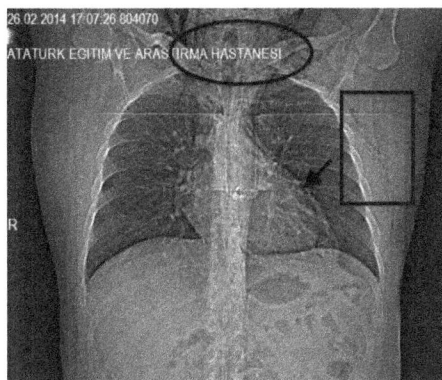

FIGURE 1: Subcutaneous air in the neck (oval) and in the axilla (rectangle) and air around the heart (arrow).

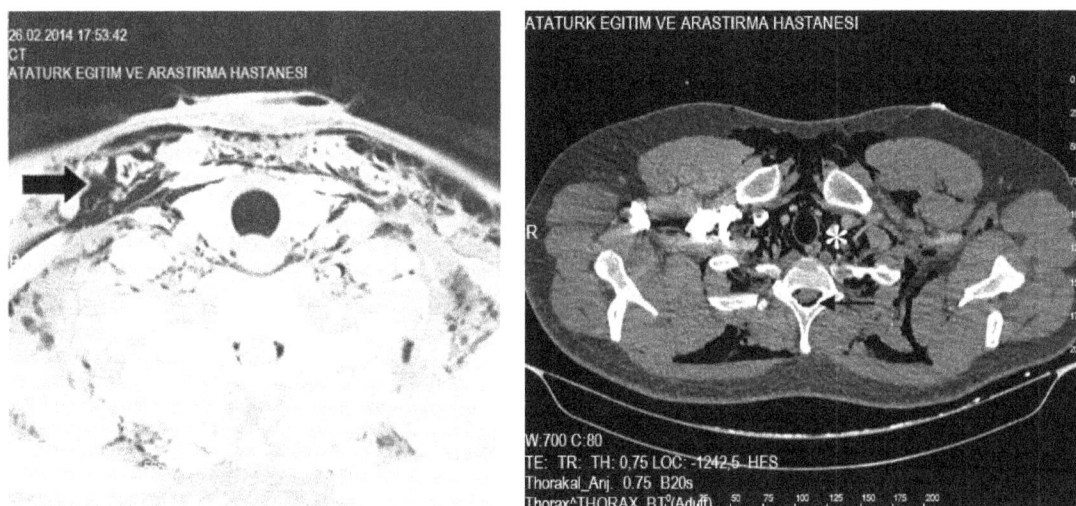

FIGURE 2: Diffuse subcutaneous emphysema (thick arrow), free air in the mediastinum (asterisk), and free air in the spinal canal (thin arrow).

physical examination, the patient was conscious, oriented, and cooperative but seemed agitated; subcutaneous crepitations were palpated in the jaw, neck, and upper chest area; his skin was sweaty. Breath sounds were natural and equal bilaterally on auscultation; on cardiac examination heart sounds were rhythmic and tachycardic; there was no additional heart sound or murmur; no significant lateralized motor findings were detected on neurological examination. Other systemic physical examinations were normal. The electrocardiogram revealed sinus tachycardia. The patient was given 5 mg diazepam intravenously for agitation. The patient's blood pressure and tachycardia returned to normal, after his agitation declined.

His chest X-ray revealed air in the subcutaneous tissue of the left axilla, the neck, and around the heart (Figure 1).

When computed tomography (CT) imaging of the neck and chest was obtained, diffuse subcutaneous emphysema, pneumomediastinum, and pneumorrhachis were detected; no rib fractures were observed (Figure 2).

The patient was consulted with thoracic surgery and neurosurgery departments. During the follow-up in the emergency department, upon increase of dyspnea and swelling on the neck, the thoracic surgeon applied a skin incision over the suprasternal notch and provided free air drainage. Conservative follow-up by neurosurgery was recommended for pneumorrhachis. The patient was transferred to the intensive care unit of the thoracic surgery department. He was treated with oxygen and analgesics. The patient was discharged after 10 days of follow-up with no additional complications.

## 3. Discussion

The toxic effects of cocaine depend on the increased central and peripheral catecholamine activity. In our patient sinus tachycardia and agitation were observed and were treated with diazepam.

Cocaine inhalation has previously been linked to pneumomediastinum [3]. It occurs secondary to barotrauma, resulting in rupture of terminal alveoli into the lung interstitium and the dissection of air along the pulmonary vasculature toward the hilum and extravasation to mediastinum [3]. Over 90% of the cases present with chest pain. Neck pain, dyspnea, hoarseness, and dysphagia may also be seen. It may be associated with subcutaneous emphysema in 64% of the cases and pneumothorax in 19% of the cases [3]. Diagnosis is usually made with a posterior-anterior and lateral chest radiograph; computed tomography can help diagnosis [3]. Treatment is conservative (oxygen, analgesics) [3].

To our knowledge, this is the 3rd case in the medical literature reporting pneumorrhachis after cocaine use. The etiology of pneumorrhachis includes trauma (skull or spine injury), medical procedures (epidural anesthesia, lumbar puncture, and surgery), epidural abscess, and malignancies [4, 5]. It is found in combination with associated air distribution in other compartments and cavities of the body, particularly, in conjunction with pneumocephalus, pneumothorax, pneumomediastinum, pneumopericardium, or subcutaneous emphysema [6]. Diagnosis is usually made on chest computed tomography scan [4].

Pneumorrhachis is usually asymptomatic, does not tend to migrate, and is reabsorbed spontaneously and completely in several days without recurrence. Therefore, patients with pneumorrhachis are usually managed conservatively [6]. Same management is advised in spontaneous pneumomediastinum with and without pneumorrhachis [5].

The mechanism of cocaine-induced subcutaneous emphysema, pneumomediastinum, and pneumorrhachis is believed to be secondary to barotrauma caused by deep inhalation and valsalva maneuver done by abusers in order to increase uptake and the euphoriant effect of substance or cough triggered by the sniffed substance. Increased intra-alveolar pressure causes rupture of a distended alveolus into the lung interstitium, and air passes into the lung interstitium; air then migrates along the pulmonary vasculature toward the lung hilum and then to the posterior mediastinum and travels through the neural foramina into the epidural space [2]. Two additional mechanisms have been proposed: alveolar wall fragility caused by repeated cocaine sniffing and air leak from cocaine induced destructed nasopharyngeal structures [4].

In our case, we detected pneumorrhachis in addition to pneumomediastinum and subcutaneous emphysema. The patient was admitted to the intensive care unit and followed up conservatively, recovered, and was discharged uneventfully.

## 4. Conclusion

Since patients with complaints related to illegal substance use are often admitted to emergency departments, emergency physicians should know emergency management of their possible complications [7].

## Conflict of Interests

The authors declare that there is no conflict of interests regarding the publication of this paper.

## Acknowledgments

The work should be attributed to Ankara Atatürk Training and Research Hospital, Department of Emergency Medicine, and Yıldırım Beyazıt University Faculty of Medicine, Department of Emergency Medicine.

## References

[1] J. Lucena, M. Blanco, C. Jurado et al., "Cocaine-related sudden death: a prospective investigation in south-west Spain," *European Heart Journal*, vol. 31, no. 3, pp. 318–329, 2010.

[2] H. Malik, S. Mohandas, and D. Mukherjee, "Epidural pneumatosis as a consequence of cocaine use," *BMJ Case Reports*, vol. 2012, 2012.

[3] M. Alnas, A. Altayeh, and M. Zaman, "Clinical course and outcome of cocaine-induced pneumomediastinum," *The American Journal of the Medical Sciences*, vol. 339, no. 1, pp. 65–67, 2010.

[4] H. Jung, S. C. Lee, D. H. Lee, and G. J. Kim, "Spontaneous pneumomediastinum with concurrent pneumorrhachis," *The Korean Journal of Thoracic and Cardiovascular Surgery*, vol. 47, no. 6, pp. 569–571, 2014.

[5] E. A. Belotti, M. Rizzi, P. Rodoni-Cassis, M. Ragazzi, M. Zanolari-Caledrerari, and M. G. Bianchetti, "Air within the spinal canal in spontaneous pneumomediastinum," *Chest*, vol. 137, no. 5, pp. 1197–1200, 2010.

[6] M. F. Oertel, M. C. Korinth, M. H. T. Reinges, T. Krings, S. Terbeck, and J. M. Gilsbach, "Pathogenesis, diagnosis and management of pneumorrhachis," *European Spine Journal*, vol. 15, no. 5, pp. S636–S643, 2006.

[7] R. J. Devlin and J. A. Henry, "Clinical review: major consequences of illicit drug consumption," *Critical Care*, vol. 12, article 202, 2008.

# 17

# An Uncommon Presentation of Spontaneous Rectus Sheath Hematoma with Acute Kidney Injury due to Obstructive Uropathy and Prerenal Azotemia

**Eleni Paschou,**[1] **Eleni Gavriilaki,**[2] **Asterios Kalaitzoglou,**[2] **Maria Mourounoglou,**[3] **and Nikolaos Sabanis**[4]

[1] Department of Family Medicine, General Hospital of Pella, 58200 Edessa, Greece
[2] Medical School, Aristotle University of Thessaloniki, 54124 Thessaloniki, Greece
[3] Department of General Surgery, General Hospital of Pella, 58200 Edessa, Greece
[4] Nephrological Department, General Hospital of Pella, 58200 Edessa, Greece

Correspondence should be addressed to Eleni Paschou; el_paschou@yahoo.gr

Academic Editor: Aristomenis K. Exadaktylos

Rectus Sheath Hematoma (RSH) represents an unusual entity which is characterized by acute abdominal pain and tender palpable abdominal mass usually, among elderly patients receiving anticoagulant therapy. We report the case of an 81-year-old woman admitted to our department due to acute abdominal pain and oligoanuria. The patient had recently been hospitalized due to acute myocardial infarction (AMI) and atrial fibrillation (AF) and received both anticoagulant and antiplatelet therapies. The radiological assessments revealed an extended Rectus Sheath Hematoma and bilateral hydronephrosis. Treatment of the hematoma required cessation of anticoagulants and antiplatelet agents, immobilization, blood and fresh frozen plasma transfusion, and administration of vasopressors. The patient recovered gradually and was discharged home fifteen (15) days later.

## 1. Introduction

During the last years, anticoagulant and antiplatelet agents have been extensively used, as a treatment or prophylaxis of several conditions in increased thrombotic risk, such as venous thromboembolism, pulmonary embolism, acute coronary syndromes, atrial fibrillation and stroke. However, the benefits do not always outweigh the risks of antithrombotic therapy, since a number of adverse events have been reported. Rectus Sheath Hematoma (RSH) represents an uncommon complication of anticoagulant therapy that can be misdiagnosed because it mimics other causes of abdominal pain.

Herein, we report an interesting case of an elderly patient with abdominal pain caused by RSH who received conservative treatment in time, avoiding further complications.

## 2. Case Report

An 81-year-old Caucasian female presented to our emergency department with acute abdominal pain and oligoanuria (urinary output 100 mL/8 h). Her medical history included a recent hospitalization due to acute myocardial infarction (AMI) and atrial fibrillation (AF), treated with amiodarone intravenous infusion (amiodarone 300 mg bolus iv) and anticoagulant therapy with acenocoumarol and dual antiplatelet treatment (aspirin 100 mg per day; clopidogrel 75 mg per day). During the first hospitalization, she developed amiodarone-induced hepatotoxicity. Therefore, the treatment with acenocoumarol was interrupted and replaced with low molecular weight heparin (LMWH) (nadroparin 5700 antiXA/0.6 mL twice daily) while antiplatelet treatment continued. Eight (8) days after she was discharged

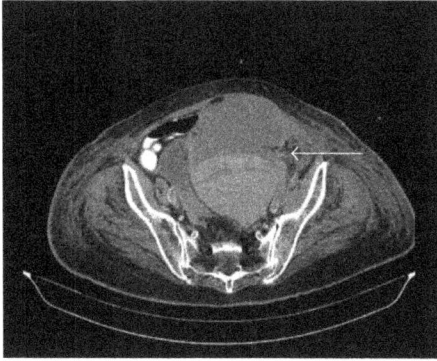

FIGURE 1: Rectus Sheath Hematoma: "hematocrit formation" point.

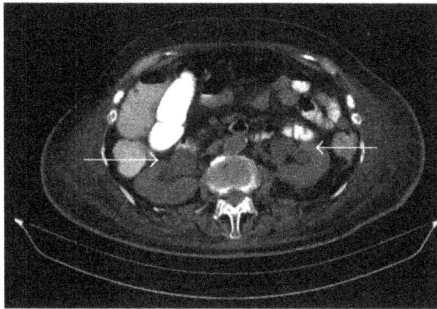

FIGURE 2: Rectus Sheath Hematoma: distension of renal pelvic system bilaterally.

home, she presented in the emergency department hemodynamically unstable (BP: 80/60 mmHg, HR: 115 bpm) with tachypnea and low grade fever. Physical examination demonstrated a painful mass extending to the lower abdomen and upper ecchymosis. Routine laboratory examinations revealed anemia, acute renal failure, hypocalcaemia, and coagulation disturbances (Table 1-Day 1). Urinalysis showed acute tubular necrosis (Specific Gravity 1027, pH 6, WBCs 0-1, RBCs 0-1, and browncast cylindroids). Both abdominal ultrasonography and abdominopelvic CT scan demonstrated an hematoma at lower abdomen, on the left rectus abdominis muscle extending to the pelvis (dimensions 11.3 × 14.6 × 10.5 cm), presented with the "hematocrit formation" point (Figure 1). Furthermore, bilateral hydronephrosis was observed due to hematoma's invasive traits. Central venous pressure (CVP) was 3 mmHg and intra-abdominal pressure (IAP), using the intravesicular method, was 21 mmHg (abdominal compartment syndrome (ACS)). Acute kidney injury correlated with acute tubular necrosis and postrenal obstructive uropathy (Figure 2).

Anticoagulant and antiplatelet agents were ceased. On day 1, in accordance with CVP, intravenous fluids (0.9% sodium chloride solution) were infused in order to restore intravascular volume. The patient received two packed red blood cells transfusions, one fresh frozen plasma transfusion and calcium gluconate (10 mL calcium gluconate 10%/8 h) because of the blood clotting mechanism's disturbances. On day 2, despite normal ranges of CVP, the patient was hemodynamically unstable and was treated with

vasopressors (dopamine 10 $\mu$g/kg/min). The above measures increased blood pressure to 120 mmHg and the urinary output improved (400 mL/8 h). The patient recovered gradually after fifteen (15) days of bed rest, without any complications, and was discharged hemodynamically stable (BP: 115/80) with normal IAP (7 mmHg), renal and liver function (Table 1-Day 15), while she had received four packed red blood cells and six fresh frozen plasma transfusions in total.

## 3. Discussion

RSH is usually a self-limiting entity that potentially can lead to severe complications. Obstructive uropathy [1] and abdominal compartment syndrome [2] are uncommon complications even though RSH is involved with other rare entities such as hemoperitoneum [3], gross hematuria [4], rectus abdominis myonecrosis [5], ileocecal perforation [6], and small bowel infraction [7].

The mortality rate has been reported at 4% in general population and up to 25% in patients under anticoagulant therapy. It is more frequent in female and elderly patients, mainly because of their decreased muscle mass [8].

RSH is a rare cause of acute abdominal pain presenting with ecchymosis and abdominal wall mass due to rupture of epigastric vessels or arteries. It occurs usually unilateral, although some rare cases of bilateral hematomas have been reported, as complications of kidney transplantation [9] and alcohol liver disease [10]. Symptoms following the appearance of RSH are mainly nonspecific and include fever, hypovolaemia, nausea, vomiting, and diarrhea. Recognition of clinical signs such as Cullen, Grey-Turner, Carnett (tenderness remains the same or increases with head raising) [11, 12], and Fothergill's sign (the abdominal mass in RSH does not cross the midline and, in contrast to an intraperitoneal mass, it remains conspicuous on tensing the abdominal wall musculature by head or leg raising) [13] may be beneficial for diagnostic approach.

The main risk factors for RSH are anticoagulant therapies, coagulation disorders, previous surgical operations [14], abdominal trauma, increased intra-abdominal pressure (cough, sneezing, strenuous exercise [15, 16], pregnancy [17], and constipation), cardiovascular diseases, and myopathies [18]. Other causes have been also described in case reports, such as acupuncture [19], subcutaneous injection, foley catheterization [20], endometriosis of rectus abdominis, transvaginal follicle aspiration during *in vitro* fertilisation [21], HCV-related mixed cryoglobulinemia [22], lymphoproliferative disease after renal transplantation [23], and tetanus [24].

The role of ultrasonography and computed tomography is crucial, although computed tomography appears to be the most accurate way of confirming the diagnosis [25].

According to Berná et al. [26] and Osinbowale and Bartholomew [13] RSH can be classified into three categories that can lead to appropriate therapeutic strategies (Table 2).

There have been reported only few cases of RSH complicated with acute kidney injury. The causes in these cases seem to be prerenal, intrarenal, or postrenal. Our patient appeared

TABLE 1: Routine laboratory examination.

| | Day 1 | Day 2 | Day 3 | Day 7 | Day 15 |
|---|---|---|---|---|---|
| WBC count ($\times 10^3/\mu$L) | 12,36 | 13,57 | 13,12 | 9,78 | 7,65 |
| Hemoglobulin (g/dL) | 7,9 | 8,6 | 8,8 | 11 | 11,5 |
| Hematocrit (%) | 24,2 | 27,7 | 29,8 | 33,5 | 36,2 |
| Platelet count ($\times 10^3/\mu$L) | 145 | 157 | 159 | 162 | 154 |
| Serum creatinine (mg/dL) | 2,73 | 2,69 | 2,14 | 1,56 | 1,12 |
| Urea (mg/dL) | 140 | 114 | 98 | 60 | 43 |
| SGOT (mg/dL) | 226 | 234 | 217 | 85 | 36 |
| SGPT (mg/dL) | 432 | 392 | 366 | 109 | 40 |
| Serum calcium (mg/dL)* | 6,7 | 6,9 | 7,1 | 7,6 | 8,2 |
| Activated partial thromboplastin time (aPTT) (sec) | 38,7 | 36,7 | 32 | 29,9 | 27,9 |
| Fibrinogen (g/L) | 1,53 | 1,66 | 2,01 | 2,6 | 2,9 |
| International normalized ratio (INR) | 1,84 | 1,67 | 1,34 | 1,27 | 1,1 |

* corrected to albumin.

TABLE 2: Berna and Osinbowale RSH classification. Computed tomography severity grades and suggested management strategy, modified and reprinted with permission from Osinbowale and Bartholomew [13].

| Grade | Anatomic extension | Symptoms | Management |
|---|---|---|---|
| I | Intramuscular, unilateral; does not dissect along fascial planes. | Mild to moderate pain. No drop in hemoglobin. | Conservative; usually outpatient follow-up only. |
| II | Bilateral; some dissection between the muscle and transversalis fascia; no extension into the prevesical space. | Minor drop in hemoglobin. | Observation, short hospital stay. May need transfusion. |
| III | Bilateral, large; dissects between the transversalis fascia and muscle into the peritoneum and prevesical space. | Significant drop in hemoglobin and hemodynamic instability. | Reversal of anticoagulants and blood transfusion. Angiographic interventions may be needed. |

with both prerenal and postrenal causes. Patient's hemodynamic instability caused prolonged renal ischemia which led to acute tubular necrosis while the bilateral obstructive uropathy caused significant raise of intratubular pressure. As a result of obstructive uropathy, renal blood flow decreased further leading to acute kidney injury.

The pathophysiological mechanisms of blood clotting disturbances in this case are complicated and involve uremia, accumulation of LMWH, and anticoagulant therapy. It is well known that uremia in patients with renal insufficiency leads to qualitative platelet abnormalities, mainly caused by A2 thromboxane reduced production due to abnormal platelet arachidonic acid metabolism [27]. In these patients, heparin levels should be reduced, especially when creatinine clearance is less than 40 mL/min [28], in order to prevent complications. The remarkable points in our case report were that the patient had also amiodarone-induced hepatotoxicity and hypocalcaemia causing further disturbances of blood clotting mechanism [29].

RSH management is mainly supportive, including immobilization, cessation of anticoagulation therapy, and transfusions. Angioembolization may be necessary [30] especially for RSHs related to LMWH [31] and surgical intervention should be reserved for cases with hemodynamic instability which resist in conventional treatment [32].

## 4. Conclusions

RSH should be in mind of physicians during differential diagnosis of acute abdominal pain, especially in elderly patients receiving anticoagulants. The causal nature remains unclear since the underlying pathophysiological pathways are complicated. Early recognition can be of great importance for patients' recovery, preventing from severe complications. Management is usually supportive although surgical intervention in some patients should be considered.

## Conflict of Interests

The authors declare that there is no conflict of interests regarding the publication of this paper.

## References

[1] J. Toyonaga, K. Tsuruya, K. Masutani et al., "Hemorrhagic shock and obstructive uropathy due to a large rectus sheath hematoma in a patient on anticoagulant therapy," *Internal Medicine*, vol. 48, no. 24, pp. 2119–2122, 2009.

[2] S. F. Jafferbhoy, Q. Rustum, and M. H. Shiwani, "Abdominal compartment syndrome—a fatal complication from a rectus sheath haematoma," *BMJ Case Reports*, 2012.

[3] O. Balafa, S. Koundouris, M. Mitsis, and K. C. Siamopoulos, "An unusual case of hemoperitoneum: spontaneous rectus sheath hematoma," *Peritoneal Dialysis International*, vol. 34, no. 1, pp. 134–135, 2014.

[4] O. Sandoval and T. Kinkead, "Spontaneous rectus sheath hematoma: an unusual cause of gross hematuria," *Urology*, vol. 82, no. 6, pp. e35–e36, 2013.

[5] L. C. Patten, S. S. Awad, D. H. Berger, and S. P. Fagan, "Rectus abdominus myonecrosis: an unrecognized complication of rectus sheath hematoma," *Journal of Trauma*, vol. 59, no. 2, pp. 475–477, 2005.

[6] A. Tsiouris, A. Falvo, J. H. Patton, and A. C. Sisley, "Rectus sheath hematoma causing ileocecal perforation," *American Surgeon*, vol. 78, no. 9, pp. 1009–1010, 2012.

[7] R. A. Dineen, N. R. Lewis, and N. Altaf, "Small bowel infarction complicating rectus sheath haematoma in an anticoagulated patient," *Medical Science Monitor*, vol. 11, no. 10, pp. CS57–CS59, 2005.

[8] W. B. Cherry and P. S. Mueller, "Rectus sheath hematoma: review of 126 cases at a single institution," *Medicine*, vol. 85, no. 2, pp. 105–110, 2006.

[9] B. Feizzadeh Kerigh and G. Maddah, "Bilateral rectus sheath hematoma in kidney transplant patient: case study and literature review," *Nephro-Urology Monthly*, vol. 5, no. 4, pp. 921–923, 2013.

[10] J. G. Docherty and A. L. Herrick, "Bilateral rectus sheath haematoma complicating alcoholic liver disease," *British Journal of Clinical Practice*, vol. 45, no. 4, article 289, 1991.

[11] H. Thomson and D. M. A. Francis, "Abdominal-wall tenderness: a useful sign in the acute abdomen," *The Lancet*, vol. 2, no. 8047, pp. 1053–1054, 1977.

[12] D. W. R. Gray, J. M. Dixon, G. Seabrook, and J. Collin, "Is abdominal wall tenderness a useful sign in the diagnosis of non-specific abdominal pain?" *Annals of the Royal College of Surgeons of England*, vol. 70, no. 4, pp. 233–234, 1988.

[13] O. Osinbowale and J. R. Bartholomew, "Rectus sheath hematoma," *Vascular Medicine*, vol. 13, no. 4, pp. 275–279, 2008.

[14] F. Procacciante, G. Diamantini, D. Paolelli, and P. Picozzi, "Rectus sheath haematoma as an early complication of laparoscopic hemicolectomy: a case report and review of the literature," *Chirurgia Italiana*, vol. 61, no. 4, pp. 481–483, 2009.

[15] Y. Choi and D. Lee, "A case of rectus sheath hematoma caused by yoga exercise," *The American Journal of Emergency Medicine*, vol. 27, no. 7, pp. 899.e1–899.e2, 2009.

[16] L. Barna, I. Toth, E. Kovacs, and E. Krizso, "Rectus sheath haematoma following exercise testing: a case report," *Journal of Medical Case Reports*, vol. 3, article 9000, 2009.

[17] M. C. Tolcher, J. F. Nitsche, K. W. Arendt, and C. H. Rose, "Spontaneous rectus sheath hematoma pregnancy: case report and review of the literature," *Obstetrical and Gynecological Survey*, vol. 65, no. 8, pp. 517–522, 2010.

[18] M. Yamagishi, S. Tajima, A. Suetake et al., "Dermatomyositis with hemorrhagic myositis," *Rheumatology International*, vol. 29, no. 11, pp. 1363–1366, 2009.

[19] S. P. Cheng and C. L. Liu, "Rectus sheath hematoma after acupuncture," *Journal of Emergency Medicine*, vol. 29, no. 1, pp. 101–102, 2005.

[20] Y. H. Choi, D. H. Lee, S. Y. Yun, and J. H. Lee, "A case of rectus sheath hematoma due to Foley catheterization after acute urinary retention," *The American Journal of Emergency Medicine*, vol. 30, no. 5, pp. 837.e3–837.e4,, 2012.

[21] J. G. Wang, M. J. Huchko, S. Kavic, and M. V. Sauer, "Rectus sheath hematoma after transvaginal follicle aspiration: a rare complication of in vitro fertilization," *Fertility and Sterility*, vol. 84, no. 1, article 217, 2005.

[22] C. M. Moschella, I. Palmieri, P. Bartolucci, M. Assenza, A. Maiuolo, and C. Modini, "Spontaneous rectus sheath haematoma in HCV mixed cryoglobulinemia requiring emergency treatment (case report)," *Il Giornale di Chirurgia*, vol. 23, no. 8-9, pp. 331–333, 2002.

[23] A. Franco, L. Jiménez, C. Muñoz, M. Chulia, P. Marco, and E. Muñoz, "Hematoma of the anterior rectus abdominis muscle as the first manifestation of lymphoproliferative disease after renal transplantation," *Nefrologia*, vol. 20, no. 6, pp. 559–562, 2000.

[24] G. M. Suhr and A. E. Green Jr., "Rectus abdominis sheath hematoma as a complication of tetanus. Diagnosis by computed tomography scanning," *Clinical Imaging*, vol. 13, no. 1, pp. 82–86, 1989.

[25] A. Moreno Gallego, J. L. Aguayo, B. Flores et al., "Ultrasonography and computed tomography reduce unnecessary surgery in abdominal rectus sheath haematoma," *British Journal of Surgery*, vol. 84, no. 9, pp. 1295–1297, 1997.

[26] J. D. Berná, V. Garcia-Medina, J. Guirao, and J. Garcia-Medina, "Rectus sheath hematoma: diagnostic classification by CT," *Abdominal Imaging*, vol. 21, no. 1, pp. 62–64, 1996.

[27] G. Remuzzi, A. Benigni, P. Dodesini et al., "Reduced platelet thromboxane formation in uremia. Evidence for a functional cyclooxygenase defect," *Journal of Clinical Investigation*, vol. 71, no. 3, pp. 762–768, 1983.

[28] P. J. Denard, J. C. Fetter, and L. R. Zacharski, "Rectus sheath hematoma complicating low-molecular weight heparin therapy," *International Journal of Laboratory Hematology*, vol. 29, no. 3, pp. 190–194, 2007.

[29] Y. Caraco, D. Raveh, M. Flugelman, and I. Raz, "Enhanced anticoagulant effect of acenocoumarol induced by amiodarone coadministration," *Israel Journal of Medical Sciences*, vol. 24, no. 11, pp. 688–689, 1988.

[30] G. Kasotakis, "Retroperitoneal and rectus sheath hematomas," *Surgical Clinics of North America*, vol. 94, no. 1, pp. 71–76, 2014.

[31] A. Smithson, J. Ruiz, R. Perello, M. Valverde, J. Ramos, and L. Garzo, "Diagnostic and management of spontaneous rectus sheath hematoma," *European Journal of Internal Medicine*, vol. 24, no. 6, pp. 579–582, 2013.

[32] A. Buffone, G. Basile, M. Costanzo et al., "Management of patients with rectus sheath hematoma: personal experience," *Journal of the Formosan Medical Association*, 2013.

# 18

# Toxic Effects of *Rhamnus alaternus*: A Rare Case Report

H. Ben Ghezala,[1] N. Chaouali,[2] I. Gana,[2] S. Snouda,[1] A. Nouioui,[2] I. Belwaer,[2] J. Ouali,[1] M. Kaddour,[1] W. Masri,[2] D. Ben Salah,[2] D. Amira,[2] H. Ghorbal,[2] and A. Hedhili[2]

[1] Teaching Department of Emergency and Intensive Care Medicine, Regional Hospital of Zaghouan, Street of Republic, 1100 Zaghouan, Tunisia
[2] Research Laboratory of Toxicology-Environment LR12SP07, Laboratory of Toxicology, Center for Emergency Medical Assistance, Montfleury, 1008 Tunis, Tunisia

Correspondence should be addressed to H. Ben Ghezala; hassen.ghezala@gmail.com

Academic Editor: Aristomenis K. Exadaktylos

In Tunisia, there are about 478 species of plants commonly used in folk medicine. Medicinal plants and herbal remedies used are responsible for 2% of intoxications listed by Tunisian National Poison Center. Most cases are related to confusion between edible plants and toxic plants lookalikes or to an excessive consumption of therapeutic plants. We report the case of a 58-year-old man admitted to the Emergency Department of the Regional Hospital of Zaghouan (Tunisia), with renal failure and rhabdomyolysis. The patient reported having daily consumption of a homemade tea based on *Mediterranean Buckthorn* roots, during the last 6 months to treat type 2 diabetes. The aim of this work was to establish an association between the consumption of the herbal remedy and the occurrence of both renal failure and rhabdomyolysis. No similar cases have been reported in recent literature.

## 1. Introduction

Herbal remedies have been used for centuries to treat a variety of diseases. *Mediterranean Buckthorn (Rhamnus alaternus)* has been used for therapeutic purposes and no toxicity effects have been documented. *Rhamnus alaternus* (Rhamnaceae) is a small tree located mainly in the north of Tunisia, where it is known as "Oud El-Khir." It has traditionally been used as a diuretic, laxative, hypotensive drug and for the treatment of diabetes, hepatic, and dermatologic complications [1, 2]. Previous phytochemical studies have shown potent antioxidant, free radical scavenging, antimutagenic and antigenotoxic activities of flavonoids and phenol isolated from *Rhamnus alaternus* roots and leaves [3, 4].

## 2. Case Report

On February 1, 2013, a 58-year-old man was admitted to the Emergency Department of the Regional Hospital of Zaghouan (Tunisia), with dizziness, weakness, anorexia, and dyspnea. His blood pressure was 130/60 mmHg. The patient has a 15-pack-year history of smoking. He was a mason by occupation. He had 20-year back history of pulmonary tuberculosis and type 2 diabetes revealed one year ago. Two days before his admission, the patient experienced nausea, vomiting, anuria, and hematuria. He reported having daily consumption of a homemade drink based on *Rhamnus alaternus* roots, during the last 6 months, to control his blood glucose levels. On physical examination, the patient had myalgia. He had no other clinical signs.

Cytological reports and sputum smear were negative (three times) for pulmonary tuberculosis. Hepatitis B and hepatitis C serology were also negative. Chest X-ray was normal; blood and urine culture were negative. In renal ultrasonography, there was a significant difference in kidney sizes and the corticomedullary differentiation was altered. Laboratory tests showed glucose 14.44 mmol/L, creatinine 1190 $\mu$mol/L, blood urea nitrogen 66.77 mmol/L, creatine phosphokinase (CPK) 2129 UI/L, pH 7.10, a CRP of 8.7 mg/L, and a normal coagulation profile (Table 1). Three dialysis sessions were performed.

*2.1. Toxicological Analyses.* Samples of the herbal decoction were obtained from the patient's wife. It was a dark brown

TABLE 1: Biochemical, hematologic, and blood gas parameters, before and after dialysis.

| Blood tests | Before dialysis | After dialysis | | | Normal ranges (adult male) |
| --- | --- | --- | --- | --- | --- |
| | | Day 4 | Day 7 | Day 9 | |
| Glucose | 14.44 | 4.74 | 4.50 | 4.55 | 3.9–6.1 mmol/L |
| Urea nitrogen | 66.77 | 46.04 | 39 | 50.99 | 2.5–7.5 mmol/L |
| Creatinine | 1190 | 756 | 853 | 811 | 60–110 $\mu$mol/L |
| Sodium | 122 | 141 | 120.5 | 128.1 | 135–145 mmol/L |
| Potassium | 4.88 | 2.44 | 3.61 | 3.81 | 3.5–4.5 mmol/L |
| Calcium | 1.4 | 1.5 | 0.92 | 1.19 | 2.20–2.55 mmol/L |
| CPK | 2129 | 2163 | 3399 | 1230 | <195 UI/L |
| CPK MB | 484.1 | 481.5 | 154.8 | 119 | 0–24 UI/L |
| Hemoglobin | 8.7 | 8.2 | 7.4 | 6.3 | 12.3–15.3 g/dL |
| WBC | 3.1 | 2.86 | 1.68 | 1.52 | $4–10 \times 10^3/mm^3$ |
| Platelets | 382.0 | 383.0 | 249.0 | 262.0 | $150.0–450.0 \times 10^3/mm^3$ |
| pH | 7.10 | 7.29 | 7.32 | 7.38 | 7.38–7.42 |
| $HCO^{3-}$ | 5.1 | 18.2 | 19.2 | 18.2 | 22–26 mmol/L |
| Anion gap | 35.8 | 25.2 | 7.21 | 20.31 | 16–18 mmol/L |
| $PaO_2$ | 88 | 91 | 88 | 86 | 95–98 mm Hg |
| $PaCO_2$ | 16.2 | 26 | 27 | 28 | 40–45 mm Hg |

suspension with fine brown deposit and a clear supernatant. It smelled a strong penetrating odor. Samples of both *Rhamnus alaternus* root and its decoction were sent to be analyzed in the Laboratory of Toxicology in the Center for Emergency Medical Assistance of Tunis in Tunisia.

*2.2. Extraction Procedures.* After the authenticity and the botanical identification of the species were confirmed according to the "Flore de la Tunisie" [6] phytochemical compounds were extracted from the medicinal decoction using routine methods including liquid-liquid extraction procedures with further analysis by gas chromatography/mass spectrometry (GC-MS). The solvents used were dichloromethane, ethyl acetate, and chloroform at different pH values (1.0, 7.0, and 9.0). The different extracts were dehydrated over anhydrous sulfate. The dry residue was diluted with 2 milliliters of ethyl acetate. One or 2 $\mu$L was analyzed by GC-MS. Dried roots of "*Rhamnus alaternus*" were reduced to small fragments and macerated in a water-methanol mixture (1 : 2) during 4 h with magnetic stirring. 24 hours later, the extract was filtered and the alcoholic layer was evaporated. The aqueous layer was collected in a separating funnel and had been alkalinized by the addition of ammonia ($NH_4OH$) and then extracted with dichloromethane by liquid-liquid extraction procedures. The organic phase was dehydrated over anhydrous sulfate and concentrated to 1 mL and then analyzed by GC-MS.

*2.3. Chromatographic Conditions.* The gas chromatograph-mass spectrometer used was a Hewlett Packard 5890-II (Agilent Technologies) fitted with a manual injector and HP5-MS (0.25-$\mu$m) capillary column (30 m long and 0.25 mm i.d.). The injection volume was 2 $\mu$L; the compounds were separated with helium (carrier gas) at a flow rate of 1 mL/min.

The operating conditions were as follows: the injector was programmed to 250°C at 10°C·s$^{-1}$ and held for 2 min. The oven was programmed from 50°C (2 min) to 100°C at 25°C·min$^{-1}$ and then to 200°C at 10°C·min$^{-1}$ (2 min). MS detection was achieved in scan mode for qualitative analysis. Run time was 16 min.

# 3. Results

Screening by GC-MS of both *Rhamnus alaternus* roots and infusion extracts revealed the presence of anthraquinone glycosides such as 4,5-dihydroxy-9,10-dioxoanthracène-2-carboxylic acid (rhein), 1,8-dihydroxy-3-(hydroxymethyl)-9,10-anthracenedione (aloe-emodin), and 1,8-dihydroxy-3-methoxy-6-methylanthracene-9,10-dione (physcion). The retention times were 8.95, 9.67, and 10.25 min, respectively (Figure 1).

Anthraquinone glycosides were detected in a dichloromethane extract and ethyl acetate extract at pH value = 9 and only in a dichloromethane extract at pH value = 7 by GC-MS analysis (Table 2).

# 4. Discussion

Blood chemistry tests performed before dialysis revealed renal nitrogen retention (serum creatinine of 1190 $\mu$mol/L and blood urea nitrogen of 66 mmol/L). Moreover, normochromic and normocytic anemia, hypocalcemia, and the loss of corticomedullary differentiation observed in our patient suggest a chronic renal insufficiency. From a biochemical point of view, major hyperglycemia (14.44 mmol/L) could be one of the underlying factors, which lead to the diagnosis of diabetic nephropathy. According to authors, this

TABLE 2: Qualitative screening by gas chromatography-mass spectrometry (GC-MS).

| | Dichloromethane extract | | | Ethyl acetate extract | | | Chloroform extract | | |
|---|---|---|---|---|---|---|---|---|---|
| | pH = 1 | pH = 7 | pH = 9 | pH = 1 | pH = 7 | pH = 9 | pH = 1 | pH = 7 | pH = 9 |
| Rhein | ND | + | + | ND | ND | + | ND | ND | ND |
| Physcion | ND | + | + | ND | ND | + | ND | ND | ND |
| Aloe-emodin | ND | + | + | ND | ND | + | ND | ND | ND |

+: detected; ND: not detected.

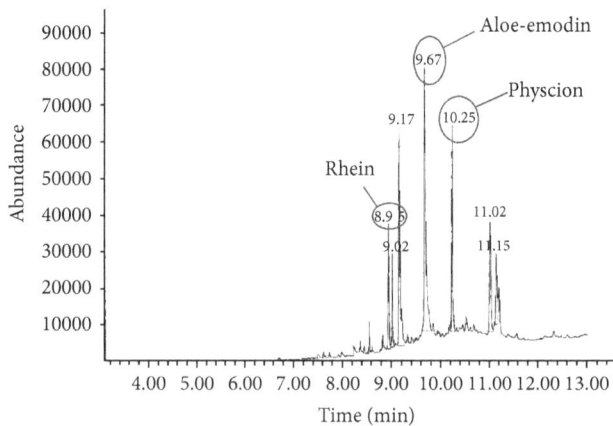

FIGURE 1: Original chromatogram of herbal tea extract (scan mode).

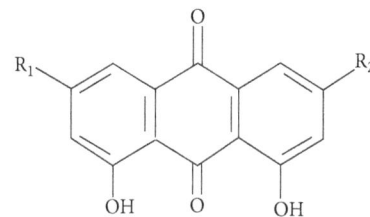

Aloe-emodin: $R_1 = CH_2OH$; $R_2 = H$

Chrysophanol: $R_1 = CH_3$; $R_2 = H$

Emodin: $R_1 = CH_3$; $R_2 = OH$

Rhein: $R_1 = COOH$; $R_2 = H$

Physcion: $R_1 = CH_3$; $R_2 = OCH_3$

FIGURE 2: Chemical structure of anthraquinone glycosides [5].

nephropathy was most likely aggravated by the potential toxic effect of anthraquinone glycosides found in *Rhamnus alaternus* infusion extract. Anthraquinones are a group of functionally diverse chemicals structurally related to anthracene, known to be present in the roots and bark of numerous plants of the genus *Rhamnus* such as senna, cascara, aloe, frangula, and rhubarb used for their laxative properties [7].

Anthraquinone glycosides including emodin, physcion, aloe-emodin, rhein, and chrysophanol are nowadays well recognized as important biologically active components (Figure 2) [8]. Recently, it was reported that anthraquinones exert a wide range of biological activities including antifungal, antimicrobial, and anticancer properties other than the well-known laxative action on the gastrointestinal apparatus [9–11]. Besides health benefits of anthraquinones, it was also reported that they have a cell toxicity effect. In fact, a study exploring anthraquinones toxicity on Sprague Dawley (S.D.) rats showed that the oral administration of these compounds for 13 weeks induced nephrotoxicity as renal tubule epithelial cells swelled and denatured in tissue slice examination. Anthraquinones were responsible for the activation of mitogen activator protein kinase (MAPK), which causes the arrest of cellular cycle, inhibits epithelial cells proliferation, and contributes to nephrotoxicity [12].

Moreover, investigations revealed increased levels of serum CPK 2129 UI/L, hyperkaliemia of 4.88 mmol/L, and widespread muscle pain on the physical examination, which constitute the diagnostic hallmark of rhabdomyolysis [13]. In the present case, rhabdomyolysis did not have an obvious explanation; there was no ischemia, trauma, or drug intake that could explain it. Nevertheless, we know that one of the

rare causes of rhabdomyolysis is metabolic disorders; rhabdomyolysis has been described in chronic hypophosphatemia and hyponatremia, and the most common cause is chronic hypokalemia as it can be seen during treatment with diuretics, in hyperemesis gravidarum or during acute diarrhea episodes [14–17].

In the reported case, the patient has experienced an episode of acute diarrhea one week before his admission to the hospital; rhabdomyolysis could be related to a severe hypokalemia that results from the rapid loss of extracellular potassium losses via gastrointestinal route. In fact anthraquinone glycosides have a strong potential to deplete potassium by stimulating the intestinal secretion of water and electrolytes ($K^+$, $Na^+$, $Cl^-$, etc.) [18], and these glycosides are poorly absorbed from the gastrointestinal tract but are cleaved by gut bacteria to produce aglycones that are more readily absorbed and are responsible for the purgative properties of herb-based stimulant preparations [19].

Long-term therapy with anthraquinone glycosides can alter the body's normal balance of fluids and minerals, which can cause dehydration, severe hypokalemia hyponatremia, asthenia, and anorexia [20, 21]. In addition, lysis of muscle cells releases toxic intracellular components in the systemic circulation that leads to electrolyte disturbances, hypovolemia, metabolic acidosis, and acute renal failure [22, 23]. The patient experienced the same symptoms when he was admitted to hospital except hypokalemia, and the patient has hyperkaliemia because of rhabdomyolysis and the release of intracellular potassium into the plasma. Furthermore, the destruction of muscle cells results in the creation of a "third space" where substantial amounts of water and $Na^+$

are concentrated [24, 25], causing hypovolemia and acute renal failure. Organic and phosphoric acids released from the muscle cell lead to metabolic acidosis and increase the anion gap due to the overproduction of organic acids [26].

In summary, the patient who refused to take any medication to control his blood glucose levels except herbal medication has an undiagnosed diabetic nephropathy aggravated by acute renal dysfunction and rhabdomyolysis. All metabolic disorders are mainly imputed to the toxic effects of the anthraquinone glycosides. We noticed that patient completely recovered and symptoms regressed completely when stopping herbal infusion ingestion. Blood chemistry tests performed after dialysis were all normal.

## 5. Conclusion

*Rhamnus alaternus* can be toxic when used in an abusive way beside its strong antibacterial, antioxidant, and antidiabetic activities. To our knowledge, this is the first report of a case of renal failure and rhabdomyolysis which is possibly associated with a chronic consumption of *Rhamnus alaternus* roots. We present this case to illustrate the role of both clinical and biological investigations in handling cases of herbal poisonings. We aimed also to increase awareness among emergency physicians about patients presenting to the Emergency Department with unexplained symptoms (renal failure, rhabdomyolysis, etc.) requiring prompt diagnosis so that such life-threatening complications can be avoided.

## Conflict of Interests

The authors declare that there is no conflict of interests regarding the publication of this paper.

## References

[1] J. Miralles, J. J. Martínez-Sánchez, J. A. Franco, and S. Bañón, "*Rhamnus alaternus* growth under four simulated shade environments: morphological, anatomical and physiological responses," *Scientia Horticulturae*, vol. 127, no. 4, pp. 562–570, 2011.

[2] R. R. Paris and H. Moyse, *Matières Médicales Tome II*, Masson et Cie, Paris, France, 1967.

[3] R. B. Ammar, W. Bhouri, M. B. Sghaier et al., "Antioxidant and free radical-scavenging properties of three flavonoids isolated from the leaves of *Rhamnus alaternus* L. (Rhamnaceae): a structure-activity relationship study," *Food Chemistry*, vol. 116, no. 1, pp. 258–264, 2009.

[4] R. B. Ammar, I. Bouhlel, K. Valenti et al., "Transcriptional response of genes involved in cell defense system in human cells stressed by $H_2O_2$ and pre-treated with (Tunisian) *Rhamnus alaternus* extracts: combination with polyphenolic compounds and classic in vitro assays," *Chemico-Biological Interactions*, vol. 168, no. 3, pp. 171–183, 2007.

[5] P. Panichayupakaranant, A. Sakunpak, and A. Sakunphueak, "Quantitative HPLC determination and extraction of anthraquinones in *Senna alata* leaves," *Journal of Chromatographic Science*, vol. 47, no. 3, pp. 197–200, 2009.

[6] G. Pottier-Alapetite, *Flore de la Tunisie Angiospermes-Dicotylédones*, Imprimerie Officielle de la République Tunisienne, 1979.

[7] E. M. Clementi and F. Misiti, "Potential health benefits of rhubarb," in *Promoting Health*, R. R. Watson and V. R. Preedy, Eds., pp. 407–423, 2010.

[8] M. Locatelli, F. Tammaro, L. Menghini, G. Carlucci, F. Epifano, and S. Genovese, "Anthraquinone profile and chemical fingerprint of *Rhamnus saxatilis* L. from Italy," *Phytochemistry Letters*, vol. 2, no. 4, pp. 223–226, 2009.

[9] M. Locatelli, S. Genovese, G. Carlucci, D. Kremer, M. Randic, and F. Epifano, "Development and application of high-performance liquid chromatography for the study of two new oxyprenylated anthraquinones produced by *Rhamnus* species," *Journal of Chromatography A*, vol. 1225, pp. 113–120, 2012.

[10] H. Matsuda, T. Morikawa, I. Toguchida, J.-Y. Park, S. Harima, and M. Yoshikawa, "Antioxidant constituents from rhubarb: structural requirements of stilbenes for the activity and structures of two new anthraquinone glucosides," *Bioorganic and Medicinal Chemistry*, vol. 9, no. 1, pp. 41–50, 2001.

[11] S. K. Agarwal, S. S. Singh, S. Verma, and S. Kumar, "Antifungal activity of anthraquinone derivatives from *Rheum emodi*," *Journal of Ethnopharmacology*, vol. 72, no. 1-2, pp. 43–46, 2000.

[12] M. Yan, L.-Y. Zhang, L.-X. Sun, Z.-Z. Jiang, and X.-H. Xiao, "Nephrotoxicity study of total rhubarb anthraquinones on Sprague Dawley rats using DNA microarrays," *Journal of Ethnopharmacology*, vol. 107, no. 2, pp. 308–311, 2006.

[13] P. A. Gabow, W. D. Kaehny, and S. P. Kelleher, "The spectrum of rhabdomyolysis," *Medicine*, vol. 61, no. 3, pp. 141–152, 1982.

[14] T. Zenone and Q. Blanc, "Rhabdomyolysis with major hypokalemia secondary to chronic glycyrrhizic acid ingestion," *La Revue de Médecine Interne*, vol. 30, no. 1, pp. 78–80, 2009.

[15] L. M. Criddle, "Rhabdomyolysis. Pathophysiology, recognition, and management," *Critical Care Nurse*, vol. 23, no. 6, pp. 14–22, 2003.

[16] A. L. Huerta-Alardín, J. Varon, and P. E. Marik, "Bench-to-bedside review: rhabdomyolysis—an overview for clinicians," *Critical Care*, vol. 9, no. 2, pp. 158–169, 2005.

[17] A. Chubachi, H. Wakui, K. Asakura, S. Nishimura, Y. Nakamoto, and A. B. Miura, "Acute renal failure following hypokalemic rhabdomyolysis due to chronic glycyrrhizic acid administration," *Internal Medicine*, vol. 31, no. 5, pp. 708–711, 1992.

[18] P. M. Copeland, "Renal failure associated with laxative abuse," *Psychotherapy and Psychosomatics*, vol. 62, no. 3-4, pp. 200–202, 1994.

[19] National Toxicology Program, "NTP toxicology and carcinogenesis studies of EMODIN (CAS NO. 518-82-1) feed studies in F344/N rats and B6C3F1 mice," National Toxicology Program Technical Report Series 493, 2001.

[20] M. Moulin and A. Coquerel, *Pharmacologie*, Masson, Paris, France, 2nd edition, 2002.

[21] J. Kienlen, "Rhabdomyolyse," in *Congrès National d'Anesthésie et de Réanimation*, Les Essentiels, pp. 469–476, 2007.

[22] L. Criddle, "Rhabdomyoysis. Pathophysiology, recognision, and management," *Critical Care Nurse*, vol. 23, no. 6, pp. 14–32, 2003.

[23] B. Dussol, "Equilibre potassique, hypokaliémie et hyperkaliémie," *Néphrologie et Thérapeutique*, vol. 6, no. 3, pp. 180–199, 2010.

[24] D. Singh, V. Chander, and K. Chopra, "Rhabdomyolysis," *Methods and Findings in Experimental and Clinical Pharmacology*, vol. 27, no. 1, pp. 39–48, 2005.

[25] D. J. Malinoski, M. S. Slater, and R. J. Mullins, "Crush injury and rhabdomyolysis," *Critical Care Clinics*, vol. 20, no. 1, pp. 171–192, 2004.

[26] T. A. Rusell, "Acute renal failure related to rhabdomyolysis: pathophysiology, diagnosis and collaborative management," *Nephrology Nursing Journal*, vol. 27, no. 6, pp. 567–577, 2000.

# 19

# Methamphetamine Ingestion Misdiagnosed as *Centruroides sculpturatus* Envenomation

## Joshua Strommen[1] and Farshad Shirazi[2,3]

[1]*Department of Emergency Medicine, Carl R Darnall Army Medical Center, 36000 Darnall Loop, Fort Hood, TX 76554, USA*
[2]*Arizona Poison & Drug Information Center (APDIC), University of Arizona College of Pharmacy, Tucson, AZ 85721, USA*
[3]*Arizona Emergency Medicine Research Center, University of Arizona College of Medicine, Tucson, AZ 85721, USA*

Correspondence should be addressed to Joshua Strommen; joshstrommen@gmail.com

Academic Editor: Serdar Kula

The authors present a case report of a 17-month-old female child who ingested a large amount of methamphetamine that looked very similar clinically to a scorpion envenomation specific to the southwestern United States by the species *Centruroides sculpturatus*. The child was initially treated with 3 vials of antivenom specific for that scorpion species and showed a transient, though clinically relevant neurologic improvement. Her clinical course of sympathomimetic toxicity resumed and she was treated with intravenous fluids and benzodiazepines after blood analysis showed significant levels of d-methamphetamine. This case report is to specifically underline the clinical confusion in discerning between these two conditions and the realization of limited and/or expensive resources that may be used in the process.

## 1. Introduction

Pediatric evaluation and treatment of *Centruroides sculpturatus* envenomation is well documented in recent literature. Using Centruroides (Scorpion) Immune F(ab')2 Equine Injection as a treatment for *C. sculpturatus* envenomation was shown to be consistently effective, with only minimal side effects that include vomiting, fever, and rash as the most common manifestations. The Centruroides (Scorpion) Immune F(ab')2 Equine Injection, also known as Anascorp, was used to treat over 1500 adult and pediatric patients alike, for known *C. sculpturatus* envenomation. Greater than 95% of these patients had symptom resolution within four hours after initiating Anascorp compared to a 3.1% resolution in a historical control database from 1990 to 2003 where only supportive care was given. Out of the 1500 patients mentioned above, none were diagnosed with the full serum sickness syndrome after receiving Anascorp [1]. Envenomation of pediatric patients by this specific type of scorpion, which has only been documented in the southwestern United States (US) and northern Mexico, is not uncommon. It is diagnosed by very specific characteristics, which, if not careful, can be mistaken for methamphetamine toxicity.

Unluckily, there is a predominance of methamphetamines in the same geographic area of the US, as the endemic locale of the *C. sculpturatus*. Illicit methamphetamine production and distribution in the United States has its historical origin from producers along the borders of both Mexico and California [2]. According to the United States Drug Enforcement Agency, for the calendar year 2012, just less than 11,000 kilograms of methamphetamine was seized along the Southwestern United States border with Mexico. This is the highest amount ever recorded. Arrestee data show stable rates of testing positive for methamphetamines in the western and southwestern United States versus the rest of the country, which reveals its geographic predominance and areas with higher rates of use [3].

Only two previously published case reports demonstrate cases of misdiagnosis of *C. sculpturatus* envenomation with what was actually a methamphetamine ingestion [4, 5]. However, none of the prior case reports of methamphetamine ingestion involve a patient who received the recommended full dose of antivenom and then showed transient neurologic improvement. The authors report a case of a 17-month-old female who had clinical improvement in neuromuscular hyperactivity and cranial nerve involvement after three vials of Anascorp for a suspected scorpion envenomation when, in fact, the patient had a methamphetamine intoxication. This observation of clinical improvement may further complicate the process of diagnosing the correct condition, in addition to the existing diagnostic dilemma of discerning methamphetamine toxicity versus a *C. sculpturatus* envenomation in nonverbal pediatric patients.

## 2. Case

A 17-month-old female with no previous medical problems presented to a community Emergency Department (ED) in Tucson, AZ, because of acute onset irritability, twitching throughout her entire body, and diaphoresis. On arrival to the ED her triage vital signs were documented as a heart rate of 122, a respiratory rate of 24, oxygen saturation of 90%, and rectal temperature of 99.7°F. Physical examination done in the ED revealed an alert and oriented female child with agitation and tremors. Her Glasgow Coma Scale was 15 and she had no derangement in her blood glucose. Pupils were equally reactive with 5-6 mm of mydriasis along with rotary nystagmus. Extraocular movements were intact. The patient's oral exam was consistent with excessive salivation, although there were no pooling secretions in the pharynx. The patient was in sinus tachycardia with no obvious murmurs and had clear breath sounds bilaterally with tachypnea. There were no obvious lesions, bruises, bites, abrasions, or erythema noted on skin exam.

The patient had presenting symptoms of abnormal eye movements, excessive salivation, and tachypnea, all of which are direct indications per the package insert for Anascorp to initiate administering the antivenom [1]. Along with the concomitant geographic setting of an Emergency Department in the Southwest US, *C. sculpturatus* envenomation was suspected as a possible diagnosis. Upon questioning, the patient's mother stated that she had seen scorpions multiple times within their home. Based on the concern for envenomation, the recommended three vials of Anascorp were given to the patient after consulting with the local Poison Center within minutes of the initial evaluation. Since scorpion envenomation was the presumed diagnosis and Anascorp was given, benzodiazepines were withheld for her agitation at this time. Both subjective and objective improvement was noted in the clinical condition of the patient within 30–40 minutes. Her nystagmus and secretions resolved, though she continued having generalized tremors.

However, the patient remained tachycardic and developed a rectal temperature of 102.0°F. Upon further questioning of the patient's mother, she revealed a history of methamphetamines being present and used at the caretaker's home in the past. While the route of ingestion for the child was unknown, the ingestion itself was confirmed by a positive urinalysis for methamphetamines. An expansive set of toxicology labs and routine chemistries were obtained and evaluated, in addition to the urine drug screen, all of which

showed no clinically pertinent abnormalities. The patient was then transferred to a tertiary care facility due to her continued symptoms of fever, tachycardia, agitation, and tremors.

At the tertiary care center, the patient remained with a sympathomimetic toxidrome. Evaluation by the toxicology team showed no clonus, rigidity, fasciculation, excessive salivation, or nystagmus. Per the parents, the patient never exhibited any behavior consistent with severe, localizing, extremity, or truncal pain typical for scorpion envenomation. Nor did the exam of the child on arrival show any direct or indirect skin findings consistent with a scorpion sting. The patient remained tachycardic, hypertensive, febrile, irritable, with mydriasis, and diaphoresis intermittently for 48 hours after admission. A noncontrast brain CT was completed to rule out the presence of spontaneous bleeding, which can be associated with severe methamphetamine ingestion. She had no clinically apparent seizure activity and had a negative EEG. The only pertinent lab abnormality was a creatine kinase of 1467 IU/L, but the patient never developed acute kidney injury during her hospital course. The patient was treated symptomatically with benzodiazepines and intravenous fluids until she returned to baseline. She was discharged on hospital day 8. Her extended stay was contributed to her workup, her treatment with several days worth of benzodiazepines, and social work services. Several weeks later lab results from the initial Emergency Department evaluation revealed blood levels consistent with d-methamphetamine greater than 61,000 ng/mL and amphetamine levels greater than 21,000 ng/mL. The patient was never readmitted with any further sequelae from this ingestion per our documentation and records.

## 3. Discussion

There have been four reported cases documented in two separate case reports in peer-reviewed literature of methamphetamine ingestion by a toddler, appearing clinically similar to a scorpion envenomation and initially being treated as such [4, 5]. *C. sculpturatus* venom contains a number of substances including neurotoxin, acetylcholinesterase, serotonin, histamine, protease inhibitors, phospholipases, hyaluronidase, and mucopolysacharides [6]. When present at toxic levels, the neurotoxin causes sodium channel inactivation, allowing an open state of the sodium channel, causing a prolonged action potential at the axonal membrane. This repeated depolarization results in an abundance of acetylcholine in the neuromuscular junction in both the central and peripheral nervous system. Cranial nerve abnormalities, bulbar dysfunction, neuromuscular hyperactivity, and dysautonomias are sensitive criteria for diagnosing this condition. Very specific findings reported by Suchard and Curry include tongue fasciculation, hypersalivation, slow and conjugate roving eye movements, and purposeless, uncoordinated motor agitation [7].

Methamphetamines have a distinct characteristic of enhancing both the central and peripheral nervous system excitatory pathways. There are two stereoisomers of methamphetamine, D-methamphetamine and L-methamphetamine. The L isomer is mostly a peripherally acting substance with alpha-adrenergic activity. It has been used in a number of products that serve as decongestants. The D isomer is the substance that has a central nervous system stimulant effect over 3–5 times more potent than that of its L counterpart. In addition when comparing the half-life of D-methamphetamine to another substance of abuse, cocaine, D-methamphetamine has a half-life of 10–12 hours versus two hours for cocaine [2]. The excitatory pathways are initiated when centrally located presynaptic monoamine reuptake transporters bind methamphetamine and release substances, which include dopamine, norepinephrine, and serotonin into the synapse.

Movement disorders from increased methamphetamine use or excessive nervous system stimulation can be associated with repetitive, stereotyped choreoathetoid movements, seizures, and tremors. Catecholamines are also significantly elevated from the adrenal medulla and postganglionic sympathetic nerve stimulation, which are responsible for causing tachycardia, mydriasis, and hypertension. The abnormal behavioral components of intoxication include aggression, psychosis, hypersexuality, and hallucinations [8]. They all stem from the dopaminergic and serotonergic alterations of the central nervous system.

Astute clinical observation and history of present illness, along with blood and/or urine toxicology screen, have revealed the true identity of the inciting agent in all reported cases. In this case, the patient had decreased cranial nerve dysfunction within 40 minutes after giving the Anascorp. The neuromuscular dysfunction of shaking, jerking, and tremors of the extremities remained however. It is plausible that this finding is due to the Anascorp administration, as a typical response time for antivenom is 30–60 minutes. The mechanism of action of Anascorp is by equine derived, venom-specific F(ab′)2 fragments of immunoglobulin G, which bind to specific toxins within bark scorpion venom. Usually four hours after administration of the antivenom, all symptoms should be resolved if the true etiology is bark scorpion envenomation [1].

In all previous case reports, only one vial of antivenom was given which yielded no clinical response, hence the mandatory search for an alternate diagnosis, whereas in this case the patient received the entire three recommended vials. Understandably, the etiology is not scorpion venom, but methamphetamine. Though as previously stated, the patient had reversal of some of her symptoms. Most notable was the disappearance of her rotary nystagmus and her oral secretions with the antivenom at a dose of three full vials. Additionally, there were also no adverse signs or symptoms to include rash, vomiting, or anaphylaxis after receiving the Anascorp.

The authors postulate that there was some amount of protein binding by the F(ab′)2 present in the blood, with the methamphetamine, causing a decrease in symptoms and clinical severity of the existing catecholamine surge. The authors realize certain questionable aspects of this theory. The most obvious incongruences are that the F(ab′)2 antibody is supposed to bind a protein which is magnitudes of size larger than the size of a methamphetamine molecule. There is also a huge discrepancy in cost between Anascorp and benzodiazepines. So to suggest that if this pharmacological interaction does exist between Anascorp and methamphetamine, we

actually suggest its use would not be economically sensible. Currently there is an ongoing study in mice looking into this interaction with Anascorp and methamphetamine toxicity by one of the coauthors. The underlying point of this case and its findings are to highlight for the emergency medicine physician and pediatrician the ease with which these two clinical scenarios may be confused and some specific findings that are useful in detecting which problem actually exists.

## Conflict of Interests

There is no conflict of interests to disclose.

## References

[1] Rare Disease Therapeutics, Anascorp Centruroides (Scorpion) Immune F(ab')2 (Equine) Injection, http://www.anascorp-us.com/.

[2] D. Ciccarone, "Stimulant abuse: pharmacology, cocaine, methamphetamine, treatment, attempts at pharmacotherapy," *Primary Care: Clinics in Office Practice*, vol. 38, no. 1, pp. 41–58, 2011.

[3] US Department of Justice and Drug Enforcement Agency, "2013 national drug threat assessment summary," 2013, http://www.justice.gov/dea/resource-center/DIR-017-13%20NDTA%20Summary%20final.pdf.

[4] P. Kolecki, "Inadvertent methamphetamine poisoning in pediatric patients," *Pediatric Emergency Care*, vol. 14, no. 6, pp. 385–387, 1998.

[5] A. R. Nagorka and P. S. Bergeson, "Infant methamphetamine toxicity posing as scorpion envenomation," *Pediatric Emergency Care*, vol. 14, no. 5, pp. 350–351, 1998.

[6] A. B. Skolnik and M. B. Ewald, "Pediatric scorpion envenomation in the United States: morbidity, mortality, and therapeutic innovations," *Pediatric Emergency Care*, vol. 29, no. 1, pp. 98–103, 2013.

[7] J. R. Suchard and S. C. Curry, "Methamphetamine toxicity," *Pediatric Emergency Care*, vol. 15, no. 4, p. 306, 1999.

[8] P. Grant, "Evaluation of children removed from a clandestine methamphetamine laboratory," *Journal of Emergency Nursing*, vol. 33, no. 1, pp. 31–41, 2007.

# 20

# Intravenous Lipid Emulsion Therapy for Acute Synthetic Cannabinoid Intoxication: Clinical Experience in Four Cases

**Gökhan Aksel,**[1] **Özlem Güneysel,**[2] **Tanju Taşyürek,**[1] **Ergül Kozan,**[2] **and Şebnem Eren Çevik**[1]

[1]*Umraniye Training and Research Hospital, Emergency Medicine Clinic, Istanbul, Turkey*
[2]*Dr. Lutfi Kirdar Kartal Education and Research Hospital, Emergency Medicine Clinic, Istanbul, Turkey*

Correspondence should be addressed to Gökhan Aksel; aksel@gokhanaksel.com

Academic Editor: Aristomenis K. Exadaktylos

There is no specific antidote for intoxication with synthetic cannabinoids. In this case series, we considered the efficiency of intravenous lipid emulsion therapy in four cases, who presented to emergency department with synthetic cannabinoid (bonzai) intoxication. The first patient had a GCS of 3 and a left bundle branch block on electrocardiography. The electrocardiography revealed sinus rhythm with normal QRS width after the treatment. The second patient had bradycardia, hypotension, and a GCS of 14. After intravenous lipid emulsion therapy, the bradycardia resolved, and the patient's GCS improved to 15. The third patient presented with a GCS of 8, and had hypotension and bradycardia. After the treatment, not only did the bradycardia resolve, but also the GCS improved to 15. The fourth patient, whose electrocardiography revealed accelerated junctional rhythm, had a GCS of 13. The patient's rhythm was sinus after the treatment. Cardiovascular recovery was seen in all four cases, and neurological recovery was also seen in three of them. Based on the fact that intravenous lipid emulsion is beneficial in patients intoxicated with lipophilic drugs, unstable patients presenting to the emergency department with acute synthetic cannabinoid intoxication may be candidates for intravenous lipid emulsion treatment.

## 1. Introduction

Since their introduction in 2004, synthetic cannabinoid (SC) receptor agonists have become increasingly popular as an abused substance, especially among adolescents [1, 2]. Although they are most commonly named as "spice" collectively, "bonzai" is new and the most commonly preferred definition in Turkey [3, 4].

There is no specific antidote for SCs, and the treatment is mainly supportive. Popularity of intravenous lipid emulsion (ILE) therapy as a rescue antidote for the treatment of local anaesthetic toxicities has increased recently [5, 6]. ILE seems to be a new, safe, and promising treatment choice for SC intoxications.

In this case series, we aimed to discuss the efficiency of ILE therapy through the examination of four cases presented to the emergency department (ED) after bonzai (spice) consumption, which is known to be a lipophilic toxin.

## 2. Case 1

A thirty-five-year-old man who was found lying on the floor unconscious with empty "bonzai" bags near him was brought to the ED by his family. His medical history revealed that he had been a bonzai and heroin user for a while. The family refused the possibility of a suicide attempt and stated that the patient may have used heroin in addition to bonzai, but no other drugs. His Glasgow Coma Scale (GCS) was 3, pupils were miotic, and no anisocoria was observed. Arterial blood pressure (ABP) was measured as 110/75 mmHg, pulse rate was 95 beats/minute, body temperature was 36,9°C, and $O_2$ saturation was 65%. His first electrocardiography (ECG) revealed a left bundle branch block (LBBB) (QRS complex width = 150 milliseconds) and sinus rhythm at a rate of 100 beats/minute (Figure 1). In the venous blood gases analyses (VBG) a respiratory acidosis was noted with a pH of 6.9 and $paCO_2$ of 125 mmHg. Liver

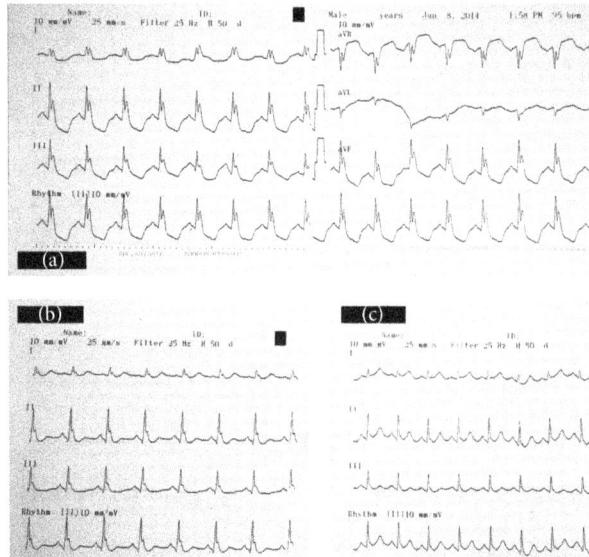

FIGURE 1: (a) Initial (before ILE treatment) electrocardiography of Case 1 with left bundle branch block. (b) Electrocardiography of Case 1 after bolus administration of intravenous lipid emulsion (5th minute of ILE). (c) Electrocardiography of Case 1 after intravenous lipid emulsion infusion (60th minute of ILE).

enzymes were elevated (aspartate transaminase = 806 U/L and alanine aminotransferase = 477 U/L) and so were the renal function tests (creatinine = 2,05 mg/dL, blood urine nitrogen = 53,5 mg/dL). White blood cell count was 25,6 K/uL and the international normalized ratio (INR) was 1,32. Other laboratory tests were normal.

As soon as the patient was intubated, a 1,5 mL/kg bolus of 20% lipid was administered intravenously, followed by an infusion of a 0,25 mL/kg/minute for 60 minutes (total dose of 1155 mL). Just after the bolus administration of ILE (5 minutes), narrowing of QRS complexes was observed. When the ILE infusion finished, the QRS complex was totally normal with width of 90 milliseconds (Figure 1). Despite the change in width of QRS, clinical improvement was not observed. Based on the suspicion of heroin use, naloxone was indicated, but we did not have the drug, nor did other hospitals in the city. After admission to the intensive care unit, the patient's renal function tests, liver enzymes, and coagulation parameters were all continued, increasing progressively. Acute respiratory distress syndrome (ARDS) also developed, and despite adequate fluid resuscitation, he became hypotensive and needed positive inotropic agents to maintain normal arterial pressure. He died two days later due to ARDS and multiorgan failure.

## 3. Case 2

A nineteen-year-old-man presented to the ED with a complaint of confusion after smoking bonzai. On examination, he had ABP of 70/30 mmHg, body temperature of 36,7°C, pulse rate of 42 beats/minute, GCS of 14, and he had no orientation and cooperation. His ECG revealed sinus bradycardia at a

rate of 41 beats/minute (Figure 2). Other physical examination findings and laboratory tests were unremarkable. After infusion of 2000 mL of normal saline, hypotension persisted, and a 1,5 mL/kg bolus of 20% lipid, followed by an infusion of a 0,25 mL/kg/minute for 60 minutes, was administered (total dose of 990 mL). After bolus infusion of ILE (5 minutes) bradycardia started to resolve with a pulse rate of 50–55 beats/minute. When the infusion finished, the bradycardia had completely resolved, ABP was measured 110/70 mmHg, and the patient's GCS improved to 15 two hours after infusion. ILE was the only treatment performed for the symptomatic bradycardia. When he was completely conscious, his medical history was detailed and he confessed to the consumption of bonzai. He was discharged in good health after 24 hours of observation with no complications.

## 4. Case 3

A fifteen-year-old unconscious man presented to the ED via ambulance. His medical history revealed that he became unresponsive after smoking bonzai. Both the patient and his friends denied use of other drugs or ingestion of any other substance. His ABP was 80/40 mmHg, pulse rate was 36 beats/minute, body temperature was 37,1°C, and O$_2$ saturation was 94%. His initial GCS was 8 and pupils were mydriatic. His physical examination findings were totally normal except bradycardia, hypotension, and a low GCS score. His laboratory results were normal. The ECG showed a sinus bradycardia at a rate of 36/minute (Figure 3). We decided to give ILE when no response was observed after 2000 mL of normal saline solution. 1.25 mL/kg bolus of %20 lipid was administered and it was followed with infusion of 0.50 mL/kg/minute for 60 minutes (total dose of 2100 mL). No other drugs were given in addition to ILE. After ILE infusion, not only did the bradycardia resolve in five minutes, but also his GCS improved to 15 in two hours. The patient was observed for 24 hours in the ED and had no complications during this period. He was discharged in good health after the follow-up period.

## 5. Case 4

A seventeen-year-old man with confusion after cannabinoid consumption transferred to our ED from a rural hospital. His ABP was 115/68 mmHg, pulse rate was 80 beats/minute, O$_2$ saturation was 98%, body temperature was 36,7°C, and he was disoriented with a GCS score of 13. Other physical examination findings were normal, and laboratory results were unremarkable. His ECG revealed accelerated junctional rhythm at a rate of 70 bpm concomitant with bigeminy ventricular extrasystoles (VES). We thought bonzai might be responsible from the abnormalities in ECG, and the patient was treated with 1.5 mL/kg bolus of 20% lipid intravenously, followed by an infusion of a 0.25 mL/kg/minute for 60 minutes (total dose of 990 mL). On the fifth minute of ILE infusion, it was observed that the frequency of VES decreased, and after finishing the ILE infusion (at 60th minute of treatment), the patient's rhythm was sinus at a rate

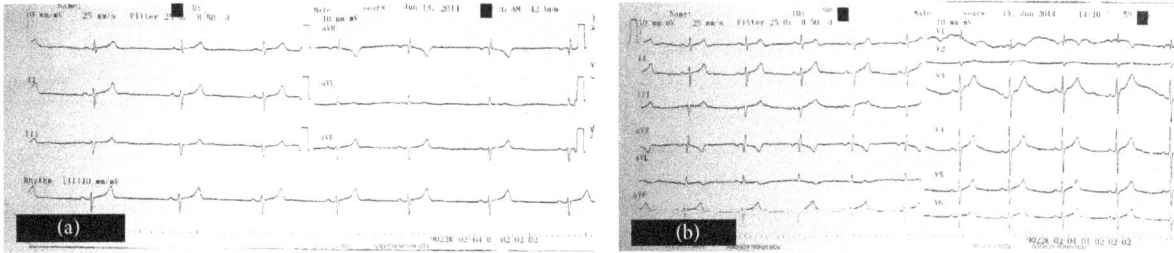

FIGURE 2: (a) Initial electrocardiography of Case 2 with sinus bradycardia. (b) Electrocardiography of Case 2, 45 minutes after initiation of intravenous lipid emulsion infusion.

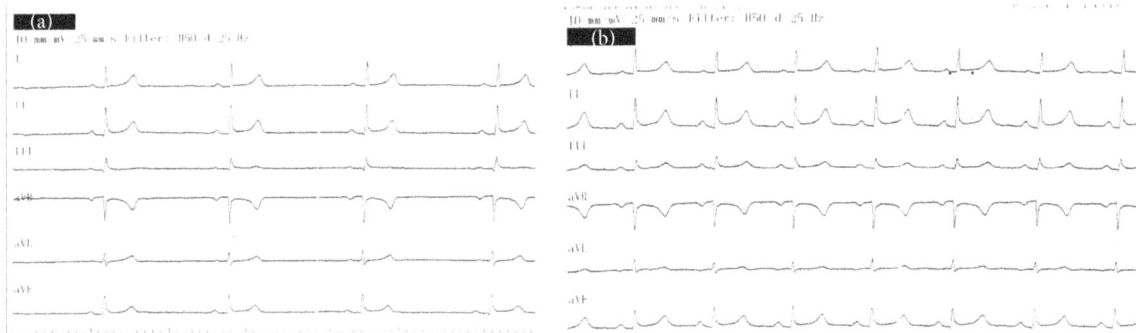

FIGURE 3: (a) Initial (before ILE treatment) electrocardiography of Case 3 with sinus bradycardia. (b) Electrocardiography of Case 3 after bolus infusion (5th minute of ILE) of intravenous lipid emulsion.

of 74 beats/minute with no VES (Figure 4). His GCS also improved to 15 four hours after ILE infusion. He was discharged in good health after 24 hours of observation without any complications.

## 6. Discussion

Synthetic cannabinoid receptor agonists are smokable herbal mixtures, marketed as legal marijuana in some countries [4]. They are commonly marketed as "legal highs." SCs have increased in popularity, owing to their low costs and not being detected on traditional urine drug screens [7]. SC products have several street and commercial names such as spice, aroma, barely legal, Yucatan fire, dream, fusion galaxy, pep spice, gorilla, K2, and K3. Bonzai and Jamaican gold are the most popular names of SCs in Turkey [2–4]. In our four cases, all patients and their relatives named the SC used as bonzai.

Users report that "spice" has a stronger psychotropic effect than marijuana. The potency of being high on JWH-018 is 5 times that of THC, while AM-694 has 500 times more potency [3]. SCs are not detected in routine, traditional drug screens; this makes them popular in adolescents [8]. Yet, newer immunoassays with high sensitivity and specificity for rapid screening of SCs in human urine are developing due to the growing need for detecting new synthetic cannabinoids [9].

Synthetic cannabinoids can cause either decreased anxiety or dysphoric reactions, including anxiety and panic. Arterial hypertension and tachycardia are the most common cardiovascular side effects, but hypotension and bradycardia were also reported. The effects are seen after 0.5–2 hours of consumption, and the duration is prolonged [3, 10]. Two of our cases had bradycardia and hypotension, while ABPs and pulse rates of the other two were in normal range. GCSs of all four patients were under 15.

ILE has been reported to reverse cardiovascular collapse in overdoses of local anaesthetic agents, and it is endorsed as an antidote for systemic toxicity of local anaesthetics by many authors [11, 12]. Advanced Cardiac Life Support guidelines also recommend ILE for cardiac arrest, secondary not only to local anaesthetics, but also to beta blockers when conventional resuscitative therapies have failed. ILE is also thought to be an effective antidote for other lipophilic drug poisonings [13–15].

While ILE's exact mechanism is not known, the first and most widely accepted mechanism is "the lipid sink" theory. This was first presented by Weinberg et al. in 1998. Drugs that are free in the intravascular space are thought to be trapped within the ILE and this reduces the concentration and toxicity of the drug. Distribution of lipid soluble drugs from tissue to a circulating lipid phase also occurs [12, 16, 17]. In vitro studies support the lipid sink theory, while competing hypotheses and some in/ex vivo small animal studies suggest that a positive inotropic or metabolic effect underlies the dramatic effects of lipid therapy [18]. Some newer publications also have identified sink-independent effects and put forward alternative mechanisms such as hemodilution [19]. ILE not only does recover cardiovascular collapse but also reverses neurologic signs and symptoms of lipophilic drug intoxication [15].

We know that all four patients inhaled bonzai, and only in the first case did the patient have an uncertain history of

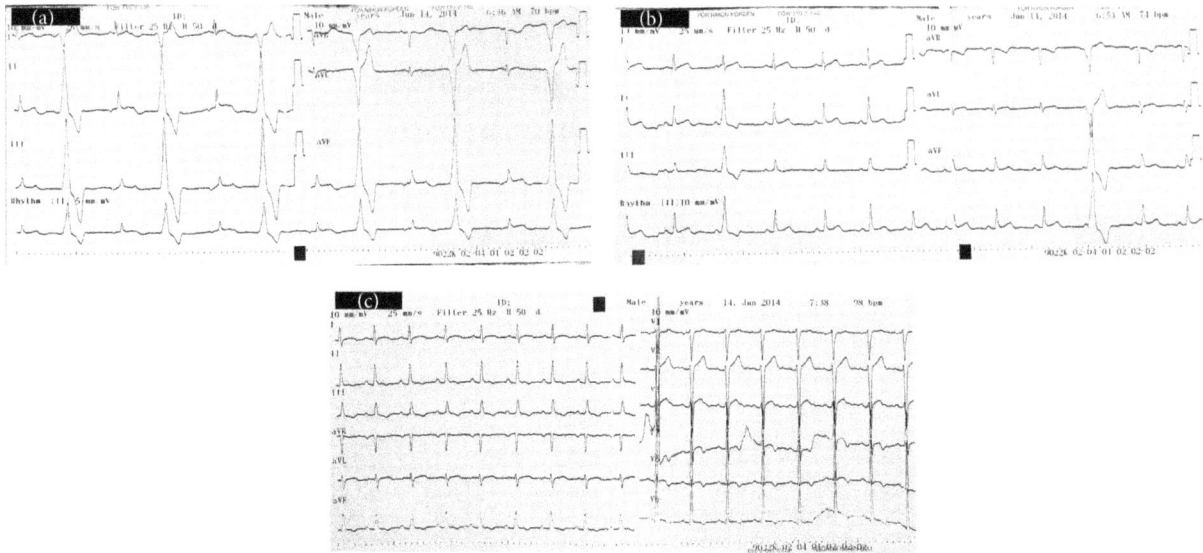

FIGURE 4: (a) Initial (before ILE treatment) electrocardiography of Case 4 with accelerated junctional rhythm concomitant with bigeminy ventricular extrasystoles. (b) Electrocardiography of Case 4 after bolus administration of intravenous lipid emulsion (5th minute of ILE). (c) Electrocardiography of Case 4 after intravenous lipid emulsion infusion (60th minute of ILE).

heroin use in addition to bonzai. Both heroin and cannabinoids are extremely lipid soluble [10, 20]. Based on the fact that ILE is beneficial in intoxicated patients with lipophilic drugs we decided to treat these patients with ILE. In the previous literature, only Cevik et al. reported successful ILE treatment of a bonzai user with hypotension and a low GCS score [21]. Two of our patients with bradycardia, hypotension and low GCS scores, had normal pulse rates, ABPs, and GCSs soon after the ILE treatment. The ECG in Case 4 showed normal sinus rhythm after ILE treatment, while his initial ECG revealed junctional rhythm with bigeminy ventricular extrasystoles. His GCS was also improved from 8 to 15. Both cardiac and neurologic signs and symptoms of the 3 patients resolved after ILE therapy.

Only one of the four patients (Case 1) died despite ILE therapy. This patient had a different history of suspicious use of heroin in addition to bonzai. The major problem with the herbal compounds named as spice or bonzai is the uncertainty of what exactly they include. Gurdal et al. reported that 98.3% of 1200 herbal compounds named as bonzai contained synthetic cannabinoids. In their study, it is also stated that 1.7% of the herbal compounds included other psychoactive substances [4]. Furthermore, there may be many other unknown or little known chemicals in those herbal compounds. A recently published article on an internet news site about a synthetic cannabinoid cooker warns about the many risks users take with questionably made substances. According to the report, agents found rat poison among the ingredients the culprit used to make his own variety of the drugs [22]. We believe, in our first case, the patient might have died due to not only bonzai use, but also use of heroin or other chemicals whose ingredients he had little to no knowledge about. It is also known that ILE treatment has some complications like pancreatitis, acute lung injury, ARDS, and laboratory interference induced by lipemia [6].

ILE might have been responsible for ARDS developing in Case 1, but it is difficult to clinically discern whether ARDS is the result of the lipid or it is the result of critical illness. The patient was critically ill with a GCS score of 3 and deep respiratory acidosis. Even so, we saw the contribution of ILE treatment improved the ECG of the patient. His dramatically narrowed QRS complex demonstrated that administration of ILE might have helped the collapsed cardiovascular system to recover.

## 7. Conclusion

Based on the fact that ILE is beneficial to patients intoxicated with lipophilic drugs, unstable patients presented to the ED with acute SC intoxication may be candidates for ILE treatment.

## Conflict of Interests

The authors declare that there is no conflict of interests regarding the publication of this paper.

## References

[1] C. O. Hoyte, J. Jacob, A. A. Monte, M. Al-Jumaan, A. C. Bronstein, and K. J. Heard, "A characterization of synthetic cannabinoid exposures reported to the National Poison Data System in 2010," Annals of Emergency Medicine, vol. 60, no. 4, pp. 435–438, 2012.

[2] C. R. Harris and A. Brown, "Synthetic cannabinoid intoxication: a case series and review," Journal of Emergency Medicine, vol. 44, no. 2, pp. 360–366, 2013.

[3] N. Hohmann, G. Mikus, and D. Czock, "Effects and risks associated with novel psychoactive substances: mislabeling and

sale as bath salts, spice, and research chemicals," *Deutsches Arzteblatt International*, vol. 111, no. 9, pp. 139–147, 2014.

[4] F. Gurdal, M. Asirdizer, R. G. Aker et al., "Review of detection frequency and type of synthetic cannabinoids in herbal compounds analyzed by Istanbul Narcotic Department of the Council of Forensic Medicine, Turkey," *Journal of Forensic and Legal Medicine*, vol. 20, no. 6, pp. 667–672, 2013.

[5] C. Jamaty, B. Bailey, A. Larocque, E. Notebaert, K. Sanogo, and J.-M. Chauny, "Lipid emulsions in the treatment of acute poisoning: a systematic review of human and animal studies," *Clinical Toxicology*, vol. 48, no. 1, pp. 1–27, 2010.

[6] M. Levine, A. B. Skolnik, A.-M. Ruha, A. Bosak, N. Menke, and A. F. Pizon, "Complications following antidotal use of intravenous lipid emulsion therapy," *Journal of Medical Toxicology*, vol. 10, no. 1, pp. 10–14, 2014.

[7] E. G. Aoun, P. P. Christopher, and J. W. Ingraham, "Emerging drugs of abuse: clinical and legal considerations," *Rhode Island Medical Journal*, vol. 96, pp. 41–45, 2014.

[8] R. Vandrey, M. W. Johnson, P. S. Johnson, and M. A. Khalil, "Novel drugs of abuse: a snapshot of an evolving marketplace," *Adolescent Psychiatry*, vol. 3, no. 2, pp. 123–134, 2013.

[9] M. Jang, W. Yang, H. Choi et al., "Monitoring of urinary metabolites of JWH-018 and JWH-073 in legal cases," *Forensic Science International*, vol. 231, no. 1–3, pp. 13–19, 2013.

[10] C. H. Ashton, "Pharmacology and effects of cannabis: a brief review," *British Journal of Psychiatry*, vol. 178, pp. 101–106, 2001.

[11] G. Foxall, R. Mccahon, J. Lamb, J. G. Hardman, and N. M. Bedforth, "Levobupivacaine-induced seizures and cardiovascular collapse treated with Intralipid," *Anaesthesia*, vol. 62, no. 5, pp. 516–518, 2007.

[12] G. Cave, M. Harvey, and A. Graudins, "Intravenous lipid emulsion as antidote: a summary of published human experience," *Emergency Medicine Australasia*, vol. 23, no. 2, pp. 123–141, 2011.

[13] T. L. Vanden Hoek, L. J. Morrison, M. Shuster et al., "Part 12: cardiac arrest in special situations: 2010 American heart association guidelines for cardiopulmonary resuscitation and emergency cardiovascular care," *Circulation*, vol. 122, no. 18, supplement 3, pp. S829–S861, 2010.

[14] R. Garrett, V. Kaura, and S. Kathawaroo, "Intravenous lipid emulsion therapy—the fat of the land," *Trends in Anaesthesia and Critical Care*, vol. 3, no. 6, pp. 336–341, 2013.

[15] L. Rothschild, S. Bern, S. Oswald, and G. Weinberg, "Intravenous lipid emulsion in clinical toxicology," *Scandinavian Journal of Trauma, Resuscitation and Emergency Medicine*, vol. 18, no. 1, article 51, 2010.

[16] G. L. Weinberg, T. VadeBoncouer, G. A. Ramaraju, M. F. Garcia-Amaro, and M. J. Cwik, "Pretreatment or resuscitation with a lipid infusion shifts the dose-response to bupivacaine-induced asystole in rats," *Anesthesiology*, vol. 88, no. 4, pp. 1071–1075, 1998.

[17] P. T. Engels and J. S. Davidow, "Intravenous fat emulsion to reverse haemodynamic instability from intentional amitriptyline overdose," *Resuscitation*, vol. 81, no. 8, pp. 1037–1039, 2010.

[18] I. Kuo and B. S. Akpa, "Validity of the lipid sink as a mechanism for the reversal of local anesthetic systemic toxicity: a physiologically based pharmacokinetic model study," *Anesthesiology*, vol. 118, no. 6, pp. 1350–1361, 2013.

[19] M. R. Fettiplace, B. S. Akpa, R. Ripper et al., "Resuscitation with lipid emulsion: dose-dependent recovery from cardiac pharmacotoxicity requires a cardiotonic effect," *Anesthesiology*, vol. 120, no. 4, pp. 915–925, 2014.

[20] R. Majdzadeh, A. Feiz-Zadeh, Z. Rajabpour et al., "Opium consumption and the risk of traffic injuries in regular users: a case-crossover study in an emergency department," *Traffic Injury Prevention*, vol. 10, no. 4, pp. 325–329, 2009.

[21] S. E. Cevik, T. Tasyurek, and O. Guneysel, "Intralipid emulsion treatment as an antidote in lipophilic drug intoxications: a case series," *The American Journal of Emergency Medicine*, vol. 32, no. 9, pp. 1103–1108, 2014.

[22] 2014, http://www.al.com/news/tuscaloosa/index.ssf/2014/06/police_synthetic_marijuana_tra.html.

# 21

# Late Onset Traumatic Diaphragmatic Herniation Leading to Intestinal Obstruction and Pancreatitis: Two Separate Cases

**Tolga Dinc, Selami Ilgaz Kayilioglu, and Faruk Coskun**

*Department of General Surgery, Ankara Numune Training and Research Hospital, Anafartalar Mah, Talatpasa Boulevard No. 5, Genel Cerrahi AD, 2. Kat B216, Altındağ, 06100 Ankara, Turkey*

Correspondence should be addressed to Tolga Dinc; tolga_dr@hotmail.com

Academic Editor: Vasileios Papadopoulos

Although diaphragmatic injuries caused by blunt or penetrating trauma are rare entities, they are the most commonly misdiagnosed injuries in trauma patients and occur in approximately 3–7% of all abdominal or thoracic traumas. Acute pancreatitis secondary to late presenting diaphragmatic hernia is very rare. Here we present two separate cases: one with acute bowel obstruction and the other with acute pancreatitis secondary to late onset traumatic diaphragmatic hernia (three and twenty-eight years after chest trauma, resp.).

## 1. Introduction

Although diaphragmatic injuries caused by blunt or penetrating trauma are rare entities, they are the most commonly misdiagnosed injuries in trauma patients and occur in approximately 3–7% of all abdominal or thoracic traumas [1]. When these injuries are not diagnosed immediately, they present months or years after the initial trauma in about 9.5% to 61% of all cases [2]. These late presentations can result in pulmonary complications, chronic abdominal pain, or acute bowel obstruction, which might cause morbidity and mortality [3]. However, acute pancreatitis secondary to traumatic diaphragmatic hernia (TDH) is quite rare.

Here we present two separate cases: one with acute bowel obstruction and the other with acute pancreatitis secondary to late onset TDH (three and twenty-eight years after chest trauma, resp.).

## 2. Case Presentation

*Case 1.* A 33-year-old male patient presented with symptoms of abdominal pain, vomiting, and obstipation to our emergency surgery department.

His vital signs at admission were normal besides the pulse rate of 110/min. His physical examination revealed decreased breathing sounds and a healed scar on the left hemithorax. Patient had a history of penetrating thoracic trauma through the intersection of left anterior axillary line and costal arch, three years ago. The patient rejected any surgical intervention at that time and left the emergency clinic. In his current presentation initial evaluation was quite helpful in identification of the source of ileus. Laboratory levels were within normal ranges besides elevated white cell count of 18.3 ($\times 10^3/\mu L$). Abdominal plain X-ray showed elevation of left diaphragm and infiltration in the left lung. This leaded to a computed tomography (CT) of chest which demonstrated herniation of small bowel, transverse, and descending colonic segments into left hemithorax through a 4 cm defect on diaphragm.

Patient underwent an urgent laparotomy which revealed a posterolateral diaphragmatic defect of 6 cm in diameter with herniation of loops of small and large intestines into the left thoracic cavity. Intestines were not ischemic; thus no resection was performed. After reduction of the intestines to the abdomen, the diaphragmatic defect was successfully repaired primarily with a single layer of nonabsorbable sutures. Patient's postoperative recovery was uneventful. Drainage tubes of abdomen and thorax were removed on the postoperative day 4. Patient was discharged on the postoperative day 6 after the surgery.

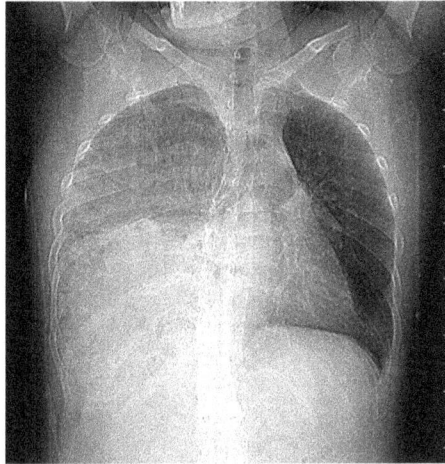

FIGURE 1: Chest X-ray. Right lung was pushed upwards and right hemithorax was filled with intestines.

*Case 2.* A forty-two-year-old male patient presented to our emergency surgery department with abdominal pain and respiratory distress. He reported that the pain started two days ago, along with respiratory distress which gradually worsened. The abdominal pain was reflecting to his back. The patient had a history of being run over by an asphalt paving cylinder 28 years earlier which resulted in paraplegia secondary to vertebral injury. His vital signs were within normal limits.

In his biochemical analysis amylase level was 2209 U/L, aspartate aminotransferase level was 135 U/L, alkaline phosphatase was 134 U/L, gamma glutamyl transferase was 1238 U/L, and total bilirubin level was 4.6 mg/dL. No gallbladder stones were detected in ultrasonography. In his chest X-ray right lung was pushed upwards and right hemithorax was filled with intestines (Figure 1). In computerized tomography it was noted that there was a 15 cm defect on the right hemidiaphragm and small bowels, ascending colon, caecum, superior mesenteric artery and its branches, pancreas, and duodenum were inside the right hemithorax (Figure 2). On his 3rd day in hospital, amylase levels started to return to normal and bilirubin levels became normal. After full recovery from acute pancreatitis, patient underwent surgical repair of the diaphragmatic defect. Despite the long history, herniated organs were easily pulled back to the abdomen without any significant adhesions and the defect was sutured. His postoperative course was uneventful and the right lung fully expended after removal of the chest tube (Figure 2).

## 3. Discussion

Diaphragmatic tear can occur after blunt or penetrating injury. Small diaphragmatic hernias might be realized months or even years later, when the patients become symptomatic. Physicians and surgeons should keep diaphragmatic hernia in mind in patients with a previous history of trauma with atypical abdominal and respiratory symptoms [4]. Blunt and penetrating traumas account for 68–75% and 25–32%

of traumatic diaphragmatic injuries, respectively [5]. One of our patients had a right sided TDH 28 years after blunt trauma and the other had a left sided TDH three years after a penetrating injury.

While it is rare, a delayed TDH is an important cause of bowel obstruction. In such cases, diagnosis must be made immediately, so that an operative intervention can be done to prevent tissue necrosis and other complications related with high mortality. 7% to 66% of diaphragmatic injuries in multitrauma patients remain undiagnosed [6]. When appropriate intervention is not undertaken in the acute setting, chronic diaphragmatic hernia and strangulation may occur in some patients, subsequently. This is the exact sequence that occurred in our first case.

Blunt trauma may cause injury in any part of the diaphragm, but the majority of injuries occur in the posterolateral aspect of the left side of the diaphragm [7]. Our second case who had a past history of blunt trauma contradicts with this fact, as the patient had a large right sided defect.

The cases in medical literature about acute pancreatitis after diaphragmatic herniation of the pancreas are mainly related to hiatal hernias or congenital hernias. Nevertheless, even this is an extremely rare presentation with no more than 7 cases described in literature [8–10]. Acute pancreatitis secondary to TDH is even rarer and we could only find one article dating back to 1952 via PubMed search, using "pancreatitis and traumatic diaphragmatic hernia" keywords [11].

There are three theories about the occurrence of acute pancreatitis in diaphragmatic hernia: (1) abnormal traction on the pancreas, total incarceration of the gland in hernia without pancreatic volvulus [12], (2) migration of the pancreas through a hernia sac and repetitive trauma as it crosses the hernia [13], and (3) ischemia associated with stretching of pancreatic vascular pedicle and intermittent folding of the main pancreatic duct [14]. In our Case 2, the pancreas was found in the right hemithorax. This displacement of the pancreas probably caused repetitive trauma and/or intermittent blockage of blood supply and pancreatic duct flow. In this case no gallbladder stones were detected. So TDH remains as the prime suspect for acute pancreatitis.

Operative intervention is the main management for delayed traumatic diaphragmatic hernias, especially if there is an acute complication like strangulation as in our first case. Although the thoracic approach has been recommended for chronic diaphragmatic hernias due to dense intrathoracic adhesions [15], abdominal or a combined chest-abdominal approach may be necessary in cases of strangulation. Laparoscopic surgery is another option in treatment of TDH; however, it can be challenging in cases with too many intra-abdominal adhesions or complicated hernias [16]. In both of our patients abdominal organs were displaced into thorax so our approach was solely abdominal. We did not encounter any thoracic complications, and reduction of hernias was relatively easy, due to absence of intrathoracic adhesions despite chronic presentation.

These two cases point out that the diagnosis of TDH can be overlooked at the initial trauma evaluation, thus stressing out the need to actively examine the diaphragm on all trauma laparotomies. The clinicians need to be vigilant,

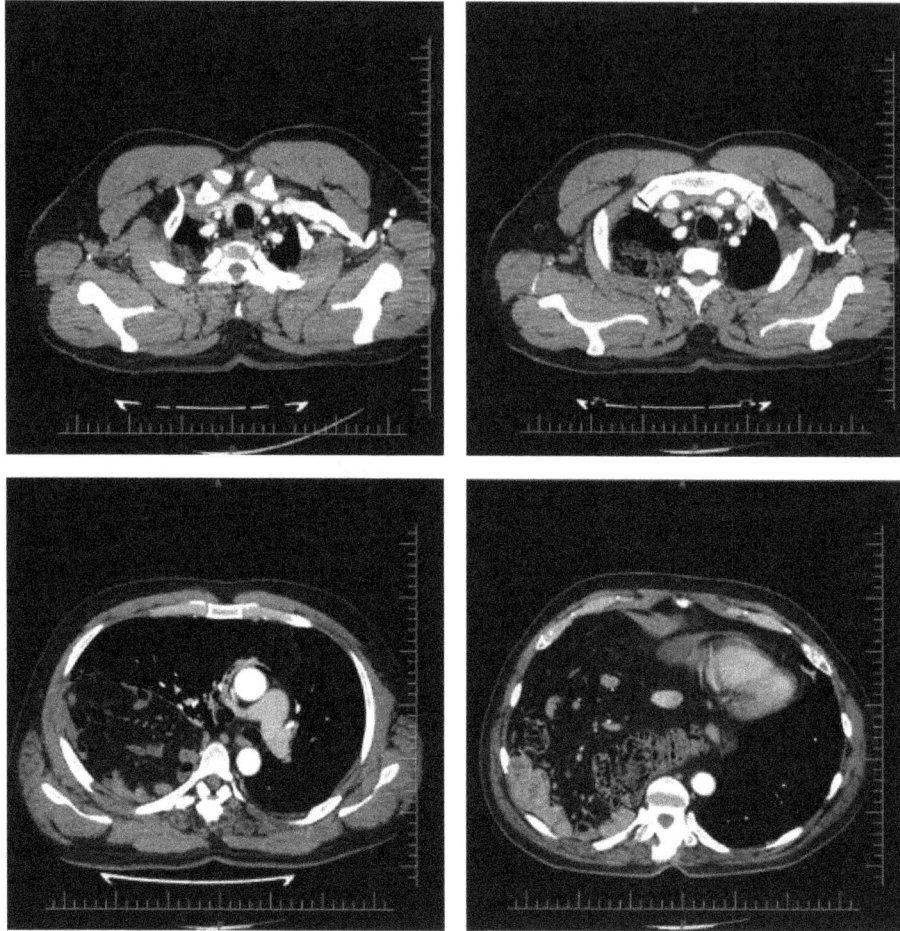

FIGURE 2: Computerized tomography scan. A defect on the right hemidiaphragm and small bowels, ascending colon, cecum, superior mesenteric artery and branches, pancreas, and duodenum were inside right hemithorax.

to maintain a high index of suspicion for the diaphragmatic injuries, whether they are immediately after the trauma or even decades after the trauma. Our case seems to be the second case in medical literature depicting acute pancreatitis after TDH.

## Conflict of Interests

The authors declare that there is no conflict of interests regarding the publication of this paper.

## References

[1] A. Reina, E. Vidaa, P. Soriano et al., "Traumatic intrapericardial diaphragmatic hernia: case report and literature review," *Injury*, vol. 32, no. 2, pp. 153–156, 2001.

[2] C. Christophi, "Diagnosis of traumatic diaphragmatic hernia: analysis of 63 cases," *World Journal of Surgery*, vol. 7, no. 2, pp. 277–280, 1983.

[3] O. Alimoglu, R. Eryilmaz, M. Sahin, and M. S. Ozsoy, "Delayed traumatic diaphragmatic hernias presenting with strangulation," *Hernia*, vol. 8, no. 4, pp. 393–396, 2004.

[4] A. Rekha and A. Vikrama, "Traumatic diaphragmatic hernia," *Sri Ramachandra Journal of Medicine*, vol. 3, no. 2, pp. 23–25, 2010.

[5] R. Shah, S. Sabanathan, A. J. Mearns, and A. K. Choudhury, "Traumatic rupture of diaphragm," *The Annals of Thoracic Surgery*, vol. 60, no. 5, pp. 1444–1449, 1995.

[6] V. Schumpelick, G. Steinau, I. Schlüper, and A. Prescher, "Surgical embryology and anatomy of the diaphragm with surgical applications," *Surgical Clinics of North America*, vol. 80, no. 1, pp. 213–239, 2000.

[7] J. M. Thillois, B. Tremblay, E. Cerceau et al., "Traumatic rupture of the right diaphragm," *Hernia*, vol. 2, no. 3, pp. 119–121, 1998.

[8] P. Chevallier, E. Peten, C. Pellegrino, J. Souci, J. P. Motamedi, and B. Padovani, "Hiatal hernia with pancreatic volvulus: a rare cause of acute pancreatitis," *American Journal of Roentgenology*, vol. 177, no. 2, pp. 373–374, 2001.

[9] P. Saxena, I. E. Konstantinov, M. D. Koniuszko, S. Ghosh, V. H. S. Low, and M. A. J. Newman, "Hiatal herniation of the pancreas: diagnosis and surgical management," *Journal of Thoracic and Cardiovascular Surgery*, vol. 131, no. 5, pp. 1204–1205, 2006.

[10] A. Coral, S. N. Jones, and W. R. Lees, "Dorsal pancreas presenting as a mass in the chest," *The American Journal of Roentgenology*, vol. 149, no. 4, pp. 718–720, 1987.

[11] F. B. Tabaka, S. J. Nigro, and E. Nora, "Traumatic diaphragmatic hernia complicated by acute traumatic pancreatitis," *The Illinois Medical Journal*, vol. 101, no. 5, pp. 269–270, 1952.

[12] N. J. Kafka, I. M. Leitman, and J. Tromba, "Acute pancreatitis secondary to incarcerated paraesophageal hernia," *Surgery*, vol. 115, no. 5, pp. 653–655, 1994.

[13] A. Henkinbrant, O. Decoster, E. Farchakh, and W. Khalek, "Acute pancreatitis caused by a giant umbilical hernia. A case report," *Acta Gastro-Enterologica Belgica*, vol. 52, no. 5-6, pp. 441–447, 1989.

[14] M. J. Oliver, A. R. M. Wilson, and L. Kapila, "Acute pancreatitis and gastric volvulus occurring in a congenital diaphragmatic hernia," *Journal of Pediatric Surgery*, vol. 25, no. 12, pp. 1240–1241, 1990.

[15] O. P. Sharma, "Traumatic diaphragmatic rupture: not an uncommon entity—personal experience with collective review of the 1980's," *Journal of Trauma*, vol. 29, no. 5, pp. 678–682, 1989.

[16] B. D. Matthews, H. Bui, K. L. Harold et al., "Laparoscopic repair of traumatic diaphragmatic injuries," *Surgical Endoscopy and Other Interventional Techniques*, vol. 17, no. 2, pp. 254–258, 2003.

# 22

# STEMI Associated with Overuse of Energy Drinks

**Daniel Solomin, Stephen W. Borron, and Susan H. Watts**

*Department of Emergency Medicine, Paul Foster School of Medicine, Texas Tech University Health Sciences Center at El Paso, El Paso, TX 79905, USA*

Correspondence should be addressed to Daniel Solomin; daniel.solomin@gmail.com

Academic Editor: Kazuhito Imanaka

Coronary artery disease (CAD) and ST-elevation myocardial infarction (STEMI) are predominantly diseases of middle-aged and older adults and when found in younger adults are usually associated with a strong family history. However, this report details the case of a nonobese 26-year-old Hispanic male who presented with an acute STEMI despite having no family history or other apparent risk factors for CAD or STEMI beyond a two pack-year smoking history and excessive energy drink consumption. The patient reported consuming between eight and ten 473 mL cans per day. Cardiac catheterization subsequently confirmed total occlusion of his left circumflex coronary artery.

## 1. Background

Energy drink consumption is a growing health concern due to limited regulation and increasing use, especially in younger demographics [1]. With substantially higher caffeine content than soft drinks or coffee beverages, in some cases, as well as other poorly studied substances, there is significant potential for harm, especially when consumed in large quantities. A review of energy drink toxicity cases in the National Poison Data System revealed moderate to major adverse effects in 15.2% of cases reported to regional poison centers, including seizures and dysrhythmias [2]. There have been two previous reports in the literature of STEMI associated with energy drink use by young people. Each patient was subsequently found to have normal coronary arteries. This report describes a novel case of a STEMI and established coronary artery disease in a young patient with no clear risk factors beyond a brief smoking history and excessive energy drink usage.

## 2. Case Presentation

The patient was a 26-year-old male who began having left-sided chest pain approximately 9 hours prior to presentation to the emergency department following drinking his usual quantity (~4L) of "Monster," "Rock Star," and other similar brands of energy drinks. The patient stated that he drank any kind of energy drink he could get access to: approximately eight to ten 473 mL drinks per day. The chest pain radiated to his left arm and his jaw but did not worsen with exertion. He also complained of numbness to his left arm, diaphoresis, nausea, and vomiting. His vital signs included a heart rate of 69, blood pressure of 132/73 mm/Hg, respiratory rate of 12, and oxygen saturation of 95% on room air. The patient was in significant distress and was diaphoretic, though not actively vomiting. The patient's heart showed regular rate and rhythm, lungs were clear to auscultation with no crackles, wheezes, or rhonchi, and the abdomen was soft and nontender without guarding or rigidity. His EKG showed significant ST-elevation in the inferior leads with reciprocal changes in the anterior leads (Figure 1). His initial troponin was 0.02 $\mu$g/L (range 0–0.08 $\mu$g/L) and CK-MB was 160.1 $\mu$mol/L (range 0–266.9 $\mu$mol/L); both tests were performed on a point-of-care testing device. The patient was taken to the cardiac catheterization lab before serial blood tests or further formal lab tests could be performed. The patient's serum caffeine concentration was not obtained, and the energy drink usage did not become known until after the patient had returned from the catheterization. The patient denied any illicit drug or stimulant use, and his urine toxicology screen was negative for any illicit drugs or stimulants, including common benzodiazepines, opiates, $\delta$-9-tetrahydrocannabinol, amphetamines, and cocaine. The

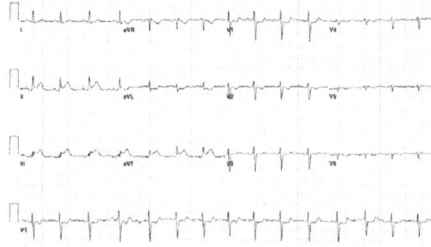

FIGURE 1: Initial electrocardiogram, showing evidence of acute inferior myocardial infarction.

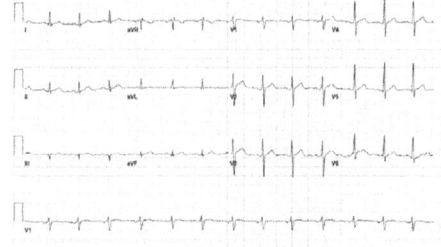

FIGURE 2: Electrocardiogram following cardiac catheterization and balloon angioplasty, showing resolution of inferior ST-elevation.

patient did however admit to smoking for the last two years, with approximately one pack (20 cigarettes) per day. The results of the patient's lipid profile were as follows: total cholesterol 5.65 $\mu$mol/L (range 1.30–5.18 $\mu$mol/L), HDL 0.96 (range 1.04–1.53 $\mu$mol/L), LDL 2.69 $\mu$mol/L (range <2.59 $\mu$mol/L), and triglycerides 4.36 $\mu$mol/L (range 0.40–1.70 $\mu$mol/L). The patient had no history of diabetes, and each blood sugar check during his hospitalization was less than 6.11 $\mu$mol/L (range 3.86–5.55 $\mu$mol/L), but HbA1C was not checked. The patient's complete blood count and complete metabolic panel were within normal limits.

The patient underwent cardiac catheterization where a 100% occlusion of the left circumflex artery was observed, so a drug-eluting stent was placed after balloon angioplasty. The catheterization report is silent on the presence of any underlying coronary artery plaque in this region. The patient had "mild irregularities" in his left anterior descending coronary artery, in addition to the left circumflex artery occlusion, but no other coronary artery disease in his other coronary vessels was noted. His ST-elevation completely resolved after the catheterization (Figure 2). He remained in the hospital for two days after stent placement and experienced no further chest pain. He was discharged with prescriptions for an antiplatelet agent, an ACE inhibitor, a beta blocker, and a statin, and he agreed to stop smoking and consuming energy drinks.

## 3. Discussion

Energy drinks in various forms have existed for more than a century, including cocaine-containing Coca Cola which was introduced at the turn of the 20th century. However, energy drinks in their current incarnation are a fairly new phenomenon, with the sale of "Red Bull" beginning in 1997. There are multiple ingredients among the common brands of energy drinks, with the most frequent being caffeine, taurine, glucuronolactone, and ginseng. A typical energy drink has approximately 0.34 mg of caffeine per mL, meaning our patient consumed between 1.2 and 1.6 g of caffeine per day, with a lethal dose of caffeine being between approximately 10 g of oral caffeine based on animal studies [3]. However, smaller doses of caffeine may be fatal. Jantos and colleagues reported a fatal case in a 25-year-old woman who had ingested energy drinks containing 8.3 g of caffeine in association with ethanol [4]. There has been increasing concern

about the safety profile of these beverages because there have been multiple case reports describing adverse effects from energy drink consumption, ranging from nausea/vomiting to palpitations and dysrhythmias. Consequently, legislation has been passed in several countries restricting the sale of energy drinks to minors, restricting the combination of these beverages with ethanol, and limiting the concentration of caffeine in these drinks. There appears to have been a decrease in suicides by caffeine following such legislation in Sweden [5].

A thorough literature review uncovered scant literature about lethal cardiac effects associated with energy drink consumption. One case of a lethal cardiac event was reported after ingestion of ecstasy (MDMA) in combination with energy drinks [6]. Two additional cases of STEMI after consumption of a large number of energy drinks have been reported in the literature. In one case, a 28-year-old male suffered cardiac arrest and ventricular fibrillation after consumption of ~7-8 cans of a "caffeinated energy drink." Though no mention is made of the specific brand, the drink was said to contain both taurine and caffeine, similar to the drinks our patient regularly ingested [7]. There is a separate published case of a 19-year-old with chest pain after drinking 2-3 cans of Red Bull per day for the week prior to his presentation. Like our patient, he also had ST-elevation on his EKG [8]. However, in these published cases, both patients had normal coronary arteries on catheterization, unlike our patient. The authors of these cases postulated that the transient STEMI was possibly due to vasospasm caused by caffeine.

Caffeine acts primarily by competitively inhibiting adenosine receptors, but it also leads to increased catecholamine release. Though caffeine alone does not appear to have a significant effect on atherosclerosis [9], energy drinks contain multiple compounds in addition to caffeine, and there have been no definitive studies of these compounds to date, either alone or in the combinations found in energy drinks. However, one placebo-controlled physiological study has examined endothelial function and platelet aggregation among healthy medical students (20–24-year-old males) who consumed a single can (250 mL) of "a sugar-free energy drink." This study reported an increase in platelet aggregation of ~14% (measured by optical aggregometry) compared to the controls, as well as a small decrease of the endothelial function [10].

We hypothesize that the significant quantity of energy drinks consumed by our patient, in the absence of any known genetic risk factors, contributed to the formation of the acute thrombus occluding the patient's coronary blood vessel. We hypothesize that vasospasm caused by excessive levels of caffeine, along with possible effects from other substances in energy drinks, reduced flow in the coronary vessel to such a degree that a thrombus was able to form. A reasonable alternative hypothesis is that of smoking related coronary artery vasospasm.

Further research into the topic of energy drink toxicity in general, as well as cardiac specific issues, is needed, and although evidence to date is scarce, it is probably prudent to recommend limited consumption of these drinks.

## Conflict of Interests

None of the authors have any conflict of interests to declare.

## Authors' Contribution

Daniel Solomin wrote the paper with editing and mentorship from Susan Watts and Stephen W. Borron.

## References

[1] F. Ali, H. Rehman, Z. Babayan, D. Stapleton, and D. D. Joshi, "Energy drinks and their adverse health effects: a systematic review of the current evidence," *Postgraduate Medicine*. In press.

[2] S. M. Seifert, S. A. Seifert, J. L. Schaechter et al., "An analysis of energy-drink toxicity in the National Poison Data System," *Clinical Toxicology*, vol. 51, no. 7, pp. 566–574, 2013.

[3] Caffeine-Toxicology Data Network, http://toxnet.nlm.nih.gov/cgi-bin/sis/search/a?dbs+hsdb:@term+@DOCNO+36.

[4] R. Jantos, K. M. Stein, C. Flechtenmacher, and G. Skopp, "A fatal case involving a caffeine-containing fat burner," *Drug Testing and Analysis*, vol. 5, no. 9-10, pp. 773–776, 2013.

[5] G. Thelander, A. K. Jönsson, M. Personne, G. S. Forsberg, K. M. Lundqvist, and J. Ahlner, "Caffeine fatalities—do sales restrictions prevent intentional intoxications," *Clinical Toxicology*, vol. 48, no. 4, pp. 354–358, 2010.

[6] S. Israelit, A. Strizevsky, and B. Raviv, "ST elevation myocardial infarction in a young patient after ingestion of caffeinated energy drink and ecstasy," *World Journal of Emergency Medicine*, vol. 3, no. 4, pp. 305–307, 2012.

[7] A. J. Berger and K. Alford, "Cardiac arrest in a young man following excess consumption of caffeinated 'energy drinks,'" *Medical Journal of Australia*, vol. 190, no. 1, pp. 41–43, 2009.

[8] M. J. Scott, M. El-Hassan, and A. A. Khan, "Myocardial infarction in a young adult following the consumption of a caffeinated energy drink," *BMJ Case Reports*, vol. 2011, Article ID bcr0220113854, 2011.

[9] J. P. Reis, C. M. Loria, L. M. Steffen et al., "Coffee, decaffeinated coffee, caffeine, and tea consumption in young adulthood and atherosclerosis later in life: the CARDIA study," *Arteriosclerosis, Thrombosis, and Vascular Biology*, vol. 30, no. 10, pp. 2059–2066, 2010.

[10] M. I. Worthley, A. Prabhu, P. de Sciscio, C. Schultz, P. Sanders, and S. R. Willoughby, "Detrimental effects of energy drink consumption on platelet and endothelial function," *The American Journal of Medicine*, vol. 123, no. 2, pp. 184–187, 2010.

# 23

# A Rare and Serious Syndrome That Requires Attention in Emergency Service: Traumatic Asphyxia

**Gultekin Gulbahar,**[1] **Tevfik Kaplan,**[2] **Ahmet Gokhan Gundogdu,**[1] **Hatice Nurdan Baran,**[3] **Burak Kazanci,**[4] **Bulent Kocer,**[5] **and Serdar Han**[2]

[1]*Division of Thoracic Surgery, Dr. Nafiz Korez Sincan State Hospital, Ankara, Turkey*
[2]*Department of Thoracic Surgery, Ufuk University School of Medicine, Ankara, Turkey*
[3]*Division of Anesthesiology and Reanimation, Dr. Nafiz Korez Sincan State Hospital, Ankara, Turkey*
[4]*Department of Neurosurgery, Ufuk University School of Medicine, Ankara, Turkey*
[5]*Division of Thoracic Surgery, Ankara Numune Teaching and Research Hospital, Ankara, Turkey*

Correspondence should be addressed to Tevfik Kaplan; tevfikkaplan@yahoo.com

Academic Editor: Ching H. Loh

Traumatic asphyxia is a rare syndrome caused by blunt thoracoabdominal trauma and characterized by cyanosis, edema, and subconjunctival and petechial hemorrhage on the face, neck, upper extremities, and the upper parts of the thorax. Traumatic asphyxia is usually diagnosed by history and inspection; however, the patient should be monitored more closely due to probable complications of thoracoabdominal injuries. Treatment is conservative, but the prognosis depends on the severity of the associated injuries. Herein we present a traumatic asphyxia due to an elevator accident in a 32-year-old male patient and discuss the diagnosis, treatment, and prognosis by reviewing the relevant literature.

## 1. Introduction

Traumatic asphyxia is a rare syndrome resulting from sudden, severe blunt trauma of the thorax and upper abdomen [1, 2]. It is characterized by cervicofacial cyanosis, edema, subconjunctival hemorrhage, and petechial eruptions on the face, neck, upper parts of the thoracic cage, and the upper extremities [3]. Commonly, thoracic injuries like pulmonary contusion, hemothorax, and pneumothorax accompany the situation [1, 2].

## 2. Case

A 32-year-old male patient was admitted to the emergency service after an industrial accident, in which an elevator cabin fell on him. The patient was conscious and had stable hemodynamic state on his initial examination. He had dyspnea, back pain, facial cyanosis, subconjunctival hemorrhage, and petechial eruptions on the anterior surface of the thoracic cage and on the left upper extremity (Figures 1(a) and 1(b)). Laboratory workup was consistent with the trauma. Bilateral pulmonary contusions, minimal pneumothorax, and fracture of the transverse processes of the first lumbar vertebrae were detected on computed axial tomography of the chest and lumbar vertebrae (Figures 2(a) and 2(b)). Chest X-ray examination of the patient revealed bilateral heterogeneous density increases (Figure 3).

The patient was hospitalized in the intensive care unit for follow-up. He was monitored in a continuous fashion. The head of the bed was elevated to 30 degrees to help overcome the increased intracranial pressure. Uninterrupted oxygen therapy was administered. Hemodynamic state of the patient, arterial blood gas analysis, oxygen saturation levels, and hematologic and biochemical parameters were checked at certain intervals. He was taken to the ward since no complication was observed on the first day of the trauma. The symptoms regressed and no complication was observed; thus he was discharged on the fifth day of hospitalization.

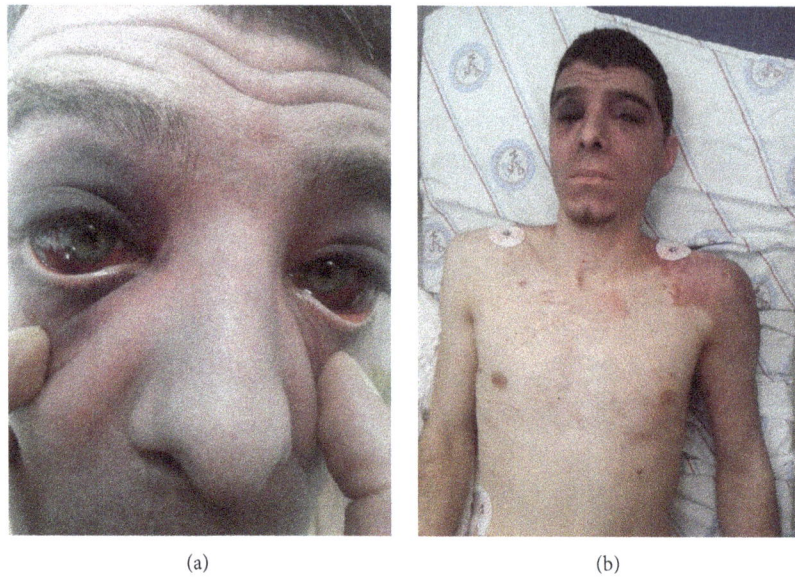

FIGURE 1: (a) The patient had bilateral subconjunctival hemorrhage. (b) The patient had facial cyanosis, petechial eruptions on the anterior surface of the thoracic cage and on left upper extremity.

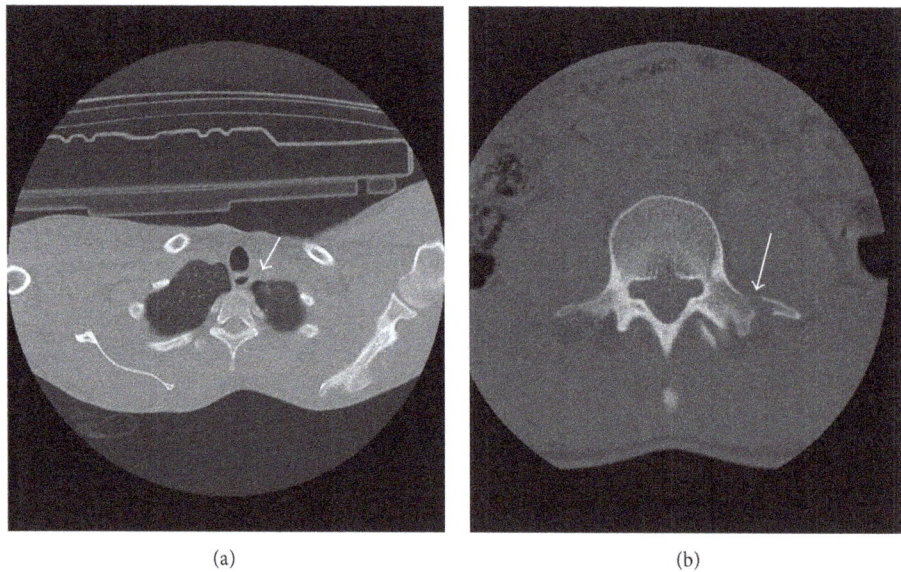

FIGURE 2: (a) Minimal pneumothorax was detected on computed axial tomography of the chest. (b) Fracture of the transverse processes of the first lumbar vertebrae was detected on computed axial tomography of the lumbar vertebrae.

## 3. Discussion

Traumatic asphyxia is quite rare [3]. In 1937, when Oliver d'Angers first defined traumatic asphyxia, he used the term "ecchymotic mask" [4]. Traumatic cyanosis, compressive cyanosis, traumatic apnea, Oliver's syndrome, and Perth's syndrome have also been used to describe the situation [5, 6]. Usually, it follows a sudden and severe thoracoabdominal trauma, but it may also be seen in asthmatic attacks, epileptic seizure episodes, excessive vomiting, and cough cases [6, 7].

Sudden increase in the intrathoracic pressure is thought to be transmitted to the venous and capillary systems in head and neck, and these yields in stasis and rupture giving rise to the characteristic findings [3, 8]. Other possible mechanism is the lack of the valve system in superior vena cava, innominate vein, and jugular veins. Deeply situated structures drain into the internal jugular veins whereas the superficial ones drain into the external jugular system. Since the valves of the external jugular system cannot prevent the backflow, the symptoms are more common in the superficial structures like

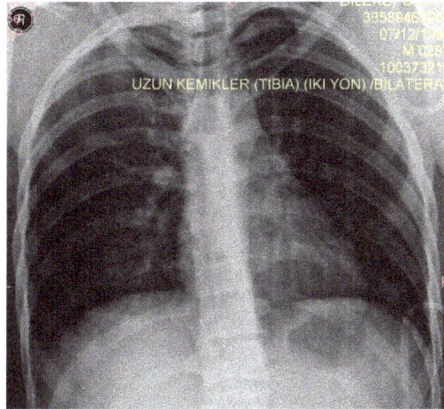

FIGURE 3: Chest X-ray of the patient.

the scalp compared to the deeper structures like brain and the respiratory tract [9]. The compressed IVC protects the lower part of the body from injury during the course of the trauma.

The extent of the signs and symptoms depend on the duration and severity of the compression that thorax and upper abdomen are exposed to [10]. Many signs may accompany the characteristic findings. Confusion, amnesia, disorientation, uneasiness, agitation, hypoxia, cerebral edema, and hemorrhage are the most common ones [6]. Other than subconjunctival hemorrhage, decreased vision, blurred vision, papillary changes, optic nerve atrophy, diplopia, and exophthalmia are the most frequent ocular findings. Epistaxes due to capillary rupture, hearing loss due to the edema of the Eustachian tubes, or hemotympanum are the other probable findings [6, 8, 9]. Severe life-threatening conditions may coexist since the traumatic asphyxia develops as a result of major trauma to thorax, mediastinum, and upper abdomen. These are thoracic and extrathoracic injuries as pulmonary contusion, hemothorax, pneumothorax, flail chest, and hepatic laceration [1, 2, 9]. Signs of pulmonary injury like dyspnea, tachypnea, and hemoptysis may be observed. In rare cases, cardiac injury may be encountered [9]. An increase in the abdominal pressure may lead to organ injury, hematemesis, and hematuria. Apnea and hypoxemia associated with prolonged thoracic compression may be life threatening and give rise to increased mortality. The results may be such severe as shock, cerebral anoxia, neurological sequelae, and sudden death [7, 9].

Although traumatic asphyxia can be diagnosed easily through short anamnesis and physical examination, other reasons like superior vena cava syndrome and skull base fractures leading to subconjunctival hemorrhage and periorbital ecchymosis must be evaluated [7]. Careful and thorough examination is necessary to detect the thoracic and extrathoracic injuries that need urgent intervention. No severe injury other than bilateral pulmonary contusion and minor pneumothorax was found in our case.

Traumatic asphyxia cases must be monitored after securing the airway and fixing the cervical spine. Oxygen inhalation therapy and intravenous fluid replacement need to be initiated and the patient shall be intubated and followed on mechanical ventilation as needed [9]. The intubation may be difficult because of the airway edema, which is seen rarely [11]. Uncomplicated cases are treated conservatively. The head of the bed is preferred to be elevated at 30 degrees and oxygen administration is essential. This procedure decreases the intracranial pressure. Continuous monitorization of the patient, arterial blood gas, oxygen saturation level examinations at certain intervals, and supportive oxygen therapy are the key factors for the management throughout the hospitalization period [6, 10].

Traumatic asphyxia has almost perfect prognosis. It heals spontaneously within weeks except the neurological and ocular signs. In cases without accompanying injuries death may occur due to prolonged compression, apnea, and hypoxia [6, 10].

## 4. Conclusion

Traumatic asphyxia is a rare entity. Prognosis usually depends on the duration of the compression and the severity of the accompanying injuries. Quick and careful evaluation of the probable life-threatening conditions in the emergency service is crucial; however oxygen inhalation therapy, efficient ventilation, intravenous hydration, and measures to prevent the increase of intracranial pressure should be initiated as soon as possible.

## Consent

Written consent form was taken from the patient for using his photographs in this scientific paper.

## Conflict of Interests

The authors declare that there is no conflict of interests regarding the publication of this paper.

## References

[1] Y. A. Karamustafaoglu, I. Yavasman, S. Tiryaki, and Y. Yoruk, "Traumatic asphyxia," *International Journal of Emergency Medicine*, vol. 3, no. 4, pp. 379–380, 2010.

[2] S. Kamali, S. Kesici, I. Gunduz, and U. Kesici, "A case of traumatic asphyxia due to motorcycle accident," *Case Reports in Emergency Medicine*, vol. 2013, Article ID 857131, 3 pages, 2013.

[3] C. Eken and Ö. Yiğit, "Traumatic asphyxia: a rare syndrome in trauma patients," *International Journal of Emergency Medicine*, vol. 2, no. 4, pp. 255–256, 2009.

[4] J. Dweek, "Ecchimotic mask," *The Journal of the International College of Surgeons*, vol. 9, pp. 257–265, 1946.

[5] N. Şenoglu, H. Oksuz, B. Zıncırcı, M. Ezberci, and A. Yasım, "Severe traumatic asphyxia: two case report and literature review," *Turkish Journal of Thoracic and Cardiovascular Surgery*, vol. 14, pp. 78–81, 2006.

[6] T. R. Hurtado and D. A. Della-Giustina, "Traumatic asphyxia in a 6-year-old boy," *Pediatric Emergency Care*, vol. 19, no. 3, pp. 167–168, 2003.

[7] J. R. Dunne, G. Shaked, and M. Golocovsky, "Traumatic asphyxia: an indicator of potentially severe injury in trauma," *Injury*, vol. 27, no. 10, pp. 746–749, 1996.

[8] J. S. Williams, S. L. Minken, and J. T. Adams, "Traumatic asphyxia-reappraised," *Annals of Surgery*, vol. 167, no. 3, pp. 384–392, 1968.

[9] E. Sertaridou, V. Papaioannou, G. Kouliatsis, V. Theodorou, and I. Pneumatikos, "Traumatic asphyxia due to blunt chest trauma: a case report and literature review," *Journal of Medical Case Reports*, vol. 6, article 257, 2012.

[10] I. Ertok, G. Kurtoglu Çelik, G. Ercan Haydar, O. Karakayali, M. Yılmaz, and T. Erşen, "Review of traumatic asphyxia syndrome with a case presentation," *Journal of Academic Emergency Medicine Case Reports*, vol. 4, no. 2, pp. 58–61, 2013.

[11] P. Ibarra, L. M. Capan, S. Wahlander, and K. M. Sutin, "Difficult airway management in a patient with traumatic asphyxia," *Anesthesia & Analgesia*, vol. 85, no. 1, pp. 216–218, 1997.

# 24

# Subclavian Artery Pseudoaneurysm Formation 3 Months after a Game of Rugby Union

**T. Evans,**[1] **S. Roy,**[2] **and M. Rocker**[1]

[1]*Department of General Surgery, Royal Glamorgan Hospital, Llantrisant CF72 8XR, UK*
[2]*Department of Orthopaedic Surgery, Royal Glamorgan Hospital, Llantrisant CF72 8XR, UK*

Correspondence should be addressed to T. Evans; tom_g_evans@hotmail.com

Academic Editor: Serdar Kula

Pseudoaneurysms of the subclavian artery remain a rare complication after fracture of the clavicle. We report a case of delayed diagnosis of a subclavian artery pseudoaneurysm after a closed fracture of the clavicle in a 15-year-old patient, 3 months after the original injury while playing rugby union. Despite several attendances to the Emergency Department with vague symptoms, the final diagnosis was confirmed by duplex ultrasound and Computed Tomography of the thorax. Surgical repair was indicated due to acute limb ischaemia from distal embolisation from a large pseudoaneurysm, with the patient making a full recovery. This case highlights the need for clinical vigilance when assessing patients, particularly on repeated occasions when their recovery appears to be impaired. A thorough history and clinical examination can raise suspicion of even rare occurrences and aid prompt management.

## 1. Case Report

A 15-year-old boy attended the Emergency Department (ED) with a short history of a pale left arm. He denied pain but complained of some altered sensation throughout his left hand. He had a significant recent medical history, having suffered a fractured midshaft of his left clavicle (see Figure 1) managed conservatively with a broad arm sling 3 months previously. Furthermore, he had 3 recent attendances to the ED with pain and "pins and needles" which felt like "a trapped nerve," the first of which was a sudden onset of clavicular pain and altered sensation on throwing a ball. At each ED visit he was assessed, reassured, and discharged with documentation stating "no neurovascular deficit."

Physical examination on his final visit revealed a warm but pale arm with no radial, ulnar, or brachial pulses palpable, but a normal capillary refill time of 2 seconds, and a reduced power in his intrinsic muscles of his left hand, but normal peripheral neurovascular examinations in remaining limbs and an electrocardiograph showing sinus rhythm. Chest X-ray confirmed no cervical ribs.

A duplex ultrasound scan showed a loss of flow in the brachial artery below the left elbow, with thrombus partially occluding the artery. Also noted was a 3 cm abnormality in the left subclavian artery that was thought to be a subclavian aneurysm that contained thrombus.

Subsequent Computed Tomography (CT) of the thorax (Figures 2 and 3) confirmed a diagnosis of a 4.5 × 3.5 × 2.5 cm false aneurysm of the subclavian artery lying on the superficial aspect of the anterior second rib and also showed evidence of the previous mid-clavicle fracture that had healed but malaligned. The CT also showed the distal end of the proximal shaft protruding posteriorly into the false aneurysm.

Transfer was arranged that day to the local acute vascular surgeon on call, where he underwent a subclavian-axillary bypass and brachial embolectomy. After 4 days of recovery as an inpatient including a heparin infusion he was discharged, symptom-free.

## 2. Discussion

The annual incidence rate of clavicular fractures is estimated to be between 30 and 60 cases per 100,000 people [1]. The most common complication following a clavicular fracture is nonunion, quoted as occurring between 6 and 15% of cases

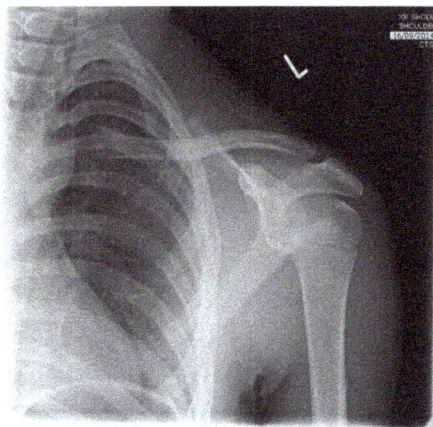

FIGURE 1: AP X-ray indicating minimally displaced mid-clavicle fracture.

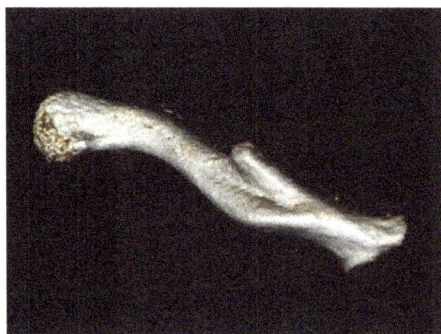

FIGURE 2: 3D reconstruction showing posterior view of clavicle.

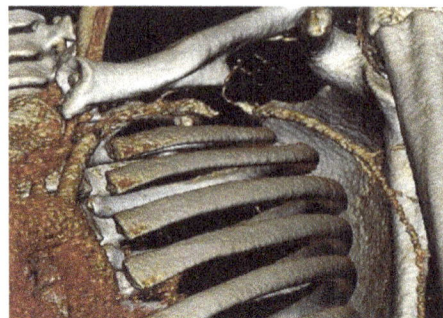

FIGURE 3: 3D reconstruction showing filling defect and pseudoaneurysms in the left subclavian artery.

[2]. Neurovascular compromise is a rare but recognised complication of clavicle fractures. While case reports commenting on similar cases exist [3–5], they remain subtle to detect clinically. Kendall et al. reported a fatality from an isolated clavicle fracture from transection of the subclavian artery [6], and while this fatality was due to a large haemothorax and subclavian artery puncture from an unwitnessed fall, it shows the life-threatening potential of these fractures. Clavicular fractures were cited as the cause of 50% of traumatic subclavian artery injuries [1]. Arterial injury can result in puncture, pseudoaneurysm formation, or occlusion. Arterial occlusion leading to acute limb ischaemia is another severe complication. A subclavian artery pseudoaneurysm is therefore regarded as a potential risk to both the life and the limb of the patient and requires prompt management.

Arterial rupture usually causes life-threatening haemorrhages and must be carefully ruled out by physical examination as well as diagnostic imaging. Physical examination of the upper limb must focus on skin color, temperature, sensation, hand function, and presence of upper limb pulses. Contrast CT represents a key diagnostic exam, while angiography offers both a diagnostic and a therapeutic approach.

In 1983 Sturm and Cicero devised five criteria that lead the examining doctor to suspect an arterial injury [7]. These criteria include first rib fracture, diminished or absent radial pulses, palpable supraclavicular hematoma, chest X-ray demonstrating a widening of the mediastinum or haematoma over the area of the subclavian artery, and brachial plexus palsy.

Management options include both surgical and endovascular techniques. Surgical management remains a challenge and generally requires either a sternotomy or a supraclavicular and infraclavicular approach for safe proximal and distal control of the vessel. This approach risks significant blood loss and injuries to nearby neurovascular structures; nonsurgical options for management have been published and endovascular procedures including covered stents seem to reduce these risks but are often not available in the acute setting [8, 9]. They do, however, seem to offer a successful method of treating this difficult and rare condition, without the need for a major intrathoracic operation. Historically, endovascular repair reduced the risks associated with a traditional surgical repair requiring wide exposure to gain access to the injured vessels. The argument against endovascular repair was the clinicians inability to exclude other injuries associated with the vascular injury since avoiding surgery also means avoiding a chance to directly see such injuries at the time of operation. However, with the increasing accuracy and availability of radiology this may well be less relevant.

## 3. Conclusions

While subclavian artery pseudoaneurysm remains a rare complication after fracture of the clavicle, this case clearly describes a prolonged series of symptoms that show how important are a detailed history and physical examination along with an open mind that can help reduce risks to patients life and limb.

## Conflict of Interests

The authors declare that there is no conflict of interests regarding the publication of this paper.

## References

[1] L. A. K. Khan, T. J. Bradnock, C. Scott, and C. M. Robinson, "Fractures of the clavicle," *The Journal of Bone & Joint Surgery Series A*, vol. 91, no. 2, pp. 447–460, 2009.

[2] R. C. McKee, D. B. Whelan, E. H. Schemitsch, and M. D. McKee, "Operative versus nonoperative care of displaced midshaft clavicular fractures: a meta-analysis of randomized clinical trials," *The Journal of Bone & Joint Surgery—American Volume*, vol. 94, no. 8, pp. 675–684, 2012.

[3] Z. T. Stockinger, M. C. Townsend, N. E. McSwain Jr., and R. L. Hewitt, "Acute endovascular management of a subclavian artery injury.," *The Journal of the Louisiana State Medical Society*, vol. 156, no. 5, pp. 262–264, 2004.

[4] G. Babatasi, M. Massetti, O. Le Page, J. Theron, and A. Khayat, "Endovascular treatment of a traumatic subclavian artery aneurysm," *The Journal of Trauma—Injury, Infection and Critical Care*, vol. 44, no. 3, pp. 545–547, 1998.

[5] R.-J. Renger, A. J. De Bruijn, H. C. Aarts, and L. G. Van Der Hem, "Endovascular treatment of a pseudo-aneurysm of the subclavian artery," *Journal of Trauma—Injury Infection & Critical Care*, vol. 55, no. 5, pp. 969–971, 2003.

[6] K. M. Kendall, J. H. Burton, and B. Cushing, "Fatal subclavian artery transection from isolated clavicle fracture," *The Journal of Trauma—Injury, Infection and Critical Care*, vol. 48, no. 2, pp. 316–318, 2000.

[7] J. T. Sturm and J. J. Cicero, "The clinical diagnosis of ruptured subclavian artery following blunt thoracic trauma," *Annals of Emergency Medicine*, vol. 12, no. 1, pp. 17–19, 1983.

[8] J. A. Hernandez, A. Pershad, and N. Laufer, "Subclavian artery pseudoaneurysm: successful exclusion with a covered self-expanding stent," *Journal of Invasive Cardiology*, vol. 14, no. 5, pp. 278–279, 2002.

[9] A. V. Patel, M. L. Marin, F. J. Veith, A. Kerr, and L. A. Sanchez, "Endovascular graft repair of penetrating subclavian artery injuries," *Journal of Endovascular Surgery*, vol. 3, no. 4, pp. 382–388, 1996.

# 25

# Unusual Presentation of Meckel's Diverticulum: Gangrene due to Axial Torsion

**Ahmet Rencuzogullari, Kubilay Dalci, and Orcun Yalav**

*Department of General Surgery, Cukurova University Medical Faculty, 01330 Adana, Turkey*

Correspondence should be addressed to Ahmet Rencuzogullari; rncz1980@gmail.com

Academic Editor: Kalpesh Jani

Meckel's diverticulum is the most common congenital anomaly of the small bowel. The majority of cases are asymptomatic; however, life-threatening complications can also take place. We present a case of a 37-year-old male who was admitted with symptoms of acute, severe abdominal pain in the right iliac fossa. The patient was operated on with the preoperative diagnosis of acute appendicitis but the operative findings were consistent with torted Meckel's diverticulum due to presence of mesodiverticular band and he was treated successfully with surgical resection.

## 1. Introduction

Meckel's diverticulum (MD) is the most common congenital anomaly of the small bowel, which was first described by Johann Friedrich Meckel in 1809. MD is a true diverticulum that develops from the obliteration of the omphalomesenteric duct during embryonic development. The incidence of this entity, in autopsy and retrospective studies, ranges from 0.14 to 4.5 percent [1]. Most commonly, MD remains asymptomatic. Complications of MD include hemorrhage associated with peptic ulceration, due to heterotopic gastric mucosa located within the diverticulum and intestinal obstruction due to banding, volvulus, intussusception, tumor formation, and axial twisting around its base [2, 3]. Preoperative diagnosis of complicated MD is challenging because the symptoms can mimic a variety of more common ailments such as appendicitis. We hereby report a case with torted Meckel's diverticulum due to presence of mesodiverticular band.

## 2. Case Report

A 37-year-old man presented to our hospital with an 8-hour history of acute, severe, and right lower abdominal pain. The physical examination of patient revealed defense and guarding in the right lower quadrant, with rebound tenderness and altered bowel sounds. The leukocyte count was elevated at $13.7 \times 10^9$/L, and a differential count demonstrated 90% segmented neutrophils. An abdominal X-ray showed minimally dilated small bowel loops. The patient was operated on with the preoperative diagnosis of acute appendicitis. The appendix, however, intraoperatively was normal; thus, the incision was extended. The torted MD was observed 60 cm proximal to the ileocecal valve and had distal necrosis (Figure 1). The rest of the bowel appeared normal. MD was resected by using a stapling device. Pathological examination confirmed the diagnosis of MD with gangrene (Figures 2(a) and 2(b)). The recovery period was uncomplicated and the patient was discharged on postoperative day 5.

## 3. Discussion

This case report describes an unusual presentation of torted MD with gangrene in a patient who was operated on with a preoperative diagnosis of acute appendicitis. Malhotra et al. in their case report published in 1998 mention only 4 adult cases and 1 pediatric case with axial torsion of MD. However, a literature review that we conducted has shown that since then an additional 19 cases have been reported [4].

MD is a true diverticulum that develops from the vestige of the omphalomesenteric duct during embryonic development and is reported to be infrequent [2]. Clinically the majority of MD is asymptomatic and is called silent

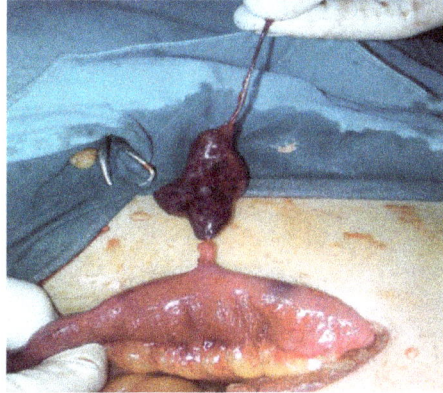

FIGURE 1: Torsion of Meckel's diverticulum around the base and necrosis.

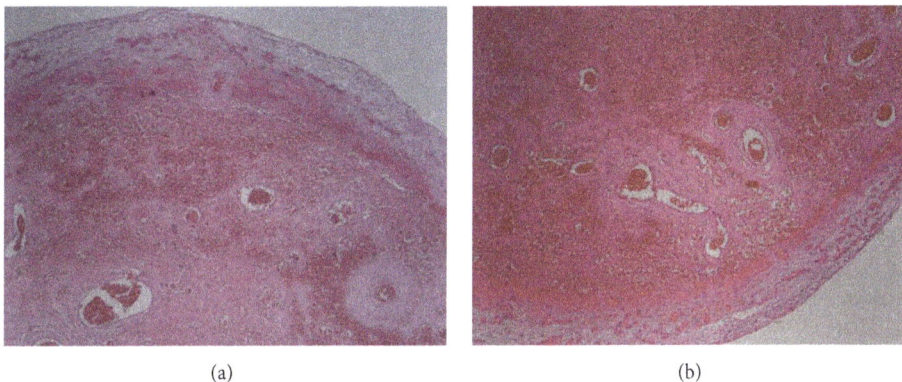

(a)                                                                                          (b)

FIGURE 2: (a) Transmural necrosis and hemorrhage (H&E staining ×100 magnification). (b) Ischemic necrosis, congestion, and hemorrhage (H&E staining ×100 magnification).

MD; however, life-threatening complications can also take place. The lifetime risk of patients with MD to develop complications was shown in a study to be 6.4% [5]. The most common of these complications is lower gastrointestinal system (GIS) bleeding, resulting from ulceration caused by ectopic gastric mucosa. Other major complications include obstruction, intussusception, diverticulitis, perforation, and development of malignancies. However, preoperatively diagnosing MD is often difficult, with only 6–12% of cases being diagnosed correctly [6]. Most commonly, the symptoms of a complicated MD simulate acute abdomen due to appendicitis; thus, appendicitis is usually the main preoperative diagnosis, while differential diagnoses include small bowel obstruction, acute cholecystitis, and liver abscess [4, 7–9]. In our case, similarly the preoperative diagnosis was acute appendicitis. Previous reports have put forth that despite improvements in radiodiagnostics, only 4% of such cases are accurately diagnosed [1]. As mentioned before, axial torsion is already the rarest complication and development of gangrene in this clinical context is even rarer. Our literature review has identified only 9 [4, 6, 7].

The mechanism of axial torsion of MD has not yet been described successfully. One explanation could be the MD having a wide body but narrow base and the presence of mesodiverticular band [4]. The macroscopic appearance of our case's MD supports this conjecture. Other possible risk factors for torsion have also been reported in the literature. A neoplasm arising within MD is one of the rare presentations mentioned despite being exceptionally rare [8].

The treatment of symptomatic MD is surgical resection. Wedge resection usually suffices; however, under some circumstances, segmental ileum resection with end-to-end anastomosis may be indicated. Resection for incidental asymptomatic MD cases is questionable. However, in any case, resection of fibrous bands is recommended to prevent further complications such as torsion and obstruction [6]. Increasing number of reports has begun recommending use of laparoscopy for treatment [10].

## 4. Conclusion

Meckel's diverticulum complications should be considered in the differential diagnosis of an acute appendicitis case, especially when intraoperatively a normal appendix is identified. Imaging has not been shown to be effective in identifying a torted MD; therefore, surgical vigilance, suspicion, and consideration are vital to recognize.

## Consent

Written informed consent was obtained from patient for publication of this case report and accompanying images.

## Conflict of Interests

The authors declare that there is no conflict of interests regarding the publication of this paper.

## References

[1] F.-E. Ludtke, V. Mende, H. Kohler, and G. Lepsien, "Incidence and frequency of complications and management of Meckel's diverticulum," *Surgery Gynecology and Obstetrics*, vol. 169, no. 6, pp. 537–542, 1989.

[2] W. C. Mackey and P. Dineen, "A fifty year experience with Meckel's diverticulum," *Surgery Gynecology and Obstetrics*, vol. 156, no. 1, pp. 56–64, 1983.

[3] D. A. Guss and D. B. Hoyt, "Axial volvulus of Meckel's diverticulum: a rare cause of acute abdominal pain," *Annals of Emergency Medicine*, vol. 16, no. 7, pp. 811–812, 1987.

[4] S. Malhotra, D. A. Roth, T. H. Gouge, S. R. Hofstetter, G. Sidhu, and E. Newman, "Gangrene of Meckel's diverticulum secondary to axial torsion: a rare complication," *The American Journal of Gastroenterology*, vol. 93, no. 8, pp. 1373–1375, 1998.

[5] J. J. Cullen, K. A. Kelly, C. R. Moir, D. O. Hodge, A. R. Zinsmeister, and L. Joseph Melton III, "Surgical management of Meckel's diverticulum: an epidemiologic, population-based study," *Annals of Surgery*, vol. 220, no. 4, pp. 564–569, 1994.

[6] G. P. Moore and F. M. Burkle Jr., "Isolated axial volvulus of a meckel's diverticulum," *The American Journal of Emergency Medicine*, vol. 6, no. 2, pp. 137–142, 1988.

[7] C. Limas, K. Seretis, C. Soultanidis, and S. Anagnostoulis, "Axial torsion and gangrene of a giant Meckel's diverticulum," *Journal of Gastrointestinal and Liver Diseases*, vol. 15, no. 1, pp. 67–68, 2006.

[8] U. A. Almagro and L. Erickson Jr., "Fibroma in Meckel's diverticulum: a case associated with axial and ileal volvulus," *The American Journal of Gastroenterology*, vol. 77, no. 7, pp. 477–480, 1982.

[9] G. Kiyak, E. Ergul, S. M. Sarikaya, and A. Kusdemir, "Axial torsion and gangrene of a giant Meckel's diverticulum mimicking acute appendicitis," *Journal of the Pakistan Medical Association*, vol. 59, no. 6, pp. 408–419, 2009.

[10] S. W. Schmid, M. Schäfer, L. Krähenbühl, and M. W. Büchler, "The role of laparoscopy in symptomatic Meckel's diverticulum," *Surgical Endoscopy*, vol. 13, no. 10, pp. 1047–1049, 1999.

# 26

# Noncardiogenic Pulmonary Edema after Amlodipine Overdose without Refractory Hypotension and Bradycardia

**M. Hedaiaty, N. Eizadi-Mood, and A. M. Sabzghabaee**

*Clinical Toxicology Department, Isfahan Clinical Toxicology Research Center, Noor Hospital, Isfahan University of Medical Sciences, Isfahan 81458-31451, Iran*

Correspondence should be addressed to N. Eizadi-Mood; izadi@med.mui.ac.ir

Academic Editor: Kazuhito Imanaka

Amlodipine overdose can be life-threatening when manifesting as noncardiogenic pulmonary edema. Treatment remains challenging. We describe a case of noncardiogenic pulmonary edema without refractory hypotension and bradycardia after ingestion of 500 milligram amlodipine with suicidal intent. Mechanical ventilation, dexamethasone, atrovent HFA (ipratropium), pulmicort inhalation, and antibiotic therapy were used for the management. Length of hospital stay was 11 days. The patient was discharged with full recovery.

## 1. Introduction

Amlodipine, a dihydropyridine group of calcium channel blockers (CCBs), constitutes the leading form of cardiovascular drug overdose and has been implicated in several deaths resulting from such overdose [1, 2]. It has half-life of 30–50 hours with a large volume of distribution (21 liter per kilograms) [1]. It has also a low metabolic clearance with the advantage of using a once-daily dosage [3].

Treating patients with amlodipine overdose can be challenging [4]. Patients severely poisoned can develop profound refractory bradycardia, hypotension, acute kidney injury, and either cardiogenic or noncardiogenic pulmonary edema [5].

Here we report a case of amlodipine overdose with noncardiogenic pulmonary edema without refractory hypotension and bradycardia which was managed supportively.

## 2. Case Report

A 36-year-old woman was admitted to our poisoning emergency department with recurrent vomiting and generalized muscular pain 11 hours after ingestion of 100 tablets of amlodipine five milligram. She had a suicidal intent. She had gone to a local health center three hours after the consumption. Gastric decontamination had been performed for her at that center. Then she had been discharged with her own consent.

On admission, she had a blood pressure of 95/60 mm Hg in the supine position with a pulse rate of 99 per minute and respiratory rate of 21 per minute (Table 1). She was afebrile, conscious, and anxious. Other cardiac and respiratory manifestations were normal. Pulse oximetry ($SpO_2$) showed 93% on room air. She denied concomitant consumption of alcohol or any other drugs. Comprehensive toxicology analysis of urine was negative for opioids, morphine, alcohols, amphetamines, and so forth. There were no signs of head trauma or focal neurologic signs. She was hospitalized in an intensive care unit with respect to high toxic ingestion. Routine laboratory tests on admission were as follows: white blood cells ($12.6 \times 10^9$ per liter; normal range: $4$–$10 \times 10^9$ per liter); 90% neutrophil; serum urea (BUN) 21 milligrams per deciliter (mg/dL); creatinine (Cr) 1.6 mg/dL; serum calcium 8.4 mg/dL; phosphorus 5.8 mg/dL; and glucose plasma level 184 mg/dL. Liver function tests, sedimentation rate (ESR), and serum electrolytes were within the normal limits. Venous blood gas analysis showed respiratory alkalosis (pH 7.54, carbon dioxide tension 18 millimeter of mercury, Bicarbonate 15.1 milimol per liter) (Table 2). Electrocardiography demonstrated sinus tachycardia with normal PR, QRS, and Q-T intervals. Chest X-ray performed immediately after admission was normal.

After four hours, blood pressure decreased to 85/50 millimeter of mercury (mm Hg). She received one-liter normal

TABLE 1: Vital signs (systolic and diastolic blood pressure, respiratory rates, and pulse rate) of patient during hospitalization (on admission and at 8.00 a.m. each day).

| Time of hospitalization (day) | Systolic blood pressure (mmHg) | Diastolic blood pressure (mmHg) | Pulse rate (per min) | Respiratory rates (per min) |
|---|---|---|---|---|
| On admission | 95 | 60 | 99 | 21 |
| 1 | 90 | 50 | 108 | 21 |
| 2 | 90 | 54 | 104 | v |
| 3 | 105 | 55 | 100 | v |
| 4 | 101 | 59 | 75 | v |
| 5 | 115 | 56 | 104 | v |
| 6 | 105 | 55 | 96 | v |
| 7 | 116 | 67 | 85 | v |
| 8 | 98 | 59 | 88 | v |
| 9 | 113 | 75 | 80 | v |
| 10 | 112 | 78 | 91 | v |
| 11 | 103 | 60 | 61 | v |
| 12 | 115 | 75 | 73 | 18 |

min: minutes; mmHg: millimeters of mercury; v: treatment with mechanical ventilation.

TABLE 2: Different variables of the patient (on admission and at 8.00 a.m. each day): intake and output volume, blood urea nitrogen (normal value ranges: 9–20 mg/dL), creatinine (normal value ranges: 0.7–1.4 mg/dL), peripheral venous blood gases including partial pressure of carbon dioxide (normal value ranges: 40–52 mmHg), venous blood pH (normal value ranges: 7.31–7.41), bicarbonate (normal value ranges: 22–27 mEq/L), and saturation of peripheral oxygen (normal present ranges: 90–100%).

| Time of hospitalization (day) | Volume intake (mL) | Volume output (mL) | Blood urea nitrogen (mg/dL) | Creatinine (mg/dL) | $PCO_2$ (mmHg) | PH | $HCO_3$ (mEq L) | $SpO_2$% |
|---|---|---|---|---|---|---|---|---|
| On admission | — | — | 21 | 1.6 | 18 | 7.54 | 15.1 | 93 |
| 1 | 2250 | 700 | 24 | 1.3 | 18 | 7.54 | 15 | 84 |
| 2 | 3950 | 250 | 37 | 2.3 | 26 | 7.24 | 15.2 | 85 |
| 3 | 3100 | 1000 | 45 | 1.4 | 24 | 7.44 | 15.9 | 89 |
| 4 | 4850 | 1200 | 32 | 1.2 | 27 | 7.46 | 18.6 | 98 |
| 5 | 3650 | 2300 | 27 | 0.8 | 29 | 7.49 | 21.4 | 94 |
| 6 | 3400 | 2100 | 18 | 0.6 | 29 | 7.49 | 38 | 96 |
| 7 | 3850 | 5400 | 12 | 0.6 | 37 | 7.50 | 28.3 | 99 |
| 8 | 3850 | 8150 | 14 | 0.6 | 51 | 7.45 | 34.6 | 100 |
| 9 | 4300 | 3700 | 14 | 0.8 | 41 | 7.50 | 31.2 | 96 |
| 10 | 3900 | 5800 | | — | 42 | 7.40 | 31.3 | 95 |
| 11 | 3100 | 2950 | 8 | 0.8 | 42 | 7.49 | 31.3 | 97 |
| 12 | 3100 | 2900 | | — | — | | | |

mg/dL: milligram per deciliter; mEq/L: milliequivalents per liter; mmHg: millimeters of mercury; mL: milliliter; $PCO_2$: partial pressure of carbon dioxide; $HCO_3$: bicarbonate; $SpO_2$: saturation of peripheral oxygen.

saline as bolus infusion. Hourly urine output was initially below 0.5 milliliter per kilograms (mL/kg) body weight but it improved after infusion of crystalloid intravenous (IV) fluids and vasopressors (dopamine hydrochloride drip at a rate of 5–10 micrograms per kilograms per minute) for ten hours. She had recovered from renal failure within 48 hours.

Next day she began to experience gradual respiratory distress including developed tachycardia, tachypnea (respiratory rates = 25) (Table 1), and mild agitation. Fine inspiratory crackles in both lungs at auscultation were present. Arterial blood gas (ABG) showed hypoxia arterial oxygen tension = 62 mm Hg and oxygen saturation of 85%. The $FiO_2/PaO_2$ ratio was less than 200. Central vein pressure was within normal range (14 centimeter of water). Chest X-ray revealed bilateral fluffy shadows in the lower zones of both lung fields without cardiomegaly. Echocardiography was performed and ejection fraction was 60%. No evidence of diastolic dysfunction was observed.

She was intubated under sedation with midazolam (0.1 milligram per kilograms) and ventilated (initial settings:

synchronized intermittent mechanical ventilation (SIMV) mode, Fraction of Inspired Oxygen (FiO$_2$) = 70%; tidal volume 6–8 mL/kg; positive end expiratory pressure (PEEP) = 5 cm H$_2$O; respiratory rate (RR) = 10/minute; pressure support (PS) = 10 mm Hg). After 10 hours, she presented with acute respiratory distress syndrome (ARDS) and the setting was adjusted to: FiO$_2$ = 40%, PEEP = 10 cm H$_2$O, RR = ten per minute, and PS = 15 cm H$_2$O. The patient received dexamethasone (8 mg, three times daily), ipratropium bromide inhalation aerosol (three milliliter vial, three times daily), and pulmicort inhalation (one milligram per day). The results regarding the vital signs, O$_2$ saturation, VBG, BUN, and Cr during hospitalization in an intensive care unit have been reported in Tables 1 and 2. Chest X-ray on day three showed typical batwing appearance without cardiomegaly which was suggestive of ARDS.

After 11 days of hospitalization she was extubated and transferred to the ward. She underwent psychiatric evaluation and was discharged without any complications.

## 3. Discussion

There are no standardized guidelines for managing severe amlodipine intoxication because of limitation in the number of describing surveys [4, 6–10].

Gastrointestinal decontamination in amlodipine overdose is beneficial when used within the one hour of consumption [11]. Also activated charcoal had been effective when given during the first 24 hours after drug ingestion [12]. In our case gastrointestinal decontamination for three hours and activated charcoal for 11 hours after ingestion were started.

Different pharmacologic therapies available for amlodipine overdose with persistent hypotension or myocardial depression include inotropic support with adrenergic agents, glucagon, IV infusion of calcium, hyperinsulinemia-euglycemia therapy, and extracorporeal membrane oxygenation in refractory shock [4, 7, 10, 11, 13]. In this case, she had mild hypotension without cardiac conduction defects; therefore, she received only crystalloid and dopamine infusion and stabilized in a short time period.

Our patient developed noncardiogenic pulmonary edema on day three. Amlodipine is a dihydropyridine that selectively blocks L-type calcium channels in smooth muscle and myocardial depressant activity at toxic levels so patients may present with cardiogenic pulmonary edema [13, 14]. Some studies also reported cases with catastrophic shock and noncardiogenic pulmonary edema [9, 10, 15]. The mechanism of noncardiogenic pulmonary edema in patients with CCB overdose is not well known. Excessive pulmonary capillary transudation due to selective precapillary vasodilatation causes an increase in transcapillary hydrostatic pressure and ultimately interstitial edema [16, 17].

In our case severe hypotension was not observed, so interstitial edema may be caused by other ways such as blocking other types of calcium channels, the cytochrome P450 isoenzyme system effects [18, 19], or P-glycoprotein-mediated transport [20]. Also cardiac ejection fraction was 60%; therefore, fluid overload could not be reason of pulmonary edema.

Considering age, sex, serum urea, creatinine level, and glomerular filtration rate, she suffered from mild and transient kidney injury. So kidney injury could not be reason of pulmonary edema.

Severe CCB poisoning is often associated with significant hyperglycemia due to L-type calcium channel in pancreatic $\beta$-cells [21], as well as dysregulation of the insulin-dependent or phosphatidylinositol three-kinase pathway [22]. However, in this case glucose plasma levels were between 151 and 184 mg/dL for initial four days that may show a role in the ultimate degree of toxicity.

Another finding in this case was the development of mild respiratory and metabolic alkalosis. However, metabolic acidosis has been reported in most of the reported cases [5–16]. Metabolic acidosis could be resulting from systemic hypotension and acute kidney injury.

ARDS manifests with diffuse alveolar inflammation and increased pulmonary vascular permeability resulting in hypoxemia [23]. A survey has shown mortality benefits with lower tidal volume of 6 mL/kg, keeping plateau pressure below 30 cm H$_2$O and PEEP adjusted to optimize alveolar recruitment without causing overdistention [24]. Our patient developed ARDS related to noncardiogenic pulmonary edema. She was treated with mechanical ventilation, dexamethasone, ipratropium bromide inhalation aerosol, and pulmicort inhalation which improved outcome and successful liberation from ventilator around 11 days.

Although high-dose insulin and extracorporeal life support were the interventions supported for the patients with severe CCB [25], supportive management might be useful in the treatment of noncardiogenic pulmonary edema after amlodipine overdose without refractory hypotension and bradycardia.

## Conflict of Interests

The authors declare that there is no conflict of interests regarding the publication of this paper.

## Acknowledgments

The authors would like to thank Dr. Farzad Gheshlaghi, Dr. Ahmad Yaraghi, Dr. Gholamali Dorvashy, and all ICU personnel for their valuable collaboration.

## References

[1] E. J. Stanek, C. E. Nelson, and D. DeNofrio, "Amlodipine overdose," *The Annals of Pharmacotherapy*, vol. 31, no. 7-8, pp. 853–856, 1997.

[2] W. A. Watson, T. L. Litovitz, W. Klein-Schwartz et al., "2003 annual report of the American association of poison control centers toxic exposure surveillance system," *American Journal of Emergency Medicine*, vol. 22, no. 5, pp. 335–404, 2004.

[3] D. R. Abernethy and J. B. Schwartz, "Calcium-antagonist drugs," *The New England Journal of Medicine*, vol. 341, no. 19, pp. 1447–1457, 1999.

[4] M. Onge, P. Dubé, S. Gosselin et al., "Treatment for calcium channel blocker poisoning: a systematic review," *Clinical Toxicology*, vol. 52, pp. 926–944, 2014.

[5] C. R. DeWitt and J. C. Waksman, "Pharmacology, pathophysiology and management of calcium channel blocker and β-blocker toxicity," *Toxicological Reviews*, vol. 23, no. 4, pp. 223–238, 2004.

[6] S. Ghosh and M. Sircar, "Calcium channel blocker overdose: experience with amlodipine," *Indian Journal of Critical Care Medicine*, vol. 12, no. 4, pp. 190–193, 2008.

[7] H. Azendour, L. Belyamani, M. Atmani, H. Balkhi, and C. Haimeur, "Severe amlodipine intoxication treated by hyperinsulinemiaeuglycemia therapy," *Journal of Emergency Medicine*, vol. 38, no. 1, pp. 33–35, 2010.

[8] K. Saravu and R. Balasubramanian, "Near-fatal amlodipine poisoning," *Journal of Association of Physicians of India*, vol. 52, pp. 156–157, 2004.

[9] R. Hasson, V. Mulcahy, and H. Tahir, "Amlodipine poisioning complicated with acute non-cardiogenic pulmonary oedema," *BMJ Case Reports*, vol. 2011, 3 pages, 2011.

[10] V. B. Kute, P. R. Shah, K. R. Goplani, M. R. Gumber, A. V. Vanikar, and H. L. Trivedi, "Successful treatment of refractory hypotension, noncardiogenic pulmonary edema and acute kidney injury after an overdose of amlodipine," *Indian Journal of Critical Care Medicine*, vol. 15, no. 3, pp. 182–184, 2011.

[11] H. Sanaei-Zadeh, "Treatment of amlodipine overdose," *Indian Journal of Critical Care Medicine*, vol. 16, no. 3, p. 182, 2012.

[12] G. Jürgens, L. C. Groth Hoegberg, and N. A. Graudal, "The effect of activated charcoal on drug exposure in healthy volunteers: a meta-analysis," *Clinical Pharmacology and Therapeutics*, vol. 85, no. 5, pp. 501–505, 2009.

[13] S. K. Shah, S. K. Goswami, R. V. Babu, G. Sharma, and A. G. Duarte, "Management of calcium channel antagonist overdose with hyperinsulinemia-euglycemia therapy: case series and review of the literature," *Case Reports in Critical Care*, vol. 2012, Article ID 927040, 5 pages, 2012.

[14] S. Vogt, A. Mehlig, P. Hunziker et al., "Survival of severe amlodipine intoxication due to medical intensive care," *Forensic Science International*, vol. 161, no. 2-3, pp. 216–220, 2006.

[15] K. Naha, J. Suryanarayana, R. A. Aziz, and B. A. Shastry, "Amlodipine poisoning revisited: acidosis, acute kidney injury and acute respiratory distress syndrome," *Indian Journal of Critical Care Medicine*, vol. 18, no. 7, pp. 467–469, 2014.

[16] T. A. Siddiqi, J. Hill, Y. Huckleberry, and S. Parthasarathy, "Noncardiogenic pulmonary edema and life-threatening shock due to calcium channel blocker overdose and its management: a case report and a clinical review," *Respiratory Care*, vol. 59, no. 2, pp. e15–e21, 2014.

[17] V. H. Humbert Jr., N. J. Munn, and R. F. Hawkins, "Noncardiogenic pulmonary edema complicating massive diltiazem overdose," *Chest*, vol. 99, no. 1, pp. 258–259, 1991.

[18] P. Gladding, H. Pilmore, and C. Edwards, "Potentially fatal interaction between diltiazem and statins," *Annals of Internal Medicine*, vol. 140, no. 8, article W31, 2004.

[19] D. A. Sica, "Interaction of grapefruit juice and calcium channel blocker," *The American Journal of Hypertension*, vol. 19, no. 7, pp. 768–773, 2006.

[20] D. R. Abernethy and J. B. Schwartz, "Calcium-antagonist drugs," *The New England Journal of Medicine*, vol. 341, no. 19, pp. 1447–1457, 1999.

[21] G. Devis, G. Somers, E. Van Obberghen, and W. J. Malaisse, "Calcium antagonists and islet function. I. Inhibition of insulin release by verapamil," *Diabetes*, vol. 24, no. 6, pp. 547–551, 1975.

[22] L. K. Bechtel, D. M. Haverstick, and C. P. Holstege, "Verapamil toxicity dysregulates the phosphatidylinositol 3-kinase pathway," *Academic Emergency Medicine*, vol. 15, no. 4, pp. 368–374, 2008.

[23] V. M. Ranieri, G. D. Rubenfeld, B. T. Thompson et al., "Acute respiratory distress syndrome: the Berlin definition," *The Journal of the American Medical Association*, vol. 307, no. 23, pp. 2526–2533, 2012.

[24] D. R. Hess, "Approaches to conventional mechanical ventilation of the patient with acute respiratory distress syndrome," *Respiratory Care*, vol. 56, no. 10, pp. 1555–1572, 2011.

[25] M. St-Onge, P.-A. Dubé, S. Gosselin et al., "Treatment for calcium channel blocker poisoning: a systematic review," *Clinical Toxicology*, vol. 52, no. 9, pp. 926–944, 2014.

# 27

# Speaking Tracheostomy Tube and Modified Mouthstick Stylus in a Ventilator-Dependent Patient with Spinal Cord Injury

Eiji Mitate,[1,2] Kensuke Kubota,[2] Kenji Ueki,[3] Rumi Inoue,[2] Ryosuke Inoue,[4] Kenta Momii,[2] Hiroshi Sugimori,[5] Yoshihiko Maehara,[2] and Seiji Nakamura[1]

[1]Section of Oral and Maxillofacial Oncology, Division of Maxillofacial Diagnostic and Surgical Sciences, Faculty of Dental Science, Kyushu University, 3-1-1 Maidashi, Higashi-ku, Fukuoka 812-8582, Japan
[2]Emergency and Critical Care Center, Kyushu University Hospital, 3-1-1 Maidashi, Higashi-ku, Fukuoka 812-8582, Japan
[3]Department of Integrated Therapy for Chronic Kidney Disease, Faculty of Medical Sciences, Kyushu University, 3-1-1 Maidashi, Higashi-ku, Fukuoka 812-8582, Japan
[4]Special Patient Oral Care Unit, Kyushu University Hospital, 3-1-1 Maidashi, Higashi-ku, Fukuoka 812-8582, Japan
[5]Cerebrovascular Center, Saga-Ken Medical Centre Koseikan, 400 Oaza Nakabaru, Kasemachi, Saga 840-8571, Japan

Correspondence should be addressed to Eiji Mitate; mitate@dent.kyushu-u.ac.jp

Academic Editor: Aristomenis K. Exadaktylos

Communication is a serious problem for patients with ventilator-dependent tetraplegia. A 73-year-old man was presented at the emergency room in cardiopulmonary arrest after falling from a height of 2 m. After successful resuscitation, fractures of the cervical spine and cervical spinal cord injury were found. Due to paralysis of the respiratory muscles, a mechanical ventilator with a tracheostomy tube was required. First, a cuffed tracheostomy tube and a speaking tracheostomy tube were inserted, and humidified oxygen was introduced via the suction line. Using these tubes, the patient could produce speech sounds, but use was limited to 10 min due to discomfort. Second, a mouthstick stylus, fixed on a mouthpiece that fits over the maxillary teeth, was used. The patient used both a communication board and a touch screen device with this mouthstick stylus. The speaking tracheostomy tube and mouthstick stylus greatly improved his ability to communicate.

## 1. Introduction

The number of patients with traumatic spinal cord injury (SCI) has increased over the past three decades [1]. The incidence of SCI in Japan is 40.2 per million [2]. Patients with ventilator-dependent tetraplegia resulting from cervical SCI suffer from stress and medical problems. In particular, communication disorders cause frustration and anxiety. Approximately 1 in 5 patients with SCI have depression [3].

Many communication devices to assist patients with tetraplegia have been reported and available on the market [4, 5]. The speaking tracheostomy tube makes phonation possible, but it can only be used for a few minutes without discomfort. With a mouthstick stylus, patients can use a communication board and touchscreen devices, but they often become fatigued due to the need for constant biting. Some modification is needed.

In this paper, the efficacy of a speaking tracheostomy tube and "modified" mouthstick stylus for a patient with ventilator-dependent tetraplegia due to cervical SCI is reported.

## 2. Case Description and Results

A 73-year-old male who fell from a height of 2 m was admitted to the hospital in cardiopulmonary arrest. His medical history included hypertension and urolithiasis. After successful resuscitation, fractures of the cervical spine (C1, C5, C6, and C7) and cervical SCI (C1 and C2) were found on examination by computed tomography (CT) and magnetic resonance imaging (MRI) (Figure 1). He became tetraplegic and required mechanical ventilator support. He underwent a tracheotomy with a cuffed tracheostomy tube (Blue Line

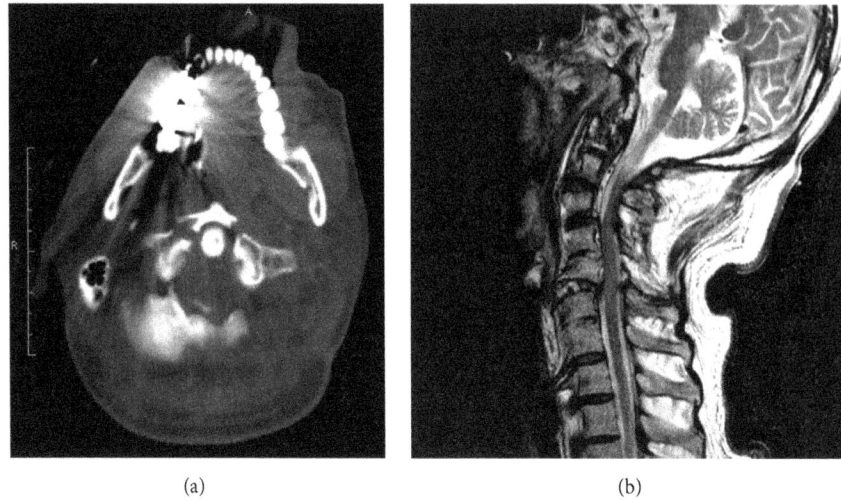

(a)                                                    (b)

FIGURE 1: Computed tomography (CT) and magnetic resonance imaging (MRI) examination on arrival. (a) shows a Jefferson fracture. (b) shows a sagittal T2-weighted MRI of the cervical spinal cord injury (C1 and C2).

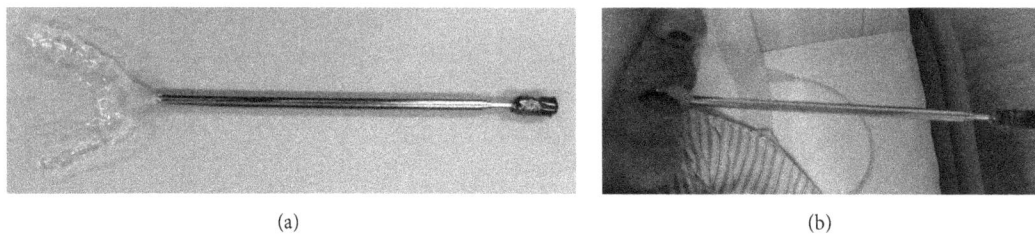

(a)                                                    (b)

FIGURE 2: Modified mouthstick stylus. (a) shows an overview of the modified mouthstick stylus. (b) shows the mouthstick stylus fixed on the maxillary teeth. The patient can use this stylus without biting.

Profile Cuff; Smiths Medical, Inc.), and soon had difficulty with communication and became depressed. First, he spoke in a hoarse whisper, assisted with 5 L/min of humidified oxygen gas via the suction line. This method could only be used for a few minutes and caused discomfort. Second, a speaking tracheostomy tube (Vocalaid; Smiths Medical, Inc.) was inserted. He could talk for up to 10 min using this tube, but with fatigue. Moreover, speaking with the tracheostomy tube was inadequate for communication.

The mouthstick stylus is also commercially available. However, the constant biting required for its operation left him fatigued. Thus, a stylus fixed on a mouthpiece of maxillary teeth with dental self-curing resin (UNIFAST III; GC Dental, Japan) was applied. The mouthpiece was made with a 2 mm thick polyethylene terephthalate glycol-modified thermoforming plate (Erkodur; ERKODENT Erich Kopp GmbH, Germany). The stylus was made with a rod antenna and conductive urethane foam for electrostatic discharge (ESD form F-10-A; Hozan Tool Ind. Co., Ltd., Japan) (Figure 2). This modified mouthstick stylus was fixed on the maxilla without the need for biting and could be used with both a communication board and a capacitive iPad touchscreen. The length of the stylus was adjustable. As this provided the patient with a method for communication, he can communicate with us.

## 3. Discussion

SCI prevention should focus on sports and motorcycle accidents involving young people, traffic accidents involving adults, and falling accidents involving aged people [2]. Traumatic SCI drastically affects the quality of life. In particular, cervical SCI may cause tetraplegia, which requires a tracheostomy with a mechanical ventilator.

Our modified mouthstick stylus firmly fixed on the maxillary teeth can be used for communication boards, keyboards, and capacitive touchscreen interfaces such as the iPhone and iPad with little risk of being dropped. 69.2% of patients with SCI use a computer; of those, 94.2% access the Internet [6]. Many assistive devices for patients with SCI are currently available, one of which is the mouthstick stylus [7]. Our stylus will be of great help to patients with tetraplegia.

The speaking tracheostomy tube for patients with tetraplegia was first reported in 1967 and it has been in routine use since then [8]. Warm and humidified oxygen or air passing the vocal cords via a suction catheter makes a hoarse whisper only for a few minutes.

The speaking tracheostomy tube has some advantages. Continuous oxygen insufflation prevents aspiration during feeding, airway obstruction, and pulmonary infection [9]. On the other hand, there are some disadvantages such as pain, discomfort, and emphysema reported [10, 11]. Oxygen misconnected to the tracheostomy cuff punctured the cuff [12]. All locations of potential tube must be checked to protect against the adverse events.

## Consent

A written informed consent was obtained from patient for publication of this case report and accompanying images.

## Disclosure

No previous presentation of the paper or abstract in any form was done.

## Conflict of Interests

The authors declare that there is no conflict of interests regarding the publication of this paper.

## References

[1] J. C. Furlan, B. M. Sakakibara, W. C. Miller, and A. V. Krassioukov, "Global incidence and prevalence of traumatic spinal cord injury," *Canadian Journal of Neurological Sciences*, vol. 40, no. 4, pp. 456–464, 2013.

[2] H. Shingu, M. Ohama, T. Ikata, S. Katoh, and T. Akatsu, "A nationwide epidemiological survey of spinal cord injuries in Japan from January 1990 to December 1992," *Paraplegia*, vol. 33, no. 4, pp. 183–188, 1995.

[3] C. H. Bombardier, "Depression and spinal cord injury," *Archives of Physical Medicine and Rehabilitation*, vol. 95, no. 2, pp. 413–414, 2014.

[4] X. Huo, C. Cheng, and M. Ghovanloo, "Evaluation of the tongue drive system by individuals with high-level spinal cord injury," in *Proceedings of the Annual International Conference of the IEEE Engineering in Medicine and Biology Society (EMBC '09)*, pp. 555–558, IEEE, Minneapolis, Minn, USA, September 2009.

[5] H. A. Caltenco, L. N. S. A. Struijk, and B. Breidegard, "Tongue-Wise: Tongue-computer interface software for people with tetraplegia," in *Proceedings of the 32nd Annual International Conference of the IEEE Engineering in Medicine and Biology Society (EMBC '10)*, pp. 4534–4537, Buenos Aires, Argentina, September 2010.

[6] N. Goodman, A. M. Jette, B. Houlihan, and S. Williams, "Computer and internet use by persons after traumatic spinal cord injury," *Archives of Physical Medicine and Rehabilitation*, vol. 89, no. 8, pp. 1492–1498, 2008.

[7] M. A. Frankel, J. Hawkesford, and J. Simonson, "A new pattern mouth stick," *Paraplegia*, vol. 13, no. 1, pp. 66–69, 1975.

[8] R. M. Whitlock, "A means of speaking for patients with cuffed tracheostomy tubes," *The British Medical Journal*, vol. 3, article 547, 1967.

[9] Y. Naito, H. Mima, T. Itaya, K. Yamazaki, and H. Kato, "Continuous oxygen insufflation using a speaking tracheostomy tube is effective in preventing aspiration during feeding," *Anesthesiology*, vol. 84, no. 2, pp. 448–450, 1996.

[10] N. Yahagi, H. Tanigami, Y. Watanabe, and K. Kumon, "A problem with an infant speaking tracheostomy tube," *Anaesthesia*, vol. 50, no. 1, pp. 91–92, 1995.

[11] T. M. Akhtar and M. Bell, "'Vocalaid' and surgical emphysema," *Anaesthesia*, vol. 48, no. 3, pp. 272–273, 1993.

[12] R. O. Feneck and W. E. Scott, "Misconnexion of a cuffed 'speaking' tracheostomy tube. A report of the consequences, and recommendations for future use of similar tracheostomy tubes," *Anaesthesia*, vol. 38, no. 1, pp. 47–51, 1983.

# 28

# Recurrent Coagulopathy after Rattlesnake Bite Requiring Continuous Intravenous Dosing of Antivenom

**Charles W. Hwang and F. Eike Flach**

*Department of Emergency Medicine, University of Florida College of Medicine, 1329 SW 16th Street, P.O. Box 100186, Gainesville, FL 32610-0186, USA*

Correspondence should be addressed to Charles W. Hwang; c7places@ufl.edu

Academic Editor: Aristomenis K. Exadaktylos

*Context.* Snakebite envenomation is common and may result in systemic coagulopathy. Antivenom can correct resulting laboratory abnormalities; however, despite antivenom use, coagulopathy may recur, persist, or result in death after a latency period. *Case Details.* A 50-year-old previously healthy man presented to the emergency department after a rattlesnake bite to his right upper extremity. His presentation was complicated by significant glossal and oropharyngeal edema requiring emergent cricothyrotomy. His clinical course rapidly improved with the administration of snake antivenom (FabAV); the oropharyngeal and upper extremity edema resolved within several days. However, over the subsequent two weeks, he continued to have refractory coagulopathy requiring multiple units of antivenom. The coagulopathy finally resolved after starting a continuous antivenom infusion. *Discussion.* Envenomation may result in latent venom release from soft tissue depots that can last for two weeks. This case report illustrates the importance of close hemodynamic and laboratory monitoring after snakebites and describes the administration of continuous antivenom infusion, instead of multidose bolus, to neutralize latent venom release and correct residual coagulopathy.

## 1. Introduction

The Crotalinae subfamily of snakes (family Viperidae), commonly known as pit viper snakes, include rattlesnakes (*Crotalus* species), pygmy rattlesnakes (*Sistrurus* species), and moccasins (*Agkistrodon* species) [1]. Pit viper envenomations are not uncommon in the United States. Annually, approximately 2,700 envenomations in the United States lead to hospital presentation; half of them receive the antidote for Crotalinae envenomation, Crotalidae Polyvalent Immune Fab (Ovine) (FabAV) (CroFab, Protherics, Nashville, TN) [1, 2].

Snakebite envenomation causes not only localized tissue damage, but also systemic derangements. One of the well-known sequelae after snakebites is the systemic coagulopathy due to enzymes within the venom, which result in laboratory abnormalities, including elevated d-dimer, hypofibrinogenemia, prolonged prothrombin time (PT), prolonged activated partial thromboplastin time (aPTT), and thrombocytopenia. The use of antivenom can correct these laboratory abnormalities; however variable response has also been observed; the coagulopathy may recur, persist, or result in death after a latency period [3, 4]. Therefore, the administration of antivenom must be tailored to each patient's clinical and laboratory presentation and venom exposure [1].

The manufacturer and the local poison center recommend initial boluses of CroFab with subsequent maintenance boluses as needed until initial control is achieved. In this case report, we describe a patient with recurrent coagulopathy after a snakebite that ultimately required 51 vials of Crofab. Furthermore, the coagulopathy resolved only after a continuous intravenous infusion of CroFab was administered.

## 2. Case Presentation

A previously healthy 50-year-old intoxicated man was driving on a road on a May afternoon when he attempted to move a snake off the road with a stick to prevent it from being run over. He was bitten on the dorsum of his right

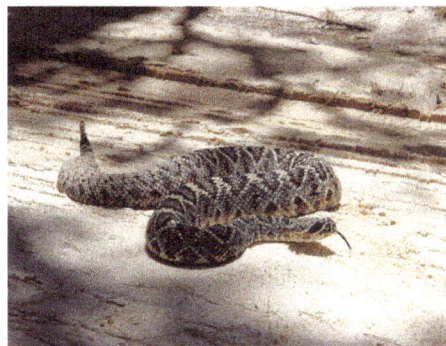

FIGURE 1: Photograph of the eastern diamondback rattlesnake (*Crotalus adamanteus*) taken by the patient's wife after the patient's snakebite.

hand by a positively identified 6-foot long diamondback rattlesnake (Figure 1). He immediately called his wife who called emergency medical services (EMS) while he drove home. When EMS arrived, he was found to be confused, nauseated, and vomiting, with altered mental status and intermittent combativeness. Once in the transport vehicle, an intravenous line was established and he was given 25 mg of intravenous (IV) diphenhydramine.

Upon arrival in the emergency department (ED) less than one hour after the initial injury, the patient was noted to be tachycardic (HR 131), hypotensive (92/79), and stridorous. On physical examination, he had decreased mental status, voice change, and significant perioral, pharyngeal, and marked glossal edema. Rapid sequence intubation (RSI) was initiated due to impending complete upper airway obstruction. The patient was pretreated with 100 mcg of phenylephrine IV to prevent hemodynamic decompensation during RSI. During video-assisted laryngoscopy, pronounced epiglottal and cord edema was noticed, and multiple attempts of passing a styletted endotracheal tube and gum elastic bougie failed. Bag valve mask ventilation was difficult despite use of an oral airway with a decline in his oxygen saturation to 78%. Thus the decision was made to proceed with emergency cricothyrotomy using a bougie-assisted landmark-guided technique, which was successful on its first attempt. A cuffed 6-0 endotracheal tube was passed over the bougie, with good chest rise and end-tidal capnography. At the time of securing the airway, the patient's oxygen saturation had returned to 100% secondary to continued uninterrupted two-person oral airway assisted bag valve mask ventilation.

Initial arterial blood gas analysis showed a pH of 7.03, $pCO_2$ of 56.1 mmHg, and $pO_2$ of 174.0 mmHg on 60% $FiO_2$. He received 125 mg IV methylprednisolone and 1 L Plasma-Lyte A with improvement of his blood pressure to 119/76.

His right upper extremity was noted to have fang marks 2.5 cm apart in the first dorsal webspace (Figure 2). There was severe amount of edema over the palmar and dorsal surface of the right hand extending proximally to the wrist with mottling and ecchymoses of the right hand. The compartments remained compressible, capillary refill remained brisk, and oxygen saturation remained 95–99% $SpO_2$ in all five fingers. Orthopedic surgery was consulted by the emergency

physicians for the evaluation of progressive swelling and potential compartment syndrome; no surgical intervention was performed as the patient maintained a radial pulse by Doppler signal and brisk capillary refill.

The state's poison center was simultaneously consulted in the ED; an initial bolus of 6 vials of FabAV (CroFab) was administered. Initial pre-FabAV laboratory findings from the emergency department demonstrated consumptive coagulopathy: thrombocytopenia (platelets $20 \times 10^3$ mm$^{-3}$), d-dimer > 20 $\mu$g mL$^{-1}$, fibrinogen < 35 mg dL$^{-1}$, INR > 8, PTT > 240 sec, and PT > 150 sec. The patient was subsequently admitted to the medical intensive care unit for further management.

The state's poison control recommended boluses of CroFab per their protocol, which initially corrected his coagulopathy. His coagulation panel at the time of administration of FabAV throughout his hospitalization is shown in Table 1. The first week of his hospitalization was uneventful. The edema of his right upper extremity stabilized within 24 hours and did not require surgical intervention. He was successfully extubated on day 5.

On day 8 of his hospitalization, his fibrinogen and platelet count trended downwards, and his PT and INR trended upwards. He remained hemodynamically stable with no drop in his blood pressure, hemoglobin, or hematocrit and did not exhibit signs or symptoms of bleeding from his coagulopathy. There was no recurrence of swelling. Hematology was consulted, and decision was made to start him on FabAV infusions each over 6 hours instead of 1 hour. After six vials of FabAV were infused over 6 hours each, his coagulopathy resolved. The resolution of his coagulopathy is demonstrated in Table 1. His coagulopathy resolved by day 12 and he was subsequently discharged from the hospital.

## 3. Discussion

Snakebite envenomation is not an uncommon occurrence in the United States. In the United States, 8,000 poisonous snakebites occur annually, which result in 9 to 15 fatalities [5]. Envenomation causes localized tissue damage, which may manifest as fang puncture, pain, tissue edema, erythema, ecchymosis, bullae formation, and lymphadenopathy. In addition, systemic effects after envenomation include panic and fear, nausea, vomiting, diarrhea, lymphadenopathy, syncope, tachycardia, hemorrhage, hypotension, tachypnea, respiratory distress and failure, coagulopathy, and encephalopathy [4–7].

The toxic effects of venom assist in its function to obtain food for the snake. The enzymes it contains help to decrease digestive time and to immobilize the snake's prey. These enzymes alter the endothelial lining, break down plasma membranes, and promote edema and hemorrhage. Therefore, when humans are subjected to snake venom, hypovolemic shock, pulmonary edema, tissue necrosis, and renal failure ensue [5].

For many years, the coagulopathy after snakebites has been observed in vivo and in vitro, resulting in hemorrhagic and thrombotic events, with or without laboratory perturbations, due to activation of specific anticoagulant and/or

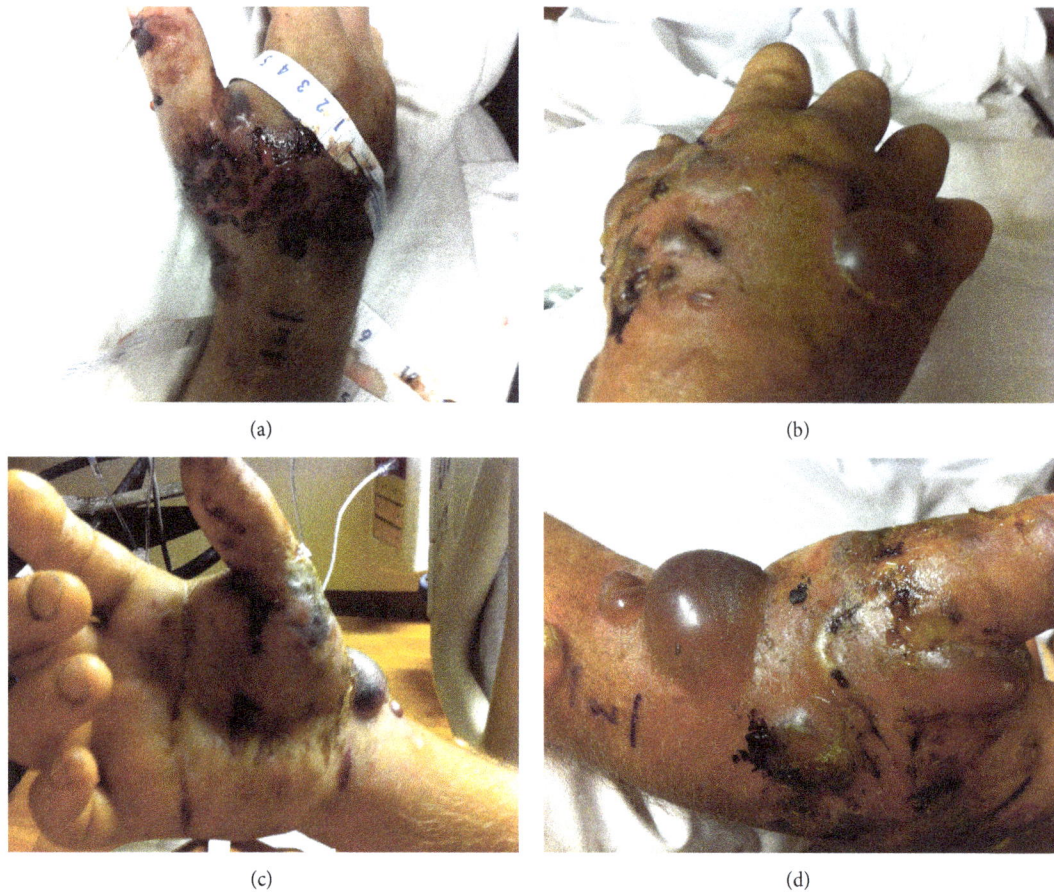

FIGURE 2: Fang marks located on the patient's right upper extremity with local tissue damage, edema, ecchymoses, and mottling.

TABLE 1: Serial coagulation panel.

| Day | 1 | 2 | | | | 3 | | 4 | 5 | | | | | | 6 | |
|---|---|---|---|---|---|---|---|---|---|---|---|---|---|---|---|---|
| Time | 1600 | 2259 | 0557 | 1415 | 2037 | 0411 | 1620 | 0004 | 0800 | 1535 | 2150 | 0353 | 1300 | 2359 | 0607 | 1210 |
| Platelets $\times 10^3$ mm$^{-3}$ | 20 | 493 | 528 | 416 | 352 | 293 | | | 200 | 263 | 335 | 341 | 219 | 141 | 115 | 116 |
| PT, sec | 150 | 29.8 | 16.9 | 15.5 | 15.6 | 15 | 14.6 | 15 | 15.5 | 15.1 | 15 | 14.6 | 14.3 | 15.7 | 15 | 14.5 |
| INR | 8 | 2.9 | 1.4 | 1.5 | 1.2 | 1.5 | 1.1 | 1.2 | 1.2 | 1.2 | 1.2 | 1.1 | 1.1 | 1.2 | 1.2 | 1.1 |
| Fibrinogen, mg dL$^{-1}$ | 35 | 35 | 104 | 167 | 176 | 166 | 158 | 164 | 151 | 129 | 156 | 150 | 189 | 232 | 291 | 319 |
| D-dimer, $\mu$g mL$^{-1}$ | 20 | 20 | 20 | | | | 16.93 | 12.58 | 17.27 | 20 | 20 | 17.05 | 12.38 | 8.8 | 10.16 | 10.9 |
| CroFab, time, and vials | 1700 12 / 2036 6 / 2246 6 | | 0715 2 / 1220 2 | 1845 2 | | | | | 1342 4 | 1939 4 | 0152 2 | 0658 2 | | | 1048 1 | 1628 1 / 2229 1 |

| Day | 7 | | 8 | | | 9 | | 10 | | 11 | | | 12 | 19 |
|---|---|---|---|---|---|---|---|---|---|---|---|---|---|---|
| Time | 0005 | 1215 | 0000 | 1145 | 2005 | 0410 | 1246 | 0405 | 1810 | 0535 | 1315 | 1715 | 0640 | 0907 |
| Platelets $\times 10^3$ mm$^{-3}$ | 97 | 97 | 91 | 77 | 67 | 43 | 48 | 60 | 109 | 128 | 150 | | 245 | 612 |
| PT, sec | 15.4 | 15 | 15.4 | 15.2 | 17.1 | 17.4 | 15.9 | 15.9 | 15.5 | 15.4 | 15.3 | 14.6 | 14.4 | 13 |
| INR | 1.2 | 1.2 | 1.2 | 1.2 | 1.4 | 1.4 | 1.3 | 1.3 | 1.2 | 1.2 | 1.2 | 1.1 | 1.1 | 1 |
| Fibrinogen, mg dL$^{-1}$ | 394 | 452 | 495 | 305 | 110 | 111 | 183 | 195 | 314 | 243 | 261 | 267 | 282 | 464 |
| D-dimer, $\mu$g mL$^{-1}$ | 8.17 | | | | | | | | | | 4.53 | | | |
| CroFab, time, and vials | | | | | | 2241 1[†] / 1048 1[†] | | 0520 1[†] | 2331 1[†] | 1100 1[†] | 2235 1[†] | | | |

[†] CroFab infusion over 6 hours.

procoagulant pathways [3, 8]. Thrombin-like and proteolytic enzymes contained within snake venom incompletely split the fibrinogen molecule, resulting in an unstable fibrin clot which traps platelets. Plasmin lyses these clots, resulting in a disseminated intravascular coagulopathy- (DIC-) like picture, which includes prolonged clotting times, prolonged prothrombin and activated partial thromboplastin times, hypofibrinogenemia, thrombocytopenia, and fibrin degradation products [5]. The clinical importance of coagulopathy is incompletely understood. Despite the significant, and occasionally extreme, perturbations in laboratory coagulation panels, these alterations do not always translate to hemorrhagic risk and hemorrhagic events [3, 8].

In the past, the duration of coagulopathy after snakebite has traditionally been considered short-lived and patients were routinely discharged after initial correction of coagulopathy [1]. However, recent literature has demonstrated that after adequate initial antivenom therapy, recurrence of coagulopathy may occur for up to 2 weeks [1, 3, 9]. In a retrospective study by Bogdan et al., 45% of snakebite patients had recurrent coagulopathy, including hypofibrinogenemia or thrombocytopenia [10]. Boyer et al. described 53% of FabAV treated envenomations that had recurrent, persistent, or late coagulopathy [1]. Hardy et al. reported recurrent thrombocytopenia despite initial correction of coagulopathy [11]. Other authors have reported persistent thrombocytopenia despite antivenom treatment [12–14]. Even though such a large percentage of patients demonstrated persistent or recurrent coagulopathy in these studies, none had clinically significant bleeding from the coagulopathy, nor did they have progression of local injury.

The mechanism of recurrence is unclear. The half-life of FabAV is less than 12 hours. It has been hypothesized that depots of unneutralized venom may continue to be released into the circulation after antivenom levels fall causing recurrent coagulopathy. Another hypothesized mechanism is the dissociation of antivenom-venom complexes, similar to digoxin-specific Fab dissociation, causing a recrudescence of coagulopathy [1, 3, 15].

Again, the clinical significance of recurrent late coagulopathy is unclear. Some experts believe that because the coagulopathy is a result of defibrination syndrome, patients are not at increased risk of bleeding [2]. However, other experts hypothesize that patients are one step away from a catastrophic hemorrhage [1, 8]. Kitchens and Eskin reported a case of delayed, recurrent coagulopathy that resulted in a fatality due to devastating intracerebral hemorrhage [3]. Since (1) pharmacokinetics strongly argues in favor of maintenance therapy to prevent recurrent coagulopathy, (2) the clinical significance of coagulopathy resulting in hemorrhage is unknown, and (3) a catastrophic event could cause life-threatening hemorrhage, low fibrinogen levels, and prolonged clotting times, and thrombocytopenia should be considered potentially clinically significant, and recurrence should be managed with additional antivenom [1, 2].

In this case, our patient initially received boluses of FabAV per current prescribing guidelines. His local injury was well-controlled with no progression of swelling or extension after the first 24 hours. Despite initial correction of his coagulopathy, our patient developed recurrence of his coagulopathy on day 8. He did not demonstrate any local or systemic signs or symptoms of venom toxicity, nor did he have any clinically significant hemorrhage or hemodynamic instability secondary to coagulopathy; he remained hemodynamically stable with an intact airway and no worsening of his extremity edema despite his coagulopathy. Lavonas et al. and White hypothesized that antivenom redosing and maintenance dosing may be required in order to (1) provide sufficient antivenom to neutralize initial acute venom levels and to (2) neutralize latent venom release from soft tissue depots that can last for two weeks [2, 8]. The hematology service initially recommended an infusion regimen over 12 hours; however, because of the off-label administration regimen, the medicine, hematology, and pharmacy services jointly decided to instead administer the FabAV antivenom over six hours which rectified his coagulopathy. Within one day of initiating continuous FabAV infusion, the patient's hematologic derangements improved.

Bush et al. reported a retrospective case series of five patients envenomated by rattlesnakes with similar success. Despite initial bolus dosing of FabAV, the patients experienced either transient or inadequate response with profound delayed hematologic abnormalities. After initiating a continuous FabAV infusion at 2 to 4 vials per 24 hours, the hematologic derangements improved within six to fourteen days after initial injury [16].

In summary, snakebites cause in vivo and in vitro coagulopathy, which, at this point, has uncertain clinical significance with respect to hemorrhage. This coagulopathy can persist or recur up to two weeks after injury. Therefore, despite the unknown incidence of clinically significant bleeding, patients appear to be one step away from a catastrophic hemorrhage. At this time, there are many unknowns: the bleeding risk of delayed or recurrent snakebite coagulopathy, the consequences of prolonged antivenom administration, and the optimal rate of infusion to correct coagulopathy and prevent hypothetical thromboembolic events. It is uncertain whether any downsides exist for administering FabAV using maintenance dosing; we feel it would be prudent to monitor for thromboembolic events in the setting of coagulopathy. More importantly, we demonstrate in this case that maintenance dosing in the form of an infusion is a plausible modality of administration that may be considered in the management of serious Crotalinae envenomation complicated by coagulopathy.

## Disclaimer

The authors alone are responsible for the content and writing of the paper.

## Conflict of Interests

The authors report no conflict of interests.

# References

[1] L. V. Boyer, S. A. Seifert, R. F. Clark et al., "Recurrent and persistent coagulopathy following pit viper envenomation," *Archives of Internal Medicine*, vol. 159, no. 7, pp. 706–710, 1999.

[2] E. J. Lavonas, T. H. Schaeffer, J. Kokko, S. L. Mlynarchek, and G. M. Bogdan, "Crotaline Fab antivenom appears to be effective in cases of severe North American pit viper envenomation: an integrative review," *BMC Emergency Medicine*, vol. 9, article 13, 2009.

[3] C. Kitchens and T. Eskin, "Fatality in a case of envenomation by *Crotalus adamanteus* initially successfully treated with polyvalent ovine antivenom followed by recurrence of defibrinogenation syndrome," *Journal of Medical Toxicology*, vol. 4, no. 3, pp. 180–183, 2008.

[4] B. S. Gold, R. C. Dart, and R. A. Barish, "Bites of venomous snakes," *The New England Journal of Medicine*, vol. 347, no. 5, pp. 347–356, 2002.

[5] B. S. Gold and W. A. Wingert, "Snake venom poisoning in the United States: a review of therapeutic practice," *Southern Medical Journal*, vol. 87, no. 6, pp. 579–589, 1994.

[6] L. Karalliedde, "Animal toxins," *British Journal of Anaesthesia*, vol. 74, no. 3, pp. 319–327, 1995.

[7] J. D. Hinze, J. A. Barker, T. R. Jones, and R. E. Winn, "Life-threatening upper airway edema caused by a distal rattlesnake bite," *Annals of Emergency Medicine*, vol. 38, no. 1, pp. 79–82, 2001.

[8] J. White, "Snake venoms and coagulopathy," *Toxicon*, vol. 45, no. 8, pp. 951–967, 2005.

[9] C. S. Kitchens, "Treatment of pit viper envenomation," *The Journal of the Florida Medical Association*, vol. 83, no. 3, pp. 174–177, 1996.

[10] G. M. Bogdan, R. C. Dart, S. C. Falbo, J. McNally, and D. Spaite, "Recurrent coagulopathy after antivenom treatment of crotalid snakebite," *Southern Medical Journal*, vol. 93, no. 6, pp. 562–566, 2000.

[11] D. L. Hardy, M. Jeter, and J. J. Corrigan Jr., "Envenomation by the northern blacktail rattlesnake (*Crotalus molossus molossus*): report of two cases and the $_{vitro}$ effects of the venom on fibrinolysis and platelet aggregation," *Toxicon*, vol. 20, no. 2, pp. 487–493, 1982.

[12] U. Hasiba, L. M. Rosenbach, D. Rockwell, and J. H. Lewis, "Disc like syndrome after envenomation by the snake, *Crotalus horridus horridus*," *The New England Journal of Medicine*, vol. 292, no. 10, pp. 505–507, 1975.

[13] T. G. Furlow and L. V. Brennan, "Purpura following timber rattlesnake (*Crotalus horridus horridus*) envenomation," *Cutis*, vol. 35, no. 3, pp. 234–236, 1985.

[14] W. J. Lyons, "Profound thrombocytopenia associated with Crotalus ruber ruber envenomation: a clinical case," *Toxicon*, vol. 9, no. 3, pp. 237–240, 1971.

[15] S. A. Seifert, L. V. Boyer, R. C. Dart, R. S. Porter, and L. Sjostrom, "Relationship of venom effects to venom antigen and antivenom serum concentrations in a patient with *Crotalus atrox* envenomation treated with a Fab antivenom," *Annals of Emergency Medicine*, vol. 30, no. 1, pp. 49–53, 1997.

[16] S. P. Bush, S. A. Seifert, J. Oakes et al., "Continuous IV Crotalidae Polyvalent Immune Fab (Ovine) (FabAV) for selected North American rattlesnake bite patients," *Toxicon*, vol. 69, pp. 29–37, 2013.

# 29

# A Bullet Entered through the Open Mouth and Ended Up in the Parapharyngeal Space and Skull Base

## Saileswar Goswami[1] and Choitali Goswami[2]

[1]*Department of Otolaryngology, Calcutta National Medical College, Kolkata, West Bengal 700014, India*
[2]*Department of General Emergency, Medical College, Kolkata, West Bengal 700073, India*

Correspondence should be addressed to Saileswar Goswami; sgoswami1962@gmail.com

Academic Editor: Aristomenis K. Exadaktylos

Shot from a revolver from a close range, a bullet pierced the chest of a policeman and entered through the open mouth of a young male person standing behind. The entry wound was found in the cheek mucosa adjacent to the left lower third molar. After hitting and fracturing the body and the ramus of the mandible, the bullet was deflected and was finally lodged in the parapharyngeal space and skull base, anterolateral to the transverse process of the atlas. The great vessels of the neck were not injured. The patient's condition was very critical but his life could be saved. The bullet was approached through a modified Blair's incision and was found to be lying over the carotid sheath. It was removed safely and the patient recovered completely.

## 1. Introduction

Foreign bodies in the parapharyngeal spaces are rare. Bora et al. [1] reported a case of bullet in the left parapharyngeal space at the level of C2–C4. In the present case, a bullet entered through the open mouth and after breaking the angle and ramus of the mandible on the left side, it traversed through the soft tissue of the neck. It was finally lodged in the left parapharyngeal space and skull base, just anterolateral to the transverse process of the atlas. It was surprising that the great vessels of the neck were spared and the patient survived. The reason behind reporting this case was its extreme rarity and the challenge it posed in its safe removal.

## 2. Case Presentation

In the evening, a 32-year-old man and two policemen were trying to pacify another man in a case of domestic violence. The accused took out the revolver of one of the policemen and shot him on the left side of his chest. The bullet came out through the back of the policeman and entered through the open mouth of the patient, who was standing behind him. The policeman died on the way to the hospital. The patient became unconscious and was admitted to the nearby hospital.

After initial treatment, the patient was referred to a Medical College and was admitted there. He was given supportive treatment including blood transfusion and he regained his consciousness in the next morning.

On examination, there was a huge haematoma over the left side of the face. The entry wound (Figure 1) was found in the inner aspect of the cheek adjacent to the left lower third molar. There was dental malocclusion. A fracture line could be palpated near the angle of the mandible on the left side. The patient was unable to open his mouth completely.

There was no injury in the pharynx. Airway was clear. There was an area of bruise with extra tenderness over the left infra-auricular area. On bimanual palpation, the patient complained of sharp pain and was able to feel the bullet there. The cranial nerves were normal.

Lateral view of the X-ray of the skull (Figure 2) revealed a bullet in the base of the skull on the left side at the level of the atlas. It was placed obliquely occupying an area posterior to the neck of the mandible, extending from the level of the atlas to the basiocciput. The base was directed anteroinferiorly and the tip was directed posterosuperiorly. Anteroposterior view of the X-ray of the skull (Figure 3) revealed that it was lying in a sagittal plane passing through the middle of the left

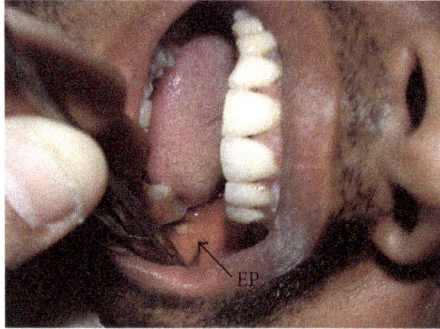

FIGURE 1: Preoperative photograph showing the entry point (EP) of the bullet (1.2 cm × 1.0 cm) on the cheek mucosa adjacent to the left lower third molar.

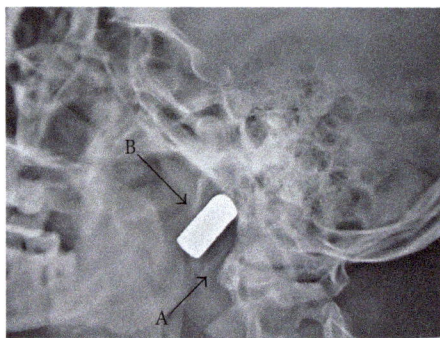

FIGURE 2: Preoperative X-ray of the skull, lateral view, showing the bullet (B) in the left parapharyngeal space at the level of the atlas (A).

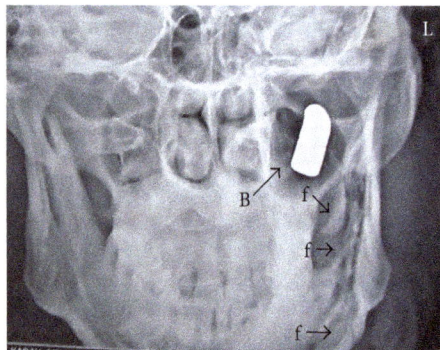

FIGURE 3: Preoperative X-ray of the skull, anteroposterior view, showing the bullet (B) lying in a sagittal plane passing through the middle of the left maxillary antrum. Note the multiple fracture fragments (f) of the mandible on the left side.

maxillary sinus. The body and ramus of the mandible were broken near its left angle with multiple fracture fragments.

CT scan revealed the bullet in the parapharyngeal space (Figure 4) about one cm anterolateral to the transverse process of the atlas on the left side. There was diffused soft tissue thickening adjacent to the foreign body with multiple air pockets, extending up to the left malar region. There were multiple fractures involving the ramus and the body of the mandible on the left side with inward displacement of the fragments (Figure 5). The bullet was found to be in close

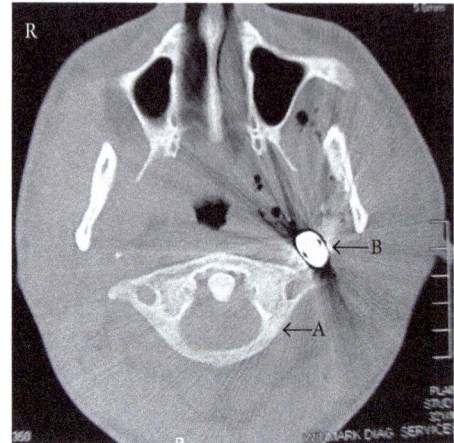

FIGURE 4: CT scan passing through the atlas, showing the bullet (B) in the left parapharyngeal space anterolateral to the transverse process of the atlas (A) with air pockets around it. Note the reflection of X-rays by the bullet.

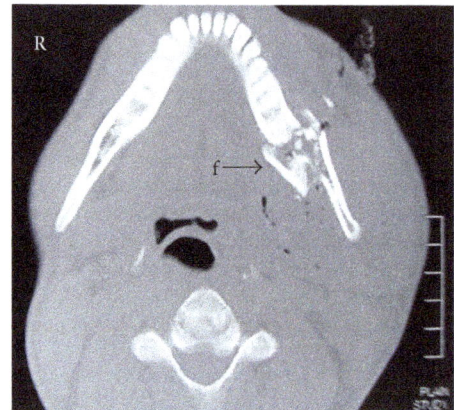

FIGURE 5: Axial CT scan showing multiple fractures of the mandible with inward displacement.

proximity to the vertebral artery and the carotid sheath. Due to reflection of the X-ray by the bullet, the image was blurred and it was not possible to assess soft tissue details.

The initial plan was to remove the bullet and manage the fractures of the mandible at the same time. However, the faciomaxillary surgeons preferred to deal with the fractures of the mandible in a second stage. The treatment plan was modified accordingly and the patient was prepared for removal of the bullet through an external approach.

The approach was made through a modified Blair's incision as in parotidectomy. The flap was elevated at the subplatysmal level. The main trunk of the facial nerve was identified first. The parotid gland along with the ramus of the mandible was retracted anterosuperiorly and the sternomastoid muscle was retracted posteriorly. Blunt dissection was carried out very carefully up to the carotid sheath but the bullet could not be found. Bimanual palpation was done with the left index finger in the dissected area and the right middle finger in the pharynx. The bullet could be felt between the fingers. Dissection was continued further medially. Finally,

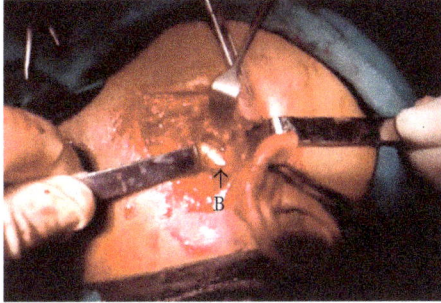

FIGURE 6: Peroperative photograph, showing the bullet (B) in the left parapharyngeal space with its tip directed posterosuperiorly.

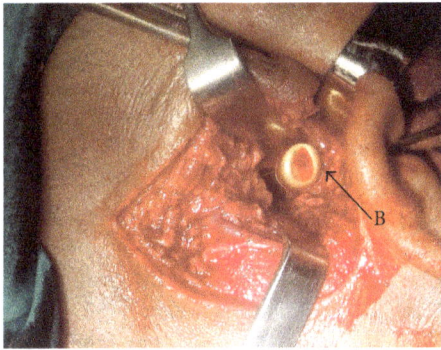

FIGURE 7: Peroperative photograph, showing the bullet (B) in the left parapharyngeal space after mobilisation of its tip.

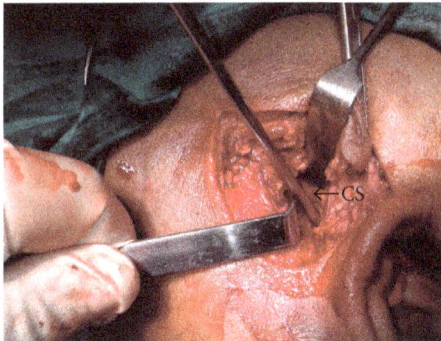

FIGURE 8: Peroperative photograph of the cavity created by the bullet with exposure of the carotid sheath (CS).

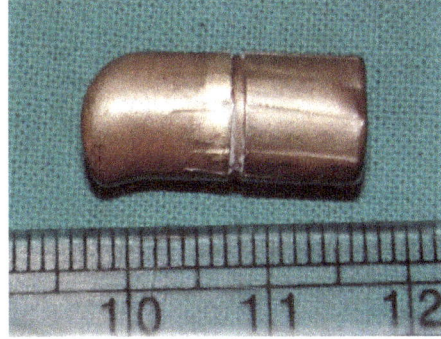

FIGURE 9: The bullet after removal (2 cm × 0.9 cm).

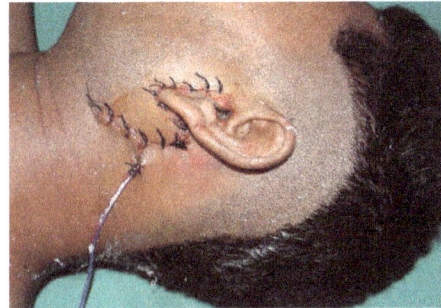

FIGURE 10: Photograph of the surgical area on the 1st postoperative day.

the bullet was found lying obliquely with its tip directed posterosuperiorly (Figure 6). It was touching the posterior surface of the carotid sheath and was pulsating with it. The tip of the bullet was mobilized from the surrounding tissue gently with the help of a blunt square hook. Surprisingly, it was very easy to free the tip as the bullet was surrounded by a cushion of air. The direction of its tip was changed outwards and upwards (Figure 7). Then, the bullet was removed by holding it with an artery forceps. The carotid sheath was found to be exposed but intact (Figure 8). Residual necrotic tissue was removed and the area was repeatedly washed with normal saline to clean the dirt. A mini-vacuum drain

was placed inside and the wound was closed in layers. The bullet was measured and was found to be 2 cm long and 0.9 cm in diameter (Figure 9). The patient recovered quickly (Figure 10) and was discharged on the eighth postoperative day.

On subsequent follow-ups, the patient's condition was found to be very good. All the wounds had healed nicely. The only problem he was having was mild difficulty in chewing, which was due to the fractures of the mandible. After going through the traumatic experience, the patient was scared and was unwilling to undergo another operation. That problem of chewing also started to be relieved gradually. OPG done three weeks after the incident (Figure 11) revealed that the fractures of the mandible had started healing. After six weeks, the patient was able to chew solid foods. Although the patient was having slight malocclusion, he was not having much problem in taking his regular diet (Figure 12).

## 3. Discussion

Foreign bodies in the parapharyngeal spaces are not common. There are reports of foreign bodies like broken toothbrush, [2] glass fragments [3, 4], and pen [5] in the parapharyngeal space. Goswami [6] reported a case of bullet in the maxillary antrum and infratemporal fossa.

Radio-opaque foreign bodies in the head and neck can easily be detected by plain X-ray. CT scan and MRI are necessary to assess the actual position of the foreign bodies.

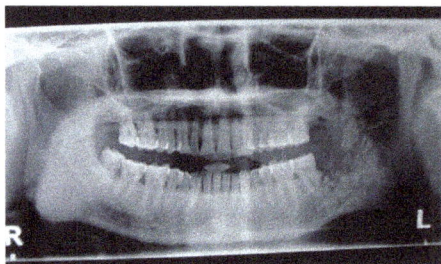

FIGURE 11: Orthopantomogram of the jaws three weeks after the injury.

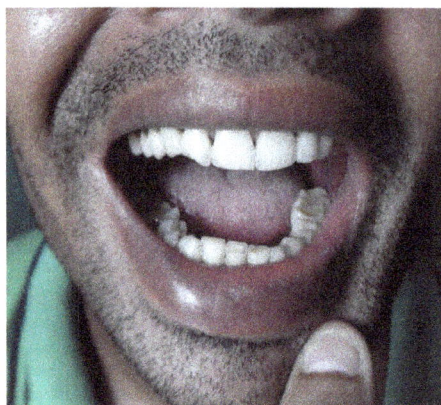

FIGURE 12: Photograph of the teeth of the patient six weeks after the injury.

Angiogram and colour Doppler study are helpful in cases of foreign bodies situated close to important vessels.

Foreign bodies in the head and neck are difficult to manage due to the presence of the great vessels, important nerves, and other vital structures. Initial management should be concentrated upon securing the airway and controlling the bleeding. In case of injury to the aerodigestive tract or major neurovascular structures, the foreign body should be removed at the earliest.

There are controversies about the time of removal of foreign bodies without any significant injury to the vital structures. A retained foreign body can lead to chronic infection, cutaneous fistula, and foreign body granuloma. It can even migrate through the common carotid artery [7] or internal jugular vein [8]. In case of a bullet, there may be lead poisoning [9]. There is a possibility of carotid artery blow-up if the bullet is situated near it.

In the present case, there was no injury in the aerodigestive tract. The patient could be taken out of the initial crisis successfully. However, as the bullet was lodged in a potentially dangerous area, it had to be removed. It was difficult to remove the bullet safely. We decided to wait for a few days so that the oedema subsided and the exploration of the bullet became easier.

There was confusion regarding the appropriate surgical approach. As the bullet was lodged in the skull base adjacent to the jugulocarotid vessels, a lateral skull base approach

like "type-A" infratemporal approach [10] could be adopted. We preferred a less extensive approach to keep the tissue dissection minimum and went for a modified parotidectomy approach. That was sufficient as the position of the bullet was accurately determined preoperatively. There was always the scope to extend the incision in case it was necessary. However, a wider approach from the beginning can be adopted, particularly when the exact position of the foreign body is not known.

## 4. Conclusion

Removal of a foreign body safely from the parapharyngeal space is a challenging task. It is very important to know its exact size, shape, and location, prior to the operation. If the situation permits, a well-planned elective procedure is preferable. A wide exposure is helpful in taking control of the great vessels of the neck. However, a less extensive approach may be sufficient if the accurate location of the foreign body is determined preoperatively.

## Conflict of Interests

The authors declare that there is no conflict of interests regarding the publication of this paper.

## References

[1] M. K. Bora, S. Narwani, P. Mishra, and A. Bhandari, "A bullet in the parapharyngeal space," Indian Journal of Otolaryngology and Head and Neck Surgery, vol. 54, no. 1, pp. 46–47, 2002.

[2] M. K. Aggarwal, G. B. Singh, R. Dhawan, and R. Kumar, "Rare case of a broken toothbrush as a parapharyngeal space foreign body," Journal of Otolaryngology—Head and Neck Surgery, vol. 38, no. 4, pp. 107–109, 2009.

[3] Y. F. Zhao, Y. Liu, L. Jiang et al., "A rare case of a glass fragment impacted in the parapharyngeal space associated with neurovascular compromise," International Journal of Oral & Maxillofacial Surgery, vol. 40, no. 2, pp. 209–211, 2011.

[4] K. Enomoto, H. Nishimura, H. Inohara et al., "A rare case of a glass foreign body in the parapharyngeal space: pre-operative assessment by contrast-enhanced CT and three-dimensional CT images," Dentomaxillofacial Radiology, vol. 38, no. 2, pp. 112–115, 2009.

[5] L. P. Rao, S. Peter, K. P. Sreekumar, and S. Iyer, "A 'pen' in the neck: an unusual foreign body and an unusual path of entry," Indian Journal of Dental Research, vol. 25, no. 1, pp. 111–114, 2014.

[6] S. Goswami, "A bullet in the maxillary antrum and infratemporal fossa," Indian Journal of Dental Research, vol. 24, no. 1, p. 149, 2013.

[7] O. A. Osinubi, A. I. Osiname, A. Pal, R. J. Lonsdale, and C. Butcher, "Foreign body in the throat migrating through the common carotid artery," Journal of Laryngology and Otology, vol. 110, no. 8, pp. 793–795, 1996.

[8] A. A. Joshi and R. A. Bradoo, "A foreign body in the pharynx migrating through the internal jugular vein," The American Journal of Otolaryngology: Head and Neck Medicine and Surgery, vol. 24, no. 2, pp. 89–91, 2003.

[9] G. E. Kikano and K. C. Stange, "Lead poisoning in a child after a gunshot injury," *Journal of Family Practice*, vol. 34, no. 4, pp. 498–504, 1992.

[10] E. Zanoletti, A. Martini, E. Emanuelli, and A. Mazzoni, "Lateral approaches to the skull base," *Acta Otorhinolaryngologica Italica*, vol. 32, no. 5, pp. 281–287, 2012.

# 30

# An Atypical Case of Methemoglobinemia due to Self-Administered Benzocaine

**Thomas M. Nappe, Anthony M. Pacelli, and Kenneth Katz**

*Department of Emergency Medicine, Lehigh Valley Hospital/USF Morsani College of Medicine, Cedar Crest Boulevard and Interstate 78, Allentown, PA 18103, USA*

Correspondence should be addressed to Thomas M. Nappe; tom.nappe@gmail.com

Academic Editor: Aristomenis K. Exadaktylos

Acquired methemoglobinemia is an uncommon hemoglobinopathy that results from exposure to oxidizing agents, such as chemicals or medications. Although, as reported in the adult population, it happens most often due to prescribed medication or procedural anesthesia and not due to easily accessed over-the-counter medications, the authors will describe an otherwise healthy male adult with no known medical history and no prescribed medications, who presented to the emergency department reporting generalized weakness, shortness of breath, headache, dizziness, and pale gray skin. In addition, the patient reported that he also had a severe toothache for several days, which he had been self-treating with an over-the-counter oral benzocaine gel. Ultimately, the diagnosis of methemoglobinemia was made by clinical history, physical examination, and the appearance of chocolate-colored blood and arterial blood gas (ABG) with cooximetry. After 2 mg/kg of intravenous methylene blue was administered, the patient had complete resolution of all signs and symptoms. This case illustrates that emergency physicians should be keenly aware of the potential of toxic hemoglobinopathy secondary to over-the-counter, nonprescribed medications. Discussion with patients regarding the dangers of inappropriate use of these medicines is imperative, as such warnings are typically not evident on product labels.

## 1. Introduction

Acquired methemoglobinemia is typically caused by oxidative stress and many prescribed medications are strongly associated with inducing methemoglobinemia (Table 1) [1, 2]. A very common presentation of this cyanotic illness is after a medical procedure, such as endoscopy or bronchoscopy, during which a liberal amount of local anesthetic, such as benzocaine spray, is used [1–3]. However, one very rarely develops methemoglobinemia from self-administering an over-the-counter medication.

It is quite unusual for a normal, healthy adult to acquire methemoglobinemia from self-administered, oral benzocaine gel. A literature review uncovered only two cases of over-the-counter benzocaine gel-related induction of methemoglobinemia. In a 2004 retrospective study of 198 adverse reactions to benzocaine reported to the FDA, only one of 132 adults with methemoglobinemia was reported to have developed it as a result of using benzocaine gel [3]. The second case was a six-year-old child, reported in 2010,

whose toothache was treated with 7.5% benzocaine gel (Baby Orajel) [4]. In fact, it is so rare for methemoglobinemia to be acquired in this fashion, that, in a 2013 study, with 576 participants, evaluating the efficacy of self-applied, over-the-counter oral benzocaine gel, there was no incidence of methemoglobinemia, even after a 1,026 mg administration by one participant in a two-hour period [5]. The reported maximum dose before inducing methemoglobinemia would be 15 mg per kilogram for a 50 kg person [5]. The authors report a rare case of an otherwise healthy adult patient who presents with methemoglobinemia after self-administering over-the-counter topical benzocaine gel. This unique case, along with a brief description of acquired methemoglobinemia and its presentation, diagnosis, and treatment, is described.

## 2. Case

A 29-year-old male of Chinese descent with no known medical history and no prescribed medications presented

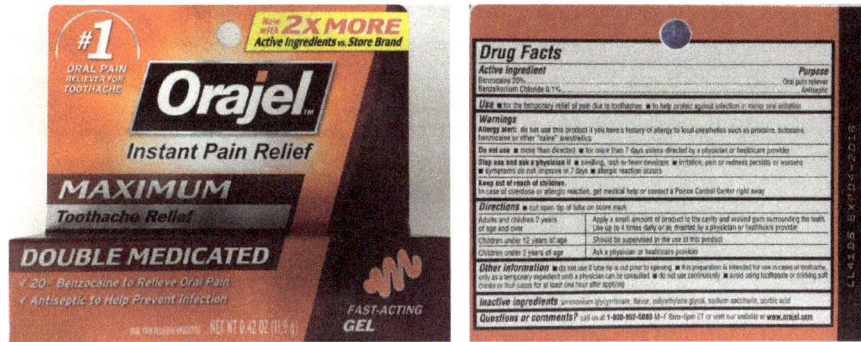

FIGURE 1: Orajel with ingredients including benzocaine 20%.

TABLE 1: Drugs known to induce methemoglobinemia (not inclusive) [1, 2].

| Amyl nitrite | Nitric oxide | Prilocaine |
|---|---|---|
| Benzocaine | Nitroglycerin | Quinones |
| Bupivacaine | Nitroprusside | (e.g., chloroquine) |
| Dapsone | Nitrofuran | Rifampin |
| Lidocaine | Phenazopyridine | Sulfonamides |
| Metoclopramide | | (e.g., sulfamethoxazole) |

to the emergency department with a chief complaint of generalized weakness since the previous evening. He also reported dyspnea, headache, and dizziness, which started the day of presentation, and his coworkers noted his skin to be pale and grayish in appearance. The patient also reported that he had a toothache for several days and was self-treating with an over-the-counter topical medication, Maximum Strength Orajel (benzocaine) (Figure 1). He stated he had been applying the gel three times per day for three days.

Physical examination revealed an alert, mildly distressed, cyanotic-appearing man. His vital signs revealed a temperature of 98.7°F, heart rate of 70 beats per minute, blood pressure of 145/68 mmHg, respirations at 16 breaths per minute, and an oxygen saturation ($SpO_2$) of 88% on six liters per minute oxygen via nasal cannula. The patient's skin displayed moderate pallor with perioral cyanosis. Upon initial venous blood draw, his blood had an abnormal chocolate-brown appearance (Figure 2).

Laboratory studies revealed an unremarkable complete blood count and comprehensive metabolic profile. An arterial blood gas with cooximetry measured pH, 7.32 (7.35–7.45); $pCO_2$, 42 mm Hg (35–48); $pO_2$, 178.0 mm Hg (83–108); $HCO_3-$, 24.3 mEq/L (21–28); $SaO_2$, 99% (95–98); total calculated hemoglobin, 17.3 g/dL; oxyhemoglobin, 71.9% (95.0–98.0); carboxyhemoglobin, 0.0% (0.5–1–5); methemoglobin, 27.4% (<3.0) with an oxygen content of 17.8 mL/dL (15.0–33.0).

The diagnosis of methemoglobinemia was made in conjunction with consultation with a medical toxicologist and 2 mg/kg intravenous methylene blue was administered. His symptoms improved within fifteen minutes and he felt markedly better within an hour. Repeat cooximetry measured

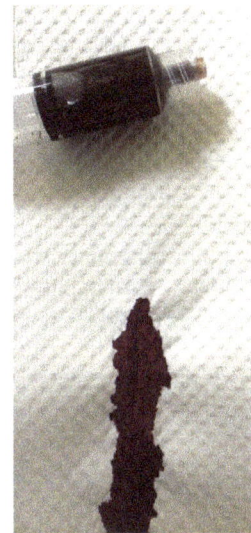

FIGURE 2: Chocolate-brown blood.

his oxyhemoglobin at 94.5% and methemoglobin at 0.9%. After a four-hour stay in the emergency department and complete resolution of his signs and symptoms, he was discharged with the instruction to discontinue the use of Orajel and seek appropriate dental care.

## 3. Discussion

Methemoglobinemia is a hemoglobinopathy that can be either inherited or acquired [1–3, 6]. Acquired methemoglobinemia is due to the exposure to an oxidizing chemical or drug (Table 1), leading to the removal of an electron from ferrous hemoglobin ($Fe^{2+}$) to create ferric hemoglobin ($Fe^{3+}$) at a rate that surpasses the endogenous reducing mechanisms, which primarily include the enzymatic activity of cytochrome b5 reductase and nicotinamide adenine dinucleotide (NADH) methemoglobin reductase [1–3, 6]. The resultant ferric hemoglobin does not release oxygen to target tissue, causing a leftward shift of the oxygen dissociation curve, leading to a functional anemia that can progress to cyanosis and even death [1–3, 6].

TABLE 2: The clinical manifestation of methemoglobinemia [1, 2].

| %MetHgb | Symptomology |
|---------|--------------|
| 0–3 | Asymptomatic and normal level in blood |
| 3–15 | Possibly asymptomatic, grayish pallor, mild cyanosis, and low oxygen saturation per pulse oximeter |
| 15–20 | Cyanosis and chocolate-brown appearance of blood |
| 20–50 | Dyspnea, fatigue, weakness, headache, dizziness, and syncope |
| 50–70 | CNS depression, lethargy, seizures, and metabolic acidosis |
| >70 | Severe cyanosis and death |

The classic presentation of a patient with methemoglobinemia is dyspnea, pallor, grayish skin, cyanosis, and hypoxia, which does not improve with supplemental oxygen administration [1, 2]. The clinical manifestation of methemoglobinemia is directly correlated to the level of measured methemoglobin, and symptoms can be worsened by extremes of age and comorbidities that may alter the levels of preexisting normal hemoglobin (Table 2) [1–3].

Diagnosis of methemoglobinemia is made by the patient's clinical presentation, with the presence of refractory hypoxemia and chocolate-colored blood and is confirmed by an arterial blood gas with cooximetry [1–3, 7, 8]. Cooximetry provides a method of differentiating between various states of hemoglobin, including measurements of total hemoglobin, oxyhemoglobin, deoxyhemoglobin, methemoglobin, carboxyhemoglobin, and sulfhemoglobin [1, 7, 8]. As present in this case, an oxygen saturation ($SaO_2$) gap is evident on ABG when compared to pulse oximetry ($SpO_2$). This means that the ABG displays a falsely normal oxygen saturation ($SaO_2$), since this is a *calculation* based on the measured serum partial pressure of oxygen ($PO_2$), given the assumption that all the patient's hemoglobin is normal (i.e., oxy- or deoxyhemoglobin); thus, the methemoglobin is included in the percentage of saturated hemoglobin in the resulting, overestimated $SaO_2$ [7, 8]. This is in contrast to pulse oximetry ($SpO_2$), which is a *measurement* of the wavelengths of oxyhemoglobin and deoxyhemoglobin, with oxyhemoglobin given as a percentage of total hemoglobin [7, 8]. Therefore, cooximetry is used as a more direct method of measurement for confirmatory testing [1, 2, 7, 8].

Treatment with oxygen and the antidote, methylene blue (1-2 mg/kg of 1% solution intravenously over five minutes), is indicated for symptomatic patients or methemoglobin levels greater than 25 to 30% [1, 2, 9]. Methylene blue accelerates the reduction of methemoglobin to hemoglobin by stimulating the activity of the nicotinamide adenine dinucleotide phosphate (NADPH) methemoglobin reductase, an enzyme that ordinarily plays a very little role in the normal reduction of methemoglobin [1]. Utilizing NADPH from the hexose monophosphate shunt, NADPH methemoglobin reductase then reduces methylene blue to leukomethylene blue, which then donates an electron to reduce methemoglobin ($Fe^{3+}$) back to hemoglobin ($Fe^{2+}$) [1, 2]. After the administration of methylene blue, improvement should be seen in minutes; otherwise, a second dose can be given within 30 to 60 minutes [1, 2]. If no improvement takes place after the second dose, other contributing factors or etiologies may be present, such as G6PD deficiency or the presence of long-acting oxidizing agents, and exchange transfusion may be considered [1].

## 4. Conclusion

Acquired methemoglobinemia is a toxic hemoglobinopathy commonly caused by prescribed medications or those administered in a hospital setting. Rarely, however, over-the-counter, self-administered medications containing benzocaine can cause methemoglobinemia in otherwise healthy adults. In this setting, emergency physicians should be keenly aware of this potentially life-threatening condition, its diagnosis and treatment, and consultation with a medical toxicologist is recommended in all cases.

## Conflict of Interests

The authors have no outside support information, conflict, or financial interests to disclose and this work has not been presented or published elsewhere.

## References

[1] A. King, N. Menke, and K. Katz, "Toxic hemoglobinopathies in the emergency department," *EM Critical Care*, vol. 3, no. 6, pp. 1–17, 2013, http://www.slremeducation.org/wp-content/uploads/2015/02/1213-Toxic-Hemoglobinopathies.pdf.

[2] J. Ashurst and M. Wasson, "Methemoglobinemia: a systematic review of the pathophysiology, detection, and treatment," *Delaware Medical Journal*, vol. 83, no. 7, pp. 203–208, 2011.

[3] T. J. Moore, C. S. Walsh, and M. R. Cohen, "Reported adverse event cases of methemoglobinemia associated with benzocaine products," *Archives of Internal Medicine*, vol. 164, no. 11, pp. 1192–1196, 2004.

[4] N.-Y. Chung, R. Batra, M. Itzkevitch, D. Boruchov, and M. Baldauf, "Severe methemoglobinemia linked to gel-type topical benzocaine use: a case Report," *Journal of Emergency Medicine*, vol. 38, no. 5, pp. 601–606, 2010.

[5] E. V. Hersh, S. G. Ciancio, A. S. Kuperstein et al., "An evaluation of 10 percent and 20 percent benzocaine gels in patients with acute toothaches: Efficacy, tolerability and compliance with label dose administration directions," *Journal of the American Dental Association*, vol. 144, no. 5, pp. 517–526, 2013.

[6] F. R. Greer, M. Shannon, Committee on Nutrition, and Committee on Environmental Health, "Infant methemoglobinemia: the role of dietary nitrate in food and water," *Pediatrics*, vol. 116, no. 3, pp. 784–786, 2005.

[7] B. Mokhlesi, J. B. Leiken, P. Murray, and T. C. Corbridge, "Adult toxicology in critical care: part I: general approach to the intoxicated patient," *Chest*, vol. 123, no. 2, pp. 577–592, 2003.

[8] A. Stolbach and R. S. Hoffman, "Respiratory principles," in *Goldfrank's Toxicologic Emergencies*, L. S. Nelson, N. A. Lewin, M. A. Howland, R. S. Hoffman, L. R. Goldfrank, and N. E. Flomenbaum, Eds., chapter 21, pp. 308–310, McGraw-Hill, New York, NY, USA, 9th edition, 2011.

[9] L. F. Rodriguez, L. M. Smolik, and A. J. Zbehlik, "Benzocaine-induced methemoglobinemia: report of a severe reaction and review of the literature," *Annals of Pharmacotherapy*, vol. 28, no. 5, pp. 643–649, 1994.

# 31

# Novel Therapies for Myocardial Irritability following Extreme Hydroxychloroquine Toxicity

**Paul B. McBeth, Perseus I. Missirlis, Harry Brar, and Vinay Dhingra**

*Division of Critical Care Medicine, University of British Columbia, Vancouver General Hospital, Vancouver, BC, Canada V5Z 1M9*

Correspondence should be addressed to Paul B. McBeth; pmcbeth@gmail.com

Academic Editor: Serdar Kula

*Introduction.* Hydroxychloroquine (HCQ) overdose is rare and potentially deadly when consumed in large doses. Management of severe HCQ toxicity is limited and infrequently reported. This report presents the case of a massive ingestion of HCQ. *Case Report.* A 23-year-old female presents following an intentional ingestion of approximately 40 g of HCQ. Within six hours after ingestion, she developed severe hemodynamic instability resulting from myocardial irritability with frequent ventricular ectopic activity leading to runs of polymorphic ventricular tachycardia (PMVT) and ventricular fibrillation (VF) requiring multiple defibrillations. Additional treatments included intravenous diazepam, epinephrine, norepinephrine, sodium bicarbonate, and magnesium sulfate. Despite the ongoing hemodynamic instability, the patient was also treated with Intralipid (ILE) and received hemodialysis. Improvements in her hemodynamics were observed after 18 hours. She survived her massive overdose of HCQ. *Conclusion.* HCQ poisoning is rare but serious because of its rapid progression to life-threatening symptoms. Hemodynamic support, gastric decontamination, electrolyte monitoring and replacement, and management of arrhythmias are the mainstays of treatment. The combined role of dialysis and ILE in the setting of massive HCQ overdose may improve outcomes.

## 1. Introduction

Hydroxychloroquine (HCQ) overdose is rare and often lethal when ingested in large doses. There exists a paucity of data on management of HCQ toxicity as it is infrequently reported. The majority of treatment recommendations are extrapolated from chloroquine (CQ) poising [1, 2]. Current management strategies are targeted at myocardial stabilization, hemodynamic support, electrolyte correction, and decontamination [1, 2]. We herein report a unique case of a massive (~40 g) ingestion of HCQ complicated by coma, hemodynamic instability, and respiratory failure treated with mechanical ventilation, vasopressor, and inotropic support, as well as hemodialysis and intravenous lipid emulsion (Intralipid) (ILE).

## 2. Case Presentation

*2.1. Clinical Presentation.* A 23-year-old female with a past medical history of depression, borderline personality disorder, obsessive compulsive disorder, psychosis NOS, and congenital hydrocephalus with VP shunt presents following ingestion of approximately 40 g of HCQ. She had been using HCQ for the treatment of pruritus. She was also being treated with risperidone, clonazepam, and zopiclone for her psychiatric disorder and fluconazole at the time of presentation for the treatment of a vaginal yeast infection. At presentation, she had a Glasgow Coma Score (GCS): 15/15, temperature: 37.1°C, blood pressure (BP): 92/60 mmHg, pulse rate: 65/min, respiratory rate: 16/min, blood glucose: 3.9 mmol/L, and serum potassium: 3.0 mmol/L. The initial blood gas demonstrated a metabolic acidosis and respiratory alkalosis: pH: 7.33, $pCO_2$: 16, $pO_2$: 70, and bicarbonate: 8. Electrocardiograph performed on arrival demonstrated sinus rhythm with a widened QRS (140 ms) and QT interval (QTc 576 ms). See Figure 1. Her urine toxicology was negative for salicylates, ethanol, acetaminophen, benzodiazepines, cannabinoid, cocaine, opiates, and amphetamines. The presenting renal and hepatic laboratory values are as follows: creatinine (Cr): 133 $\mu$mol/L; albumin: 39 g/L; lipase: 113 units/L; gamma-glutamyl transpeptidase (GGT): 30 units/L; alkaline phosphatase: 55 units/L; total bilirubin:

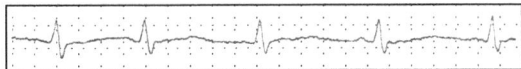

FIGURE 1: Presenting ECG tracing.

3 μmol/L; direct bilirubin: 1 μmol/L; alanine aminotransferase (ALT): 23 units/L; aspartate aminotransferase (AST): 14 units/L.

*2.2. Resuscitation and Management.* Within three hours of her overdose, the patient became obtunded requiring intubation and mechanical ventilation. Hypotension was treated with crystalloid and vasopressor support. Gastric lavage and activated charcoal for decontamination were provided. Within six hours of her overdose, she demonstrated severe hemodynamic instability resulting from myocardial irritability with frequent ventricular ectopic activity leading to runs of polymorphic ventricular tachycardia (PMVT) and ventricular fibrillation (VF) requiring 18 defibrillations with 200J with biphasic defibrillator over the first 18 hours after ingestion. Given her protracted cardiac instability, additional treatments including intravenous diazepam 60 mg followed by infusion of 6 mg/hr for calcium channel stabilization (total of 82 mg given), epinephrine 20 mcg/min, norepinephrine 30 mcg/min, sodium bicarbonate 30 mmol/hr, and magnesium sulfate 1 g/hr infusions were also initiated. The serum potassium three hours after the overdose was 1.5 mmol/L. In total, 380 mmol of potassium chloride was given over the first 18 hours administered in 20 mmol boluses. She also received intravenous sodium bicarbonate for alkalization. To treat refractory ventricular ectopy, a bolus dose of 1.5 mL/kg of 20% Intralipid ILE was initially given followed by a high dose infusion over approximately 30 minutes. A total of 500 mL of ILE was given. No further infusion of ILE was given after this initial dose. Vascular access for dialysis was established immediately after the bolus dose and thus dialysis overlapped briefly with the infusion of ILE. The runs of PMVT and VF were felt to be secondary to a preexisting channelopathy likely potentiated by fluconazole and risperidone. Ventricular pacing was reviewed but not considered indicated. The patient was started on piperacillin/tazobactam for possible aspiration pneumonia. Echocardiographic imaging revealed normal global ventricular contractility with an ejection fraction of 60%.

The patient was started on intermittent hemodialysis (IHD) in an attempt to reduce HCQ levels despite a paucity of literature regarding its use. The pharmacokinetics suggests that much of the drug is not accessible to the dialyzer, but given the severity of the overdose and the impact of hemodynamics even a small amount removed was considered favorable. Plasma HCQ level was 6425 mol/L 12 hours after ingestion. A five-hour run of hemodialysis was initiated with end points being either improved hemodynamics or of significant decrease in blood levels. A F1000 Dialyzer was used with a dialysate flow rate of 800 cc/hr. In total, 135 L of blood was processed. As noted above, concurrent with the dialysis run, an ILE infusion was administered in an effort to

create a "lipid sink" to sequester lipophilic HCQ. At 31 hours after ingestion, the plasma HCQ level was 4328 mol/L.

Improvements in her hemodynamics were observed after administration of dialysis and ILE. She was subsequently weaned from the ventilator and extubated on day 3 and discharged from ICU on postadmission day six.

## 3. Discussion

Hydroxychloroquine is sold under the trade name Plaquenil and is an aminoquinoline derivative used in the prophylaxis and treatment of malaria. It is also used as an anti-inflammatory agent in rheumatoid arthritis and complications of lupus and connective tissue disorders with an off label use in the treatment of urticaria. Hydroxychloroquine is highly toxic in overdose resulting in rapid onset of hypotension, ventricular dysrhythmias, and cardiac arrest resulting in death [1–3]. Seizures, coma, and respiratory arrest can occur in patients with severe toxicity [3].

Descriptions of HCQ overdose are limited to case reports in the literature. Given this paucity of data, the current emergency treatment is modeled on the experience of CQ overdose. The mortality rate of a CQ overdose for adults is between 10 and 30% [1]. Unlike a CQ overdose, there is no established lethal or toxic dose of HCQ. Treatments are targeted at myocardial stabilization, hemodynamic support, electrolyte correction, decontamination, and prevention of seizures. At present, there is limited data regarding the use of dialysis and to our knowledge there is no description of the use of ILE in combination with dialysis.

Hydroxychloroquine has a dose-related cardiac sodium and potassium channel blocking effect resulting in delayed repolarization and slow intraventricular conduction. This results in bradycardia, hypotension, ventricular dysrhythmias, widened QRS, and prolonged QT interval [4]. Hypokalemia appears to be due to intracellular movement of potassium via a direct effect on cell membrane.

Hydroxychloroquine is rapidly absorbed following ingestion. Peak plasma levels of HCQ occurred 2–4.5 hours after ingestion. In overdose, onset of symptoms usually occurs within 30 minutes. It is highly tissue bound with a large volume of distribution. Distributional half-life is 15–30 hours [5]. Elimination half-life ranges from 4 to 40 days. Death from cardiorespiratory arrest or refractory shock often occurs within 3 hours after ingestion. ECG changes include QRS widening and QT prolongation [3, 6]. Common dysrhythmias include ventricular ectopic beats, ventricular tachycardia, ventricular fibrillation, and torsades de pointes.

Patients presenting to health care facilities less than one-hour after ingestion should be considered for gastric decontamination with gastric lavage and activated charcoal. The use of multiple-dose activated charcoal should be considered in severe HCQ poisoning [7, 8].

Profound hypokalemia is a known effect of HCQ poisoning and appears to correlate with toxicity. The mechanism is related to reduced potassium efflux from the blockade of membrane channels. It is unknown whether HCQ causes direct cardiotoxicity or if it is partly due to the hypokalemia.

ECG findings include prolonged QT and QRS intervals leading to life-threatening ventricular arrhythmias and cardiac arrest [3, 6]. Aggressive potassium replacement is required; however, monitoring for rebound hyperkalemia [9–11] with resultant dysrhythmias is important. Diazepam infusion (1-2 mg/kg IV over 30 minutes) has been suggested to modify cardiac toxicity and improve survival based on animal experimental data [4, 12]. This has also been demonstrated in several retrospective studies in patients with acute HCQ toxicity [12–14]. The chronic use of HCQ may lead to QT prolongation [15]. Physicians prescribing HCQ to patients for extended use should consider monitoring patients for cardiac arrhythmias.

The clinical value of hemodialysis and peritoneal dialysis has not been established for the overdose of HCQ. The apparent volume of distribution for HCQ is approximately 600 L/kg. This implies that the drug rapidly becomes unavailable for removal after ingestion [1]. The extensive sequestration of HCQ by tissues limits effectiveness of hemodialysis. Despite the lack of guidelines in favor of hemodialysis in this case, it may have been helpful for the following reasons. CQ and by extension HCQ are known to interfere with potassium efflux and facilitate insulin release [16]. Hypokalemia and hypoglycemia are both known precipitants of cardiac arrest. Perhaps critical hypokalemia and hypoglycemia were averted by stabilizing plasma levels with hemodialysis. Secondly, in the face of the overwhelming overdose, the "lipid sink" provided by ILE may become saturated and thus abolish the gradient for lipophilic compounds to diffuse out from the intracellular compartment to the extracellular compartment. It is conceivable that the "lipid sink" diffusion gradient was preserved by dialysing Intralipid that had become saturated with HCQ. Extracorporeal membrane oxygenation (ECMO) has also been successfully demonstrated in an isolated case severe HCG toxicity [17]. The use of ECMO was not considered in this case.

Intravenous lipid emulsion is commercially available and termed Intralipid for treatment of local anesthetic systemic toxicity (LAST). Early basic science research by Weinberg et al. established that lipid emulsion successfully resuscitated rats and dogs from bupivacaine induced cardiac arrest [18, 19]. This work described the "lipid sink" theory of ILE, whereas ILE may act as an expanded lipid reservoir to sequester lipophilic bupivacaine away from cardiac myocytes [18]. Rosenblatt et al. described the first use of ILE for the treatment of cardiac arrest after bupivacaine and mepivacaine overdose [20]. Subsequently, Litz et al. reported the recovery of a perfusing cardiac rhythm with ILE after prolonged asystolic arrest following a ropivacaine overdose after axillary plexus block [21]. Given these promising developments, the role of ILE was expanded from the treatment of LAST to other toxic overdoses [17, 22]. Similar to bupivacaine, HCQ is lipophilic with a large volume of distribution [23] and blocks sodium channel function [24]. Experience with HCQ overdose is limited as there are few published case reports in the literature. Thus, resuscitation of HCQ overdose is managed similar to CQ overdose given their structural and toxidromal similarities [1]. A recent case report describes two cases of HCQ overdose in which ILE was utilized in the resuscitation [25]. Despite the standard resuscitation of these patients with sodium bicarbonate and diazepam, both died despite ILE infusion. The first case was a mixed overdose of HCQ and CQ in which the patient developed torsades des pointes that failed to respond to single bolus dose of 100 mL of 20% Intralipid. The second patient suffered from a cardiac arrest following a 20 mg HCQ overdose with the return of spontaneous circulation (ROSC) after cardiopulmonary resuscitation (CPR) for 5 minutes. A bolus dose of 100 mL of 10 Intralipid was given followed by 400 mL over 30 minutes. The patient subsequently developed wide complex tachycardia and cardiac arrest with ROSC after 25 minutes of CPR. Despite these interventions, the patient suffered another arrest and died. In both cases, the authors did not institute hemodialysis.

## 4. Conclusion

In conclusion, HCQ poisoning is rare but serious because of its rapid progression to life-threatening symptoms. Hemodynamic support, gastric decontamination, electrolyte monitoring and replacement, and management of arrhythmias are the mainstays of treatment. The combined role of dialysis and ILE in the setting of massive HCQ overdose may improve outcomes by extending the "lipid sink" effect of ILE and normalizing electrolyte concentrations.

## Conflict of Interests

The authors declare that there is no conflict of interests.

## Authors' Contribution

Paul B. McBeth, Perseus I. Missirlis, and Harry Brar were major contributors in writing the paper, providing the revisions, and creating the figures. Paul B. McBeth, Harry Brar, Perseus I. Missirlis, and Vinay Dhingra provided revisions and contributed to the writing and completion of the paper. Vinay Dhingra provided critical revisions and gave final approval of the version for publication. All the contributing authors have read and approved the final paper.

## References

[1] K. Marquardt and T. E. Albertson, "Treatment of hydroxychloroquine overdose," *American Journal of Emergency Medicine*, vol. 19, no. 5, pp. 420–424, 2001.

[2] P. Jordan, J. G. Brookes, G. Nikolic, and D. G. Le Counteur, "Hydroxycholoroquine overdose: toxicokinetics and management," *Journal of Toxicology. Clinical toxicology*, vol. 37, no. 7, pp. 861–864, 1997.

[3] G. K. Isbister, A. Dawson, and I. M. Whyte, "Hydroxychloroquine overdose: a prospective case series," *American Journal of Emergency Medicine*, vol. 20, no. 4, pp. 377–378, 2002.

[4] S. A. Pruchnicki, T. F. Good, and P. D. Walson, "Severe hydroxychloroquine poisoning reversed with diazepam," *Journal of Toxicology. Clinical Toxicology*, vol. 33, p. 582, 1996.

[5] D. N. Bateman, P. G. Blain, K. W. Woodhouse et al., "Pharmacokinetics and clinical toxicity of quinine overdosage: lack

of efficacy of techniques intended to enhance elimination," *Quarterly Journal of Medicine*, vol. 54, no. 214, pp. 125–131, 1985.

[6] J.-L. Clemessy, C. Favier, S. W. Borron, P. E. Hantson, E. Vicaut, and F. J. Baud, "Hypokalaemia related to acute chloroquine ingestion," *The Lancet*, vol. 346, no. 8979, pp. 877–880, 1995.

[7] D. Lockey and D. N. Bateman, "Effect of oral activated charcoal on quinine elimination," *British Journal of Clinical Pharmacology*, vol. 27, no. 1, pp. 92–94, 1989.

[8] L. F. Prescott, A. R. Hamilton, and R. Heyworth, "Treatment of quinine overdosage with repeated oral charcoal," *British Journal of Clinical Pharmacology*, vol. 27, no. 1, pp. 95–97, 1989.

[9] A. Jaeger, P. Sauder, J. Kopferschmitt, and F. Flesch, "Clinical features and management of poisoning due to antimalarial drugs," *Medical Toxicology and Adverse Drug Experience*, vol. 2, no. 4, pp. 242–273, 1987.

[10] J.-L. Clemessy, P. Taboulet, J. R. Hoffman et al., "Treatment of acute chloroquine poisoning: a 5-year experience," *Critical Care Medicine*, vol. 24, no. 7, pp. 1189–1195, 1996.

[11] J. L. Clemessy, S. W. Borron, and F. J. Baud, "Hypokalaemia and acute chloroquine ingestion—reply," *The Lancet*, vol. 347, no. 8998, pp. 404–405, 1996.

[12] J. L. Crouzette, E. Vicaut, S. Palombo, C. Girre, and P. E. Fournier, "Experimental assessment of the protective activity of diazepam on the acute toxicity of chloroquine," *Journal of Toxicology: Clinical Toxicology*, vol. 20, no. 3, pp. 271–279, 1983.

[13] J. Demaziere, J. M. Saissy, M. Vitris et al., "Effects of diazepam on mortality from acute chloroquine poisoning," *Annales Françaises d'Anesthèsie et de Rèanimation*, vol. 11, no. 2, pp. 164–167, 1992.

[14] J. Crouzette, E. Vicaut, S. Palombo, C. Girre, and P. E. Fournier, "Experimental assessment of the protective activity of diazepam on the acute toxicity of chloroquine," *Journal of Toxicology: Clinical Toxicology*, vol. 20, no. 3, pp. 271–279, 1983.

[15] F. Mongenot, Y. Tessier Gonthier, F. Derderian, M. Durand, and D. Blin, "Treatment of hydroxychloroquine poisoning with extracorporeal circulation," *Annales Francaises d'Anesthesie et de Reanimation*, vol. 26, no. 2, pp. 164–167, 2007.

[16] C.-Y. Chen, F.-L. Wang, and C.-C. Lin, "Chronic hydroxy-chloroquine use associated with QT prolongation and refractory ventricular arrhythmia," *Clinical Toxicology*, vol. 44, no. 2, pp. 173–175, 2006.

[17] L. Rothschild, S. Bern, S. Oswald, and G. Weinberg, "Intra-venous lipid emulsion in clinical toxicology," *Scandinavian Journal of Trauma, Resuscitation and Emergency Medicine*, vol. 18, no. 1, article 51, 2010.

[18] G. L. Weinberg, T. VadeBoncouer, G. A. Ramaraju, M. F. Garcia-Amaro, and M. J. Cwik, "Pretreatment or resuscitation with a lipid infusion shifts the dose-response to bupivacaine-induced asystole in rats," *Anesthesiology*, vol. 88, no. 4, pp. 1071–1075, 1998.

[19] G. Weinberg, R. Ripper, D. L. Feinstein, and W. Hoffman, "Lipid emulsion infusion rescues dogs from bupivacaine-induced cardiac toxicity," *Regional Anesthesia and Pain Medicine*, vol. 28, no. 3, pp. 198–202, 2003.

[20] M. A. Rosenblatt, M. Abel, G. W. Fischer, C. J. Itzkovich, and J. B. Eisenkraft, "Successful use of a 20% lipid emulsion to resuscitate a patient after a presumed bupivacaine-related cardiac arrest," *Anesthesiology*, vol. 105, no. 1, pp. 217–218, 2006.

[21] R. J. Litz, M. Popp, S. N. Stehr, and T. Koch, "Successful resuscitation of a patient with ropivacaine-induced asystole after axillary plexus block using lipid infusion," *Anaesthesia*, vol. 61, no. 8, pp. 800–801, 2006.

[22] A. J. Sirianni, K. C. Osterhoudt, D. P. Calello et al., "Use of lipid emulsion in the resuscitation of a patient with prolonged cardio-vascular collapse after overdose of bupropion and lamotrigine," *Annals of Emergency Medicine*, vol. 51, no. 4, pp. 412.e1–415.e1, 2008.

[23] H.-S. Lim, J.-S. Im, J.-Y. Cho et al., "Pharmacokinetics of hydroxychloroquine and its clinical implications in chemo-prophylaxis against malaria caused by *Plasmodium vivax*," *Antimicrobial Agents and Chemotherapy*, vol. 53, no. 4, pp. 1468–1475, 2009.

[24] P. F. Kolecki and S. C. Curry, "Poisoning by sodium channel blocking agents," *Critical Care Clinics*, vol. 13, no. 4, pp. 829–848, 1997.

[25] O. F. Wong, Y. C. Chan, S. K. Lam, H. T. Fung, and J. K. Y. Ho, "Clinical experience in the use of intravenous lipid emulsion in hydroychloroquine and chloroquine overdose with refractory shock," *Hong Kong Journal of Emergency Medicine*, vol. 18, no. 4, pp. 243–248, 2011.

# 32

# Rhabdomyolysis and Acute Renal Failure after Gardening

**Zeljko Vucicevic**

*Department of Internal Medicine, Intensive Care Unit, School of Medicine, "Sestre Milosrdnice" University Hospital Centre, University of Zagreb, Vinogradska Cesta 29, 10000 Zagreb, Croatia*

Correspondence should be addressed to Zeljko Vucicevic; zeljko.vucicevic@zg.t-com.hr

Academic Editor: Oludayo A. Sowande

Acute nontraumatic exertional rhabdomyolysis may arise when the energy supply to muscle is insufficient to meet demands, particularly in physically untrained individuals. We report on a psychiatric patient who developed large bruises and hemorrhagic blisters on both hands and arms, rhabdomyolysis of both forearm muscles with a moderate compartment syndrome, and consecutive acute renal failure following excessive work in the garden. Although specifically asked, the patient denied any hard physical work or gardening, and heteroanamnestic data were not available. The diagnosis of rhabdomyolysis was easy to establish, but until reliable anamnestic data were obtained, the etiology remained uncertain. Four days after arrival, the patient recalled working hard in the garden. The etiology of rhabdomyolysis was finally reached, and the importance of anamnestic data was once more confirmed.

## 1. Introduction

Acute nontraumatic exertional rhabdomyolysis may arise in individuals with normal muscles when the energy supply to muscles insufficiently meets demands [1]. Examples usually include ultramarathon races which may be aggravated by extremely hot, humid conditions particularly in physically untrained individuals [2]. Friction blisters on the palms and fingers frequently follow vigorous physical work or repetitive physical activities causing detachment of the skin epidermis. In more severe cases, particular areas of the skin can be entirely detached from the basis and blisters filled with blood. We report on a psychiatric patient who developed large bruises and hemorrhagic blisters on both hands and arms, rhabdomyolysis of both forearm muscles with a moderate compartment syndrome, and a consecutive acute renal failure following excessive work in the garden.

## 2. Case Report

A 55-year-old man was admitted to the intensive care unit because of bullae and hematomas of both hands and arms of unknown etiology (Figures 1 and 2).

Forearms were tense and swollen with large bruising of the skin. Hemorrhagic and nonhemorrhagic bullae were seen on the left palm and fingers. The patient was not capable of squeezing his left hand or of moving his fingers which was indicative of moderate compartment syndrome and nerve paresis. A few reddish skin indurations were visible on the front chest wall with no itching or burning sensation.

The patient had a history of long-term psychosis treatment with clozapine, haloperidol, alprazolam, and biperiden without other comorbidities. Upon arrival, he was alert, afebrile, eupneic, and normotensive and in a good general condition. No other abnormalities were noted at physical examination. The patient denied any trauma, hard physical work, contacts with chemicals, burns, cold, or alcohol and narcotic abuse. He also specifically denied any close contact with various kinds of plants or grasses.

Results of laboratory tests were as follows: C-reactive protein, red and white blood cell count, ECG, X-ray chest, blood sugar, electrolytes (K, Na, Cl, Ca, Mg, and P), and coagulation tests were within normal range. Results that lie outside the laboratory reference ranges are summarized in Table 1.

These laboratory findings were indicative of rhabdomyolysis and acute renal failure. The acid-base status of the capillary blood sample was still satisfying. Doppler ultrasound exam of both arms showed a normal arterial and venous

TABLE 1: The review of abnormal test results in serum (S) and urine (U).

| Test | Measured value | Reference values |
|------|----------------|------------------|
| Creatine phosphokinase (S) | 22626 U/L | <177 U/L |
| Aspartate transaminase (S) | 443 U/L | 11–38 U/L |
| Alanine aminotransferase (S) | 194 U/L | 12–48 U/L |
| Lactic acid dehydrogenase (S) | 930 U/L | <241 U/L |
| Creatinine (S) | 4.5 mg/dL<br>395 $\mu$mol/L | 0.9–1.4 mg/dL<br>79–125 $\mu$mol/L |
| Urine myoglobin (U) | 6780 $\mu$g/L | <30 $\mu$g/L |

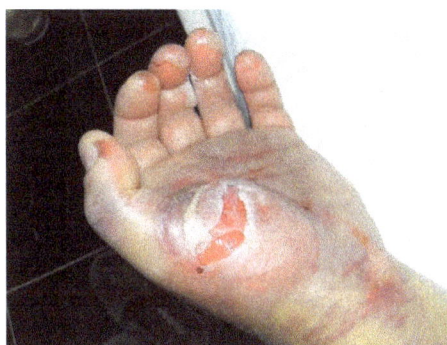

FIGURE 1: Hemorrhagic and nonhemorrhagic bullae, hematomas, and edema of the left palm.

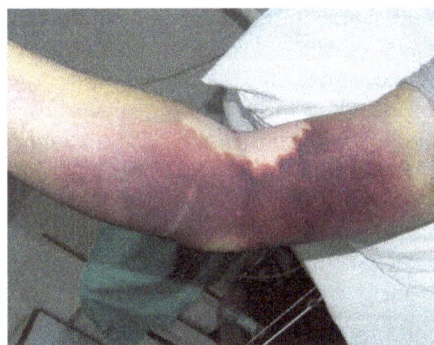

FIGURE 2: Large bruise and edema of the right arm and forearm.

blood flow. Nuclear magnetic resonance of both forearms revealed a diffuse edema of subcutaneous fat tissue and an extreme edema of forearm muscles (Figure 3).

The result of a chest and hand skin biopsy obtained later was unspecific and inconclusive. Bacteriological blister swabs were sterile. Serologic tests to antinuclear antibodies (ANA), rheumatoid factor (RF), and anti-Jo1 were negative.

The therapy consisted of an intensive fluid replacement, forced diuresis, antihistamine, and a surgical wound care.

On the fourth day of hospitalization, the patient suddenly recalled that he was pruning hedges with very small scissors and was pulling weeds with bare hands only 24 h before arrival to the hospital. On a hot day, stripped to the waist, he was entering into the bushes to reach the vegetation he wanted to cut, exposing his chest to pricking and prodding of sharp twigs and sprigs. After several hours of such a hard work, he noticed a few blisters and scratches on his hands, put the gloves on, and continued to work.

The five-day symptomatic treatment resulted in a moderate edema regression and completely restored renal function, and the patient was discharged. The full recovery occurred three weeks later.

## 3. Discussion

Bullae and blisters can be caused by various mechanical or environmental factors. One of the most known causes is friction that comes from using a various shovel or like in this case from grabbing hedges and weeds. The skin was directly traumatised and exposed to various flora, some of which

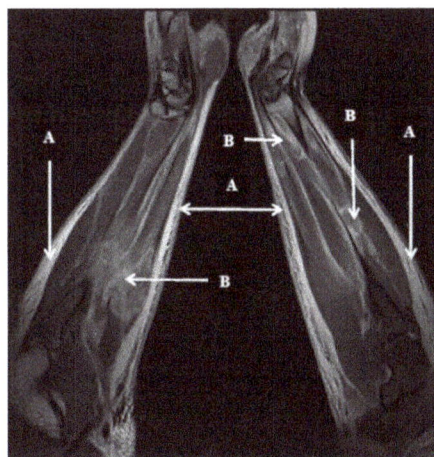

FIGURE 3: Coronal fat-suppressed proton density-weighted MR images of both forearms show diffuse hyperintensity in the subcutaneous fat tissue (A) and multifocal, confluent areas of hyperintensity in the muscles due to edema (B).

might have had toxic effect. Such an extreme physical activity is known to result in some degree of rhabdomyolysis.

Numerous causes of rhabdomyolysis can be classified into three main categories: traumatic, nontraumatic exertional (e.g., marked exertion in untrained individuals), and non-traumatic nonexertional (e.g., drugs or toxins, infections, or electrolyte disorders) [3].

Nontraumatic exertional rhabdomyolysis may follow significant physical exertion in physically untrained persons especially in extremely hot and/or humid conditions [4]. We believe that was what happened with our patient.

Hypokalemia caused by potassium loss from sweating may additionally induce impairment of muscle metabolism and contribute to muscle dysfunction [5], but in our patient the serum potassium level was normal.

Once it happens, rhabdomyolysis may lead to kidney failure. There are several mechanisms by which rhabdomyolysis impairs the glomerular filtration rate. The pathogenesis of rhabdomyolysis is based on muscle cell death, depletion of adenosine triphosphate (ATP), and an increase in free ionized calcium in the cytoplasm [6]. ATP depletion causes dysfunction of the Na/K-ATPase and $Ca^{2+}$ ATPase pumps that are essential to maintaining integrity of the myocyte.

The lesion of skeletal muscle results in subsequent release of toxic intracellular contents into the circulatory system including myoglobin, creatine phosphokinase, potassium, aldolase, lactate dehydrogenase, and glutamic-oxaloacetic transaminase [7]. Experimental evidence suggests that intrarenal vasoconstriction, direct and ischemic tubule injury, and tubular obstruction all play a role [6].

One of the possible complications of rhabdomyolysis is the compartment syndrome. If the energy-dependent transcellular pump systems fail in the traumatized tissue, the muscle cells swell. As a result, intracompartmental pressure rises and may provoke additional myocyte damage and necrosis [8].

Although more common in the anterior compartment of the lower leg, it has been described in the forearm of motocross racers [9] and in an elite flatwater sprint kayaker [10].

For the first couple of days, our patient was unable to squeeze his left hand or move his fingers as a consequence of muscle edema and nerve compression typical of the compartment syndrome.

The key problems in this case were unreliable anamnestic data taken from the psychiatric patient who lived alone and heteroanamnestic data that were not available. Since the clinical features were limited to both arms, we primarily suspected a working contact with potentially hazardous agent, but the reddish skin indurations on the front chest wall were additionally confusing. Although rather unusual after gardening, the diagnosis of rhabdomyolysis was easy to establish, but the etiology remained uncertain until reliable anamnestic data were obtained. Eliciting a reliable medical history that contributes to diagnosis requires a very careful and persistent approach when psychiatric patient is involved.

## Conflict of Interests

The author declares that there is no conflict of interests regarding the publication of this paper.

## References

[1] E. Keltz, F. Y. Khan, and G. Mann, "Rhabdomyolysis. The role of diagnostic and prognostic factors," *Muscles, Ligaments and Tendons Journal*, vol. 3, no. 4, pp. 303–312, 2013.

[2] K. P. Skenderi, S. A. Kavouras, C. A. Anastasiou, N. Yiannakouris, and A.-L. Matalas, "Exertional rhabdomyolysis during a 246-km continuous running race," *Medicine & Science in Sports & Exercise*, vol. 38, no. 6, pp. 1054–1057, 2006.

[3] A. L. Huerta-Alardín, J. Varon, and P. E. Marik, "Bench-to-bedside review: rhabdomyolysis—an overview for clinicians," *Critical Care*, vol. 9, no. 2, pp. 158–169, 2005.

[4] M. H. Trujillo and G. C. Fragachán, "Rhabdomyolysis and acute kidney injury due to severe heat stroke," *Case Reports in Critical Care*, vol. 2011, Article ID 951719, 4 pages, 2011.

[5] S. Agrawal, V. Agrawal, and A. Taneja, "Hypokalemia causing rhabdomyolysis resulting in life-threatening hyperkalemia," *Pediatric Nephrology*, vol. 21, no. 2, pp. 289–291, 2006.

[6] X. Bosch, E. Poch, and J. M. Grau, "Rhabdomyolysis and acute kidney injury," *The New England Journal of Medicine*, vol. 361, no. 1, pp. 62–72, 2009.

[7] V. Mršić, V. N. Adam, E. G. Stojčić, Ž. Rašić, A. Smiljanić, and I. Turčić, "Acute rhabdomyolysis: a case report and literature review," *Acta Medica Croatica*, vol. 62, no. 3, pp. 317–322, 2008.

[8] R. Vanholder, M. S. Sever, E. Erek, and N. Lameire, "Rhabdomyolysis," *Journal of the American Society of Nephrology*, vol. 11, no. 8, pp. 1553–1561, 2000.

[9] J. N. Goubier and G. Saillant, "Chronic compartment syndrome of the forearm in competitive motor cyclists: a report of two cases," *British Journal of Sports Medicine*, vol. 37, no. 5, pp. 452–453, 2003.

[10] D. P. Piasecki, D. Meyer, and B. R. Bach Jr., "Exertional compartment syndrome of the forearm in an elite flatwater sprint kayaker," *The American Journal of Sports Medicine*, vol. 36, no. 11, pp. 2222–2225, 2008.

# 33

# Body Packing: From Seizures to Laparotomy

**Joanna M. Janczak,**[1] **Ulrich Beutner,**[1] **and Karin Hasler**[2]

[1]*Department of General, Visceral and Transplantation Surgery, Kantonsspital St. Gallen, Rorschacherstrasse 95, 9007 St. Gallen, Switzerland*
[2]*Emergency Department, Kantonsspital St. Gallen, Rorschacherstrasse 95, 9007 St. Gallen, Switzerland*

Correspondence should be addressed to Joanna M. Janczak; joanna.janczak@kssg.ch

Academic Editor: Kalpesh Jani

Body packing is a common method for illegal drug trafficking. Complications associated with body packing can be severe and even lead to rapid death. Thus, a timely diagnosis is warranted. As most body packers initially do not show any symptoms, making a correct diagnosis can be rather challenging. We describe a case of a 41-year-old male, who was admitted with an epileptic seizure and who turned out to be a cocaine intoxicated body packer. Due to neurological and cardiovascular deterioration an emergency surgery was performed. Four bags of cocaine could be removed. We discuss the current management regimen in symptomatic and asymptomatic body packers and highlight pearls and pitfalls with diagnosis and treatment.

## 1. Introduction

Body packing refers to the practice of swallowing illegal drugs in small containers (typically plastic bags or condoms) for intestinal transport across country borders. Only a few percent of the body packers show clinical symptoms [1], but they can be associated with a broad spectrum of gastrointestinal, neurological, or cardiovascular complaints. Clinical manifestation depends on many factors such as type and amount of the drug, nature of container, duration of retention, grade of rupture, location in the gastrointestinal tract, or the general health of the courier. Diagnostic uncertainty and the lack of a medical history due to the patient's inability and unwillingness to collaborate make an accurate diagnosis in a timely fashion very challenging. Furthermore, radiological exams and laboratory tests are often inconclusive in these cases.

## 2. Case Description

A confused 41-year-old male was found in a park and brought to emergency department by the paramedics. During transit he had two generalized seizures. On the admission the patient appeared confused but conscious with a Glasgow Coma Scale of 13. He behaved aggressively and spoke neither English nor a local language. An interpreter was consulted, but the patient showed aggressive behaviour, therefore making it impossible to take a history. The physical examination was unremarkable except for a tongue bite and several bruises and scratches over the whole body. The pupils were moderately dilated and sluggishly reactive. All vital signs were stable (heart rate: 108 beats per minute, blood pressure: 123/80 mmHg, oxygen saturation: 98% at room air with a normal respiratory rate, and a body core temperature of 37.2°C). Laboratory tests revealed a leukocytosis of 25.1 G/L, elevated values for C-reactive protein (12 mg/L), creatinine kinase (2185 U/L), myoglobin (618 $\mu$g/L), creatinine (143 mmol/L), and uric acid (1344 mmol/L) suggesting renal insufficiency. Electrolytes, liver enzymes, troponin I, coagulation, and haematology were in the normal range. An electrocardiogram showed a sinus tachycardia. Neurology service was consulted because of ongoing confusion and for assessment of epilepsy. A cranial CT scan ruled out haemorrhage or other focal lesions. Lorazepam (2 mg, IV) was administered twice with no effect on his neurological status. The patient started to sweat and became hypertensive (systolic blood pressure of 180 mmHg) and more tachycardic (heart rate of 140/min). A drug screening (Triage 8) was performed, which was positive for

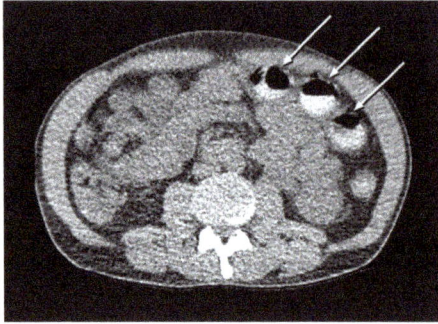

FIGURE 1: CT scan showing three of four, round, foreign bodies (arrows) in the left transverse colon.

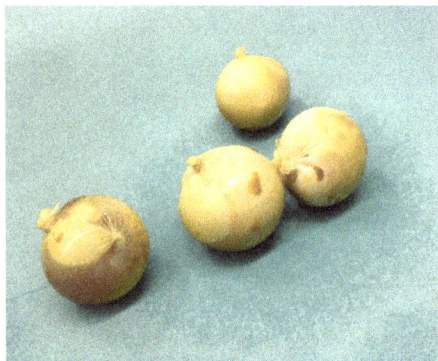

FIGURE 2: Foreign bodies removed from the colon.

cocaine. Finally he admitted the cocaine consumption but refused to give further information. Benzodiazepines as well as phentolamine were given. In order to further investigate the drug intoxication a plain abdominal dual-energy CT scan was requested. Four round, hyperdense, foreign bodies were found in the transverse colon (Figure 1).

An emergency laparotomy was indicated and carried out immediately. Following colotomy four packages (Figure 2) were removed. Thorough exploration revealed no further packages. The procedure took 60 minutes and postoperatively the patient was on observation for 24 h in the intensive care unit. The neurological signs as well as the renal insufficiency improved rapidly under conservative therapy. The further clinical course was unremarkable, and the patient was discharged six days after surgery.

## 3. Discussion

Internal concealment of illegal drugs is increasingly seen even outside bigger cities without international airports. Clinical symptoms due to complications associated with body packing are rare as 1.4 to 6.6% [2–5] probably owing to improvements in drug wrapping [6]. However, it must be highlighted that mortality can be as high as 56%, when symptoms occur [6]. Typical cardiovascular complications such as tachycardia, ventricular fibrillation, hypertension, myocardial infarction, or even cardiac arrest occur in around 75% of body packers.

Neurological signs comprise anxiety, seizures, or altered consciousness often associated with agitation and anxiety as well as coma. Gastrointestinal symptoms are mostly related to bowel obstruction occurring in 25% of cases [7]. Drug container rupture leads to rapid intestinal drug absorption with possible fatal consequences [3]. Interestingly, the number of drugs packages does not correlate with the rate of perforation [8]. The reported rate of surgical removal of drug bags due to failure of spontaneous intestinal passage is up to 5% [8]. Often patient's history is unreliable and the diagnosis of body packing is solely based on the physician's intuition. Physical examination, radiological findings, and laboratory test are mandatory in confirming or rejecting the suspected diagnosis. Physical examination should begin with the classical ABCDE survey. Although Beckley et al. [3] found that physical examination was unremarkable in 81% of the cases, a thorough neurological, abdominal, and rectal examination preceding diagnostic imaging is crucial [9]. General laboratory work including urea, electrolytes, liver enzymes as well as coagulation, and haematology should be obtained. We also performed a 12-lead ECG to detect arrhythmias or myocardial ischemia.

Plain radiography and contrast enhanced computer tomography are recommended radiological examinations. An abdominal CT scan is preferable due to the better specificity and sensitivity, especially for the detection of liquid cocaine, which is practically invisible on normal X-ray images [3, 4]. Sensitivity of plain abdominal X-rays, however, can be as low as 40% [9]. Current drug packaging made of nonradiopaque materials is generally difficult to detect radiologically [10]. False positive results were observed because of bladder stones, other calcifications, or coprostasis [8]. Low-dose CT seems to be an effective alternative to abdominal radiography [11].

Urine tests for rapid drug screening can be useful in symptomatic patients but yield false negative results in 48% of asymptomatic patients [12]. While some authors oppose urine drug tests due to their poor sensitivity of 37% [8], other authors report a sensitivity of up to 96.3% and a specificity of up to 99.8% and recommend routine use prior to radiological examinations [6].

Asymptomatic body packers should be monitored closely, preferably on an intermediate or intensive care unit, allowing for a quick response in case of complications or clinical deterioration. Asymptomatic patients should be started on activated charcoal, which reduces the lethality in oral cocaine intoxication [8]. Bowel irrigation with polyethylene glycol can be used to induce purging of the body bags [8, 13, 14].

Oily laxatives should not be applied due to the high risk of perforating the latex wrapping [8, 14]. The recommended observation time in case of extended intestinal passage varies between 72 hours and 7 days [2, 3].

One should not attempt to remove the drug containers endoscopically as this can result in ruptures [2, 8]. However, some successful gastroscopic bag recoveries from the upper gastrointestinal tract were reported [2, 8]. In the study of Schaper et al. [4] the average length of hospital stay ranged from 2.8 days for conservatively treated body packers to 10.4 days for surgically treated body packers.

Indications for surgery are signs of intoxication, bowel obstruction, and extended intestinal passage (over 48 hours and suspected leakage) [1, 2]. Immediate surgery is vital in these patients. In the study of Schaper et al. [4], only 32% of the symptomatic patients survived until the operation, and the majority died before the intervention could begin. This holds true in cases of cocaine intoxication especially, since no antidote is available [5, 7]. A relative indication for surgery is failure of intestinal passage for more than five days according to Silverberg et al. [10].

Other rare emergency situations were gastric outlet syndrome, gastrointestinal ulceration, or bleeding as well as respiratory arrest due to airway obstruction by the containers [10]. Whether preemptive surgery should be performed in asymptomatic body packers is still under debate. A prophylactic operation was recommended few years ago for unsophisticated drug containers due to the high risk of rupture [8].

According to Bogusz et al. [12] a preemptive surgery should be reserved for symptomatic patients because in asymptomatic patients the risks related to surgery outweigh the risks of conservative therapy. Intraoperative morbidity and mortality were estimated to be up to 16% and 2%, respectively [2]. The preferred surgical approach for bag retrieval is by enterotomy. The number of enterotomies correlates with the surgical site infection rate (up to 40%) [10]. If the bags are located more distally in the colon or in the rectum, they can be pushed towards and through the anus without performing an enterotomy [2, 10].

Radiological imaging should be repeated after the operation to document removal of all containers [8].

## 4. Conclusion

Diagnostic uncertainty related to the lack of a good medical history as well as the diversity of clinical symptoms challenges the clinical management of body packers. It is generally advisable to perform an abdominal CT scan while urine drug tests seem to be less reliable in confirming the suspected diagnosis. Although most body packers remain asymptomatic, a close monitoring is crucial. Clinical deterioration can be sudden and requires immediate laparotomy and enterotomy. As long as there are no official guidelines for the clinical management of body packers, every hospital should set up its own diagnostic and treatment algorithms, since any delay in treatment can be fatal.

## Conflict of Interests

The authors declare no conflict of interests regarding the publication of this paper.

## References

[1] G. M. Eisen, T. H. Baron, J. A. Dominitz et al., "Guideline for the management of ingested foreign bodies," *Gastrointestinal Endoscopy*, vol. 55, no. 7, pp. 802–806, 2002.

[2] S. A. de Beer, G. Spiessens, W. Mol, and P. R. Fa-Si-Oen, "Surgery for body packing in the Caribbean: a retrospective study of 70 patients," *World Journal of Surgery*, vol. 32, no. 2, pp. 281–285, 2008.

[3] I. Beckley, N. A. A. Ansari, H. A. Khwaja, and Y. Mohsen, "Clinical management of cocaine body packers: the Hillingdon experience," *Canadian Journal of Surgery*, vol. 52, no. 5, pp. 417–421, 2009.

[4] A. Schaper, R. Hofmann, P. Bargain, H. Desel, M. Ebbecke, and C. Langer, "Surgical treatment in cocaine body packers and body pushers," *International Journal of Colorectal Disease*, vol. 22, no. 12, pp. 1531–1535, 2007.

[5] N. Mandava, R. S. Chang, J. H. Wang et al., "Establishment of a definitive protocol for the diagnosis and management of body packers (drug mules)," *Emergency Medicine Journal*, vol. 28, no. 2, pp. 98–101, 2011.

[6] J. K. de Bakker, P. W. B. Nanayakkara, L. M. G. Geeraedts Jr., E. S. M. de Lange, M. O. MacKintosh, and H. J. Bonjer, "Body packers: a plea for conservative treatment," *Langenbeck's Archives of Surgery*, vol. 397, no. 1, pp. 125–130, 2012.

[7] N. de Prost, A. Lefebvre, F. Questel et al., "Prognosis of cocaine body-packers," *Intensive Care Medicine*, vol. 31, no. 7, pp. 955–958, 2005.

[8] S. J. Traub, R. S. Hoffman, and L. S. Nelson, "Body packing—the internal concealment of illicit drugs," *The New England Journal of Medicine*, vol. 349, no. 26, pp. 2519–2526, 2003.

[9] R.-A. Yegane, M. Bashashati, E. Hajinasrollah, K. Heidari, N.-A. Salehi, and M. Ahmadi, "Surgical approach to body packing," *Diseases of the Colon and Rectum*, vol. 52, no. 1, pp. 97–103, 2009.

[10] D. Silverberg, T. Menes, and U. Kim, "Surgery for 'body packers'—a 15-year experience," *World Journal of Surgery*, vol. 30, no. 4, pp. 541–546, 2006.

[11] P.-A. Poletti, L. Canel, C. D. Becker et al., "Screening of illegal intracorporeal containers ('body packing'): is abdominal radiography sufficiently accurate? A comparative study with low-dose CT," *Radiology*, vol. 265, no. 3, pp. 772–779, 2012.

[12] M. J. Bogusz, H. Althoff, M. Erkens, R.-D. Maier, and R. Hofmann, "Internally concealed cocaine: analytical and diagnostic aspects," *Journal of Forensic Sciences*, vol. 40, no. 5, pp. 811–815, 1995.

[13] G. Macedo and T. Ribeiro, "Esophageal obstruction and endoscopic removal of a cocaine packet," *American Journal of Gastroenterology*, vol. 96, no. 5, pp. 1656–1657, 2001.

[14] R. J. Booker, J. E. Smith, and M. P. Rodger, "Packers, pushers and stuffers-managing patients with concealed drugs in UK emergency departments: a clinical and medicolegal review," *Emergency Medicine Journal*, vol. 26, no. 5, pp. 316–320, 2009.

# 34

# A Woman with Unilateral Rash and Fever: Cellulitis in the Setting of Lymphedema

**Melissa Joseph, Marissa Camilon, and Tarina Kang**

*Department of Emergency Medicine, LAC+USC Medical Center, 1200 N. State Street, Los Angeles, CA 90033, USA*

Correspondence should be addressed to Melissa Joseph; mjoseph@dhs.lacounty.gov

Academic Editor: Kazuhito Imanaka

Cellulitis in the setting of lymphedema is an uncommon but clinically important presentation to the emergency department. Stagnant lymph is an ideal medium for bacterial growth and progression can be rapid due to decreased ability to fight infection in the affected area. Infections are commonly caused by gram-positive cocci, though blood cultures are often negative. Treatment should be aimed at rapid initiation of antibiotics targeting these species. There may be a role for antibiotic prophylaxis in recurrent cases.

## 1. Introduction

Cellulitis is a common presenting complaint to the emergency department (ED). Lymphedema cellulitis is a less common presentation of cellulitis, but it is important to recognize due to its aggressive onset, potential for recurrence, and increased risk of treatment failure [1, 2]. Patients with damaged or surgically removed lymphatic beds are at increased risk for cellulitis secondary to impairment of both lymphatic flow and elimination of phagocytosed bacteria [1, 3]. We present a case of cellulitis in the setting of previous axillary lymph node dissection and lymphedema.

## 2. Case

A 46 year-old female with a history of left breast invasive ductal carcinoma (PT 4bN3a) with axillary metastasis presented with one day of fever, chills, and a painful rash over her left arm, breast, and back (Figures 1(a) and 1(b)). Her cancer treatment consisted of axillary lymph node dissection two years prior and a breast TRAM flap reconstruction without implant. She received four cycles of Adriamycin and Cytoxan and twelve cycles of taxol in addition to radiotherapy, which was completed more than a year prior to her presentation to the ED. She was currently taking tamoxifen.

Examination revealed erythematous, warm, indurated skin over the left upper arm, chest, abdomen, and left back that did not cross the midline aside from a small portion below the umbilicus. Exam was not significant for a fluctuant mass. A bedside ultrasound did not show a focal fluid collection, or a deep venous thrombosis in her upper extremity. Her vital signs were a temperature of 39.5 C; heart rate of 105 beats per minute; and a respiratory rate of 25 breaths per minute. Serum laboratory values were significant for a WBC of 20.6 K/cumm with 94.9% neutrophils, a C-reactive protein of 145.5 mg/dL, and an erythrocyte sedimentation rate (ESR) of 49 mm/hr.

Initial differential diagnosis included cellulitis, drug eruption, necrotizing soft tissue infection, erythroderma, cutaneous T-cell lymphoma, and toxic shock syndrome. A computed tomography (CT) scan of the chest and abdomen with intravenous (IV) contrast showed inflammation adjacent to the TRAM flap reconstruction site and in the subcutaneous tissues of the anterior abdominal wall.

She was diagnosed with lymphedema cellulitis in the ED and admitted to the hospital. She was started on IV ceftriaxone and vancomycin, which was continued for five days until she was transitioned to oral ciprofloxacin and trimethoprim-sulfamethoxazole. She was discharged on hospital day #5 and completed an additional 5-day course of the oral antibiotics. Punch biopsy showed perivascular and interstitial dermatitis with neutrophils. Blood and biopsy cultures were negative for bacterial growth. At her follow-up appointment, she reported complete resolution of her symptoms.

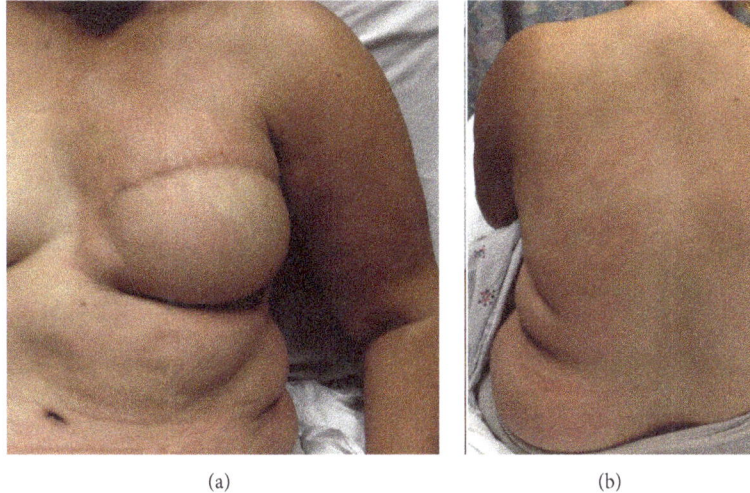

(a)                                                     (b)

FIGURE 1: Lymphedema cellulitis.

## 3. Discussion

Approximately 200 million persons worldwide suffer from lymphedema, with filariasis being the most common cause [4]. Lymphedema affects women more than men and can range from subclinical impairment of lymphatic drainage to reversible pitting edema, irreversible brawny edema, or elephantiasis. In developed nations, lymphedema is predominantly caused by lymphadenectomy [4]. Axillary lymph node dissection remains the mainstay of staging and treatment planning in patients with breast cancer, and thus damage to and/or removal of the axillary lymph nodes is not uncommon [1]. Lymphedema acts as an ideal medium for bacterial growth, likely due to decreased lymphatic flow and impaired elimination of phagocytosed bacteria [1, 3]. Patients with cellulitis complicating lymphedema can have abrupt onset of symptoms and tend to have a longer duration of the inflammatory response, manifested by fevers, erythema at the site, and tachycardia [3, 5]. Lymphedema has also been found to be an independent risk factor for cellulitis treatment failure [2].

Patients who have undergone lymph node dissection alone are at increased lifelong risk for cellulitis, and those with lymphedema are at even higher risk [1, 6]. Additional risk factors include a history of a radical hysterectomy, mastectomy, radiation therapy, or lymphatic filariasis [3]. Patients who present status post lumpectomy and radiation, which is becoming increasingly more common as cancers are detected in earlier stages, tend to develop cellulitis earlier than those who have had a mastectomy or other more aggressive initial interventions, for reasons that remain unclear [1]. Increased risk for cellulitis is seen in those with more severe lymphedema, and also in those who develop lymphedema more than one year following surgery [1]. As was seen in our patient, lymphedema and cellulitis involving the ipsilateral trunk can also develop following mastectomy secondary to the lymphatic track it shares with the axilla [7].

Patients should be counseled to avoid trauma or blood draws to the affected extremity, employ frequent handwashing, and take measures to protect against skin breaks from daily activities such as handwashing with protective gloves and liberal moisturizing [6]. Sentinel lymph node biopsy instead of initial axillary lymph node dissection may also decrease the risk of lymphedema cellulitis from occurring as it has been associated with less lymphedema overall [8].

In addition to a complete blood count, procalcitonin and C-reactive protein (CRP) have been discussed in the literature as potentially useful lab values. Procalcitonin is a polypeptide hormone that is associated with infection and inflammation in patients. [9] CRP is an inflammatory marker that has been heavily investigated due to its potential to determine disease progress and effectiveness of treatment [10].

Treatment consists of antibiotics to cover gram-positive cocci, most commonly non-group A streptococcus [1, 8]. Blood cultures are typically negative, which is thought to be due to the large numbers of cytokines and lymphokines present in lymph [3, 11]. Early initiation of antibiotics is ideal, as cessation of bacterial multiplication may help prevent further damage to the lymphatic drainage system [3]. Additionally, because much of the skin reaction and fever is thought to be secondary to the antigenic response, anti-inflammatory medications may be of benefit [11]. Hospital admission is recommended for patients with signs of sepsis, who have failed outpatient oral antibiotics, or fail to respond to first or second line antibiotics [8]. Antibiotics should be continued until all signs of infection have resolved with a minimum course of 14 days [5]. Recommended initial oral regimens include amoxicillin and clindamycin as first and second line treatments, respectively. Initial IV antibiotic regimens should cover both streptococcus and staphylococcus species [5].

Many patients with lymphedema cellulitis will have recurrent episodes [1, 3, 5, 12, 13]. Long-acting depot penicillin or daily low-dose oral clindamycin or penicillin V has been suggested as prophylactic options, though penicillin use is limited by rising resistance [5, 14, 15]. Alternatively, decongestive lymphatic therapy has been shown to significantly reduce lymphedema and cellulitis recurrence [5, 12]. A recent study also showed a reduction in recurrent lymphedema cellulitis following lymphaticovenular anastomosis [13].

In addition to increased risk of infection, the immune dysfunction associated with lymphedema can lead to malignancy. The most commonly described malignancy is an angiosarcoma, commonly called Stewart-Treves syndrome, which presents as multiple reddish-blue macules or nodules. Additional associated malignancies include Kaposi sarcoma, basal cell carcinoma, and squamous cell carcinoma [16].

In conclusion, lymphedema cellulitis is a clinically important presentation to the emergency department. Our case represents a scenario of truncal and upper extremity lymphedema and infection following axillary lymph node dissection and mastectomy for breast cancer. In addition to rapid onset of symptoms and systemic response, patients with lymphedema cellulitis are at risk for prolonged symptoms, treatment failure, and recurrent episodes.

## Conflict of Interests

The authors declare that there is no conflict of interests regarding the publication of this paper.

## References

[1] M. S. Simon and R. L. Cody, "Cellulitis after axillary lymph node dissection for carcinoma of the breast," *The American Journal of Medicine*, vol. 93, no. 5, pp. 543–548, 1992.

[2] D. Peterson, S. McLeod, K. Woolfrey, and A. McRae, "Predictors of failure of empiric outpatient antibiotic therapy in emergency department patients with uncomplicated cellulitis," *Academic Emergency Medicine*, vol. 21, no. 5, pp. 526–531, 2014.

[3] P. C. Y. Woo, P. N. L. Lum, S. S. Y. Wong, V. C. C. Cheng, and K. Y. Yuen, "Cellulitis complicating lymphoedema," *European Journal of Clinical Microbiology and Infectious Diseases*, vol. 19, no. 4, pp. 294–297, 2000.

[4] J. A. Carlson, "Lymphedema and subclinical lymphostasis (microlymphedema) facilitate cutaneous infection, inflammatory dermatoses, and neoplasia: a locus minoris resistentiae," *Clinics in Dermatology*, vol. 32, no. 5, pp. 599–615, 2014.

[5] V. Keely, P. Mortimer, J. Welsh et al., *Consensus Document on the Management of Cellulitis in Lymphoedema*, British Lymphoma Society, 2013, http://www.thebls.com/consensus.php.

[6] G. Bertelli, D. Dini, G. G. Forno, and A. Gozza, "Preventing cellulitis after axillary lymph node dissection," *The American Journal of Medicine*, vol. 97, no. 2, pp. 202–203, 1994.

[7] C. C. Roberts, J. R. Levick, A. W. B. Stanton, and P. S. Mortimer, "Assessment of truncal edema following breast cancer treatment using modified Harpenden skinfold calipers," *Lymphology*, vol. 28, no. 2, pp. 78–88, 1995.

[8] A. Husted Madsen, K. Haugaard, J. Soerensen et al., "Arm morbidity following sentinel lymph node biopsy or axillary lymph node dissection: a study from the Danish Breast Cancer Cooperative Group," *The Breast*, vol. 17, no. 2, pp. 138–147, 2008.

[9] C. Oh, S. M. Pang, M. P. Chlebicki, Z. Ho, and T. Thirumoorthy, "Cellulitis: making the right diagnosis and its management: a Singapore experience," *Hong Kong Journal of Dermatology and Venereology*, vol. 20, no. 1, pp. 13–19, 2012.

[10] C. Pitsavos, D. B. Panagiotakos, N. Tzima et al., "Diet, exercise, and C-reactive protein levels in people with abdominal obesity: the ATTICA Epidemiological Study," *Angiology*, vol. 58, no. 2, pp. 225–233, 2007.

[11] E. Martinez, A. Marcos, and P. Domingo, "Cellulitis after axillary lymph node dissection," *The American Journal of Medicine*, vol. 97, no. 2, pp. 201–202, 1994.

[12] L. M. Baddour, "Recent considerations in recurrent cellulitis," *Current Infectious Disease Reports*, vol. 3, no. 5, pp. 461–465, 2001.

[13] M. Mihara, H. Hara, D. Furniss et al., "Lymphaticovenular anastomosis to prevent cellulitis associated with lymphoedema," *British Journal of Surgery*, vol. 101, no. 11, pp. 1391–1396, 2014.

[14] M. P. Chlebicki and C. C. Oh, "Recurrent cellulitis: risk factors, etiology, pathogenesis and treatment," *Current Infectious Disease Reports*, vol. 16, no. 9, article 422, 2014.

[15] M. S. Klempner and B. Styrt, "Prevention of recurrent staphylococcal skin infections with low-dose oral clindamycin therapy," *The Journal of the American Medical Association*, vol. 260, no. 18, pp. 2682–2685, 1988.

[16] R. Lee, K. M. Saardi, and R. A. Schwartz, "Lymphedema-related angiogenic tumors and other malignancies," *Clinics in Dermatology*, vol. 32, no. 5, pp. 616–620, 2014.

# 35

# Elevated Intracranial Pressure Diagnosis with Emergency Department Bedside Ocular Ultrasound

**D. Amin, T. McCormick, and T. Mailhot**

*Department of Emergency Medicine, Los Angeles County-University of Southern California, Los Angeles, CA 90033, USA*

Correspondence should be addressed to T. McCormick; taylormccormick@gmail.com

Academic Editor: Chih Cheng Lai

Bedside sonographic measurement of optic nerve sheath diameter can aid in the diagnosis of elevated intracranial pressure in the emergency department. This case report describes a 21-year-old female presenting with 4 months of mild headache and 2 weeks of recurrent, transient binocular vision loss. Though limited by patient discomfort, fundoscopic examination suggested the presence of blurred optic disc margins. Bedside ocular ultrasound (BOUS) revealed wide optic nerve sheath diameters and bulging optic discs bilaterally. Lumbar puncture demonstrated a cerebrospinal fluid (CSF) opening pressure of 54 cm $H_2O$ supporting the suspected diagnosis of idiopathic intracranial hypertension. Accurate fundoscopy can be vital to the appropriate diagnosis and treatment of patients with suspected elevated intracranial pressure, but it is often technically difficult or poorly tolerated by the photophobic patient. BOUS is a quick and easily learned tool to supplement the emergency physician's fundoscopic examination and help identify patients with elevated intracranial pressure.

## 1. Introduction

Visual complaints are common in the emergency department (ED), and many ocular emergencies are time sensitive [1]. However, the proper diagnosis and management of ocular emergencies by emergency physicians can be limited by lack of sophisticated tools and training. Ocular ultrasound is considered to be a core indication for emergency ultrasound by the American College of Emergency Physicians [2], and bedside ocular ultrasound (BOUS) is becoming a vital aspect of the eye exam for patients with eye complaints. BOUS is sensitive for the diagnosis of retinal detachment (RD) and may have a role in excluding RD in patients presenting to the ED with "floaters," "flashes," and vision loss [3–5]. Another promising application of BOUS is the assessment of optic nerve sheath diameter in patients with suspected intracranial hypertension. A prospective study of ICU patients with intracranial pressure monitors in place showed a strong correlation between an optic nerve sheath diameter of more than 5 mm and intracranial pressure greater than 20 cm $H_2O$ [5]. We describe a case of a young female presenting with long-standing headache and vision loss. BOUS revealed widened and bulging optic nerve sheaths bilaterally, and

she was subsequently diagnosed with idiopathic intracranial hypertension.

## 2. Case Report

A 21-year-old female with no past medical history presented to the ED complaining of 2 weeks of recurrent, transient binocular vision loss. The episodes lasted approximately 30 seconds and were increasing in frequency, occurring 6 times on the day of presentation. In between episodes, the patient reported normal vision. On further questioning, the patient reported a mild throbbing headache for 4 months. The pain started in the upper neck and radiated to the top of the head and bilateral shoulders like an electric shock; it was worse with bending forward. She denied photophobia, nausea, vomiting, fevers, chills, neck stiffness, numbness, or weakness. She was taking no medications or oral contraceptives. She had no personal or family history of venous thromboembolism. On physical examination her temperature was 37.2°C, heart rate 69 beats/min, respiration rate 16 breaths/min, and blood pressure 105/69 mmHg. Finger-stick glucose was 84 mg/dL. Her corrected visual acuity was 20/25 in her right

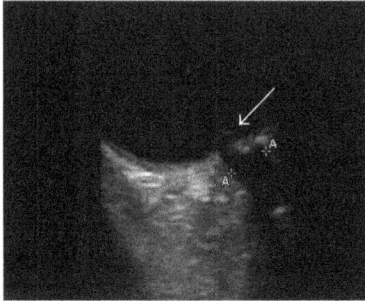

FIGURE 1: Bedside ocular ultrasound of the right eye demonstrating bulging of the optic nerve cup, indicative of papilledema.

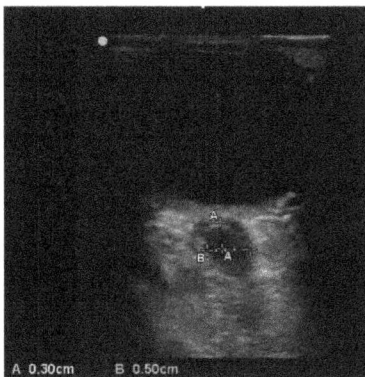

FIGURE 2: Bedside ocular ultrasound of the patient's left eye demonstrating optic nerve sheath diameter (ONSD) measurement. The measurement of the ONSD is taken 3 mm posterior to the globe and occurs perpendicular to the long axis of the optic nerve.

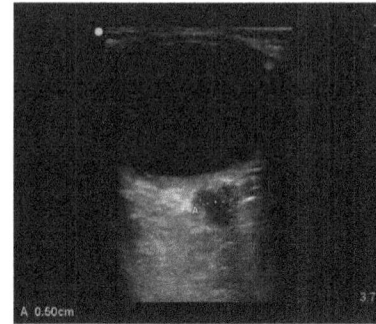

(a)

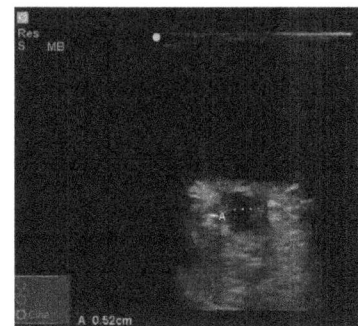

(b)

FIGURE 3: Bedside ocular ultrasound of left (a) and right (b) eyes, showing measurement of optic nerve sheath diameter. Measurements are 5 mm and 5.2 mm, respectively.

eye and 20/25 in her left eye. Her extraocular motions were intact and pupils were equally round and reactive to light and accommodation. Visual fields were intact. Fundoscopic examination was poorly tolerated due to patient discomfort; however, there appeared to be optic disc edema bilaterally. She had no nuchal rigidity, and Kernig and Brudzinski signs were negative. The remainder of her HEENT, cardiovascular, pulmonary, abdominal, and neurologic examinations were normal.

BOUS was performed using a 13–6 MHz linear array transducer (SonoSite M-Turbo, Bothell, WA). It showed a hyperechoic prominence protruding into the posterior chamber at the location of the optic nerve (Figure 1). The optic nerve sheath diameter measured 3 mm posterior to the globe was 5.0 mm in the right eye and 5.2 mm in the left eye (Figures 2 and 3). Noncontrast computed tomography of the brain was unremarkable. Opening cerebrospinal fluid pressure during lumbar puncture was 540 mm $H_2O$. The patient's headache improved significantly after the lumbar puncture. Neurology was consulted and recommended starting the patient on acetazolamide. MRI without contrast was normal and her symptoms were well controlled on acetazolamide 3 months later.

## 3. Discussion

Physical examination of the eye is significantly limited in patients who are photophobic, intubated, or unable to follow commands, and accurate detection of papilledema can be technically difficult even in a cooperative patient. Furthermore, papilledema may be delayed after elevations in intracranial pressure (ICP) by several hours to days [7]. A small prospective study of head injured patients with suspected intracranial injury found that an optic nerve sheath diameter of >5 mm was 100% sensitive (95% CI 68 to 100%) for the presence of elevated ICP [8]. These findings suggest that BOUS may have an even more important role in detecting acute increased ICP than the fundoscopic exam. However, the possibility of elevated ICP without papilledema or increased ONSD should be considered in the appropriate clinical context.

Anatomically, the optic nerve is a part of the central nervous system, which is surrounded by the dura mater, the subarachnoid space, and cerebrospinal fluid; therefore, any change in ICP affects the optic nerve sheath, changing its diameter. Helmke and Hansen first described the use of ocular ultrasound to detect increased ICP in cadavers in 1996 [9]. Blaivas et al. described close correlation between optic nerve sheath dilation and CT evidence of elevated ICP in ED patients with head trauma and spontaneous intracranial hemorrhage [10]. The relationship between ONSD and ICP has been well established and this case report contributes to the rising body of evidence that elevated ICP can be rapidly and noninvasively detected using BOUS.

Bulging of the optic nerve into the posterior chamber was also seen on BOUS in this patient. While ONSD has been studied in several prospective trials, data on optic disc bulging into the posterior chamber is limited to case reports [6, 11]. This finding may be a more direct sonographic correlate to the physical exam finding of papilledema than ONSD, but further research is needed to determine its significance.

While elevated ICP may be the most concerning and time sensitive cause of a widened ONSD and optic disc bulging for the emergency physician, inflammatory, infectious, and ischemic diseases of the optic nerve can result in similar BOUS findings [6] and should be considered in the appropriate clinic setting.

## Conflict of Interests

The authors declare that there is no conflict of interests regarding the publication of this paper.

## References

[1] G. D. Khare, R. C. Andrew Symons, and D. V. Do, "Common ophthalmic emergencies," *International Journal of Clinical Practice*, vol. 62, no. 11, pp. 1776–1784, 2008.

[2] American College of Emergency Physicians, *Emergency Ultrasound Guidelines 2008*, 2013, http://www.acep.org/.

[3] R. Yoonessi, A. Hussain, and T. B. Jang, "Bedside ocular ultrasound for the detection of retinal detachment in the emergency department," *Academic Emergency Medicine*, vol. 17, no. 9, pp. 913–917, 2010.

[4] M. Blaivas, D. Theodoro, and P. R. Sierzenski, "A study of bedside ocular ultrasonography in the emergency department," *Academic Emergency Medicine*, vol. 9, no. 8, pp. 791–799, 2002.

[5] H. H. Kimberly, S. Shah, K. Marill, and V. Noble, "Correlation of optic nerve sheath diameter with direct measurement of intracranial pressure," *Academic Emergency Medicine*, vol. 15, no. 2, pp. 201–204, 2008.

[6] S. Daulaire, L. Fine, M. Salmon et al., "Ultrasound assessment of optic disc edema in patients with headache," *American Journal of Emergency Medicine*, vol. 30, no. 8, pp. 1654.e1–1654.e4, 2012.

[7] H. Steffen, B. Eifert, A. Aschoff, G. H. Kolling, and H. E. Volcker, "The diagnostic value of optic disc evaluation in acute elevated intracranial pressure," *Ophthalmology*, vol. 103, no. 8, pp. 1229–1232, 1996.

[8] V. S. Tayal, M. Neulander, H. J. Norton, T. Foster, T. Saunders, and M. Blaivas, "Emergency department sonographic measurement of optic nerve sheath diameter to detect findings of increased intracranial pressure in adult head injury patients," *Annals of Emergency Medicine*, vol. 49, no. 4, pp. 508–514, 2007.

[9] H. C. Hansen and K. Helmke, "The subarachnoid space surrounding the optic nerves. An ultrasound study of the optic nerve sheath," *Surgical and Radiologic Anatomy*, vol. 18, no. 4, pp. 323–328, 1996.

[10] M. Blaivas, D. Theodoro, and P. R. Sierzenski, "Elevated intracranial pressure detected by bedside emergency ultrasonography of the optic nerve sheath," *Academic Emergency Medicine*, vol. 10, no. 4, pp. 376–381, 2003.

[11] M. B. Stone, "Ultrasound diagnosis of papilledema and increased intracranial pressure in pseudotumor cerebri," *The American Journal of Emergency Medicine*, vol. 27, no. 3, pp. 376.e1–376.e2, 2009.

# 36

# Herbal Weight Loss Pill Overdose: Sibutramine Hidden in Pepper Pill

**Gul Pamukcu Gunaydin,**[1] **Nurettin Ozgur Dogan,**[2]
**Sevcan Levent,**[3] **and Gulhan Kurtoglu Celik**[1]

[1]Ankara Ataturk Training and Research Hospital, Bilkent Yolu 3. Km., Ankara, Turkey
[2]Department of Emergency Medicine, Faculty of Medicine, Kocaeli University, Umuttepe Kampüsü, Kocaeli, Turkey
[3]Bilecik State Hospital, Gazipaşa Mahallesi Tevfikbey Caddesi No. 4, Bilecik, Turkey

Correspondence should be addressed to Gul Pamukcu Gunaydin; gulpamukcu@gmail.com

Academic Editor: Ching H. Loh

Supposedly herbal weight loss pills are sold online and are widely used in the world. Some of these products are found to contain sibutramine by FDA and their sale is prohibited. We report a case of a female patient who presented to the emergency department after taking slimming pills. 17-year-old female patient presented to the emergency room with palpitations, dizziness, anxiety, and insomnia. She stated that she had taken 3 pills named La Jiao Shou Shen for slimming purposes during the day. Her vital signs revealed tachycardia. On her physical examination, she was restless, her oropharynx was dry, her pupils were mydriatic, and no other pathological findings were found. Sibutramine intoxication was suspected. She was given 5 mg IV diazepam for restlessness. After supportive therapy and observation in emergency department for 12 hours there were no complications and the patient was discharged home. Some herbal pills that are sold online for weight loss have sibutramine hidden as an active ingredient, and their sale is prohibited for this reason. For people who use herbal weight loss drugs, sibutramine excessive intake should be kept in mind at all times.

## 1. Introduction

A variety of the so-called herbal pills are widely used for slimming purposes in the world. Because these pills are not considered as medicine, there is no standardization for the ingredients of them and they may have hidden ingredients [1]. Serious adverse effects even death have been reported due to herbal pills consumption.

Some slimming pills are thought to be herbal, natural, and healthy, but sibutramine has been detected as an active ingredient in them. In one study ingredients of herbal slimming pills were analyzed and sibutramine was the most often detected synthetic substance [2]. Turkish Ministry of Health has analyzed some supposedly herbal pills that are sold in Turkey (Pepper Time Capsule©, Lida Daidaihua Weight Loss Capsule©, and La Jiao Shou Shen Capsule©) and has found that these pills have contained more sibutramine than the licensed weight loss medicine. The sale of those pills is banned.

Sibutramine is a synthetic noradrenaline, dopamine, and serotonin reuptake inhibitor used for the treatment of obesity. FDA and European Medicines Agency banned it because of its cardiovascular risks [1, 3, 4]. Tachycardia, hypertension, headache, and dizziness have been reported with sibutramine overdose [1, 5].

Although products that contain sibutramine have been banned, they can be easily purchased online. We present a case that took 3 slimming pills and had findings consistent with sibutramine overdose.

## 2. Case Report

17-year-old female patient has presented to emergency room at 2:30 a.m., with palpitation, dizziness, fatigue, and insomnia. In her medical history she did not have any disease, did not have surgery, and was not on any drugs. She stated that she bought pepper capsules named La Jiao Shou Shen©

TABLE 1: Common drugs hidden in weight loss pills [1, 7].

| Appetite suppressant | Diuretic | Laxative | Other |
| --- | --- | --- | --- |
| Ephedrine Fenfluramine Mazindol Sibutramine Pseudoephedrine | Hydrochlorothiazide Spironolactone | Sennosides Phenolphthalein Anthraquinones Bisacodyl | Fluoxetine Thyroid hormones Caffeine |

online. Her neighbor who also used it for weight loss recommended the pills to her. The patient took 3 pills in the previous 24 hours. She had the box of the pills ready with her. She has taken the last pill 4 hours before she arrived at emergency room. In her vital signs her blood pressure was 98/62 mmHg, her pulse was 138/min, and her body temperature was 37.5°C. In her physical exam she had tachycardia and anxiety, her oropharyngeal mucosa was dry, and her pupils were mydriatic. There were no other pathological findings. Her EKG showed sinus tachycardia; rate was 142/dk. Complete blood count, liver enzymes, renal function tests, serum electrolytes, thyroid function tests, and creatine kinase were within normal limits. After search online, the name of the product was found to be in the banned weight loss products that were adulterated with sibutramine. Thus sibutramine intoxication was diagnosed. Because she came to the emergency room 4 hours after she took the last pill, we neither placed nasogastric tube nor performed gastric lavage. Supportive therapy was initiated with normal saline 150 mL/hour. 5 mg of diazepam was given IV for anxiety. She was observed in the emergency room for 12 hours. There were no complications, her physical exam and vital signs returned to normal, and she was discharged with instructions to not use the pills again.

## 3. Discussion

Dietary supplements are not considered medicine and therefore not rigorously tested before they are on market. Some of these pills have synthetic drugs instead of herbal supplements. Sibutramine was detected in 44% of herbal slimming products. Some of these products may have up to 35 mg of sibutramine per pill [6]. In another study 80% percent of the patients who presented with weight loss pill overdose were found to take sibutramine unintentionally and 73% percent of products had sibutramine in them [7]. Consumers are not aware of the threat in many herbal products adulterated with synthetic drugs. Some common drugs hidden in weight loss pills are displayed in Table 1.

The most commonly reported side effects of sibutramine use are headache, dry oropharyngeal mucosa, anorexia, constipation, and insomnia whereas tachycardia, hypertension, headache, and dizziness are reported for its overdose [1, 5]. Serotonin syndrome has also been reported in some cases that were on sibutramine [8]. Sibutramine overdose complications are shown in Table 2.

In two published case reports 2 female patients and a male patient that took the same particular brand of herbal weight loss pill as in our case were presented. Their symptoms were

TABLE 2: Sibutramine overdose complications [2].

(i) Cardiovascular: tachycardia, palpitations, chest pain, and hypertension

(ii) Neurological: headache, anxiety, irritation, dizziness, insomnia, paresthesia, and serotonin syndrome

(iii) Gastrointestinal: nausea, dry mouth, and constipation

attributed to capsaicin but we think these patients may also have sibutramine intoxication [9, 10].

In this case we could not test blood or urine for sibutramine or could not analyze the ingredients of the capsules unfortunately. Sibutramine intoxication was considered because the symptom onset was rapid and the patient had no disease, was not on any drugs, and her symptoms were consistent with sibutramine intoxication. FDA announced that this particular brand (La Jiao Shou Shen©) of pepper pills contains sibutramine and phenolphthalein [11]. This has also supported our diagnosis.

Some weight loss pills are banned for having sibutramine as an active ingredient but these pills can be easily bought online and sibutramine overdose should always be kept in mind in cases with herbal weight lose pills consumption.

## Disclosure

This paper has been presented in oral presentation section of 3rd Eurasian Congress on Emergency Medicine 19–22 September 2012, Antalya, Turkey.

## Conflict of Interests

The authors declare that there is no conflict of interests regarding the publication of this paper.

## References

[1] B. Ozdemir, I. Sahin, H. Kapucu et al., "How safe is the use of herbal weight-loss products sold over the Internet?" *Human and Experimental Toxicology*, vol. 32, no. 1, pp. 101–106, 2013.

[2] H. J. Kim, J. H. Lee, H. J. Park, S.-H. Cho, and W. S. Kim, "Monitoring of 29 weight loss compounds in foods and dietary supplements by LC-MS/MS," *Food Additives and Contaminants, Part A: Chemistry, Analysis, Control, Exposure and Risk Assessment*, vol. 31, no. 5, pp. 777–783, 2014.

[3] FDA Government, *FDA Drug Safety Communication: FDA Recommends against the Continued Use of Meridia (Sibutramine)*, US Food and Drug Administration, 2014, http://www.fda.gov/drugs/drugsafety/ucm228746.htm.

[4] European Medicines Agency website, Questions and answers on the suspension of medicines containing sibutramine, 2014, http://www.ema.europa.eu/docs/en_GB/document_library/ Referrals_document/Sibutramine_107/WC500094238.pdf.

[5] FDA.gov, "Meridia drug information sheet," http://www.fda .gov/downloads/Drugs/DrugSafety/PublicHealthAdvisories/ UCM130745.pdf.

[6] C. Mathon, A. Ankli, E. Reich, S. Bieri, and P. Christen, "Screening and determination of sibutramine in adulterated herbal slimming supplements by HPTLC-UV densitometry," *Food Additives and Contaminants Part A: Chemistry, Analysis, Control, Exposure and Risk Assessment*, vol. 31, no. 1, pp. 15–20, 2014.

[7] M. H. Tang, S. P. Chen, S. W. Ng, A. Y. Chan, and T. W. Mak, "Case series on a diversity of illicit weight-reducing agents: from the well known to the unexpected," *British Journal of Clinical Pharmacology*, vol. 71, no. 2, pp. 250–253, 2011.

[8] P. K. Lam, K. S. Leung, T. W. Wong, H. H. C. Lee, M. H. Y. Tang, and T. W. L. Mak, "Serotonin syndrome following overdose of a non-prescription slimming product containing sibutramine: a case report," *Human and Experimental Toxicology*, vol. 31, no. 4, pp. 414–417, 2012.

[9] O. Sogut, H. Kaya, M. T. Gokdemir, M. S. Nimetoglu, and L. Solduk, "Cardiotoxicity developed after the use of cayenne pepper pill for slimming: a report of two cases," *Turkish Journal of Emergency Medicine*, vol. 10, no. 3, pp. 133–136, 2010.

[10] O. Sogut, H. Kaya, M. T. Gokdemir, and Y. Sezen, "Acute myocardial infarction and coronary vasospasm associated with the ingestion of cayenne pepper pills in a 25-year-old male," *International Journal of Emergency Medicine*, vol. 5, no. 1, article no. 5, 2012.

[11] FDA.gov, "Public Notification: La Jiao Shou Shen Contains Hidden Drug Ingredient," 2007, http://www.fda.gov/Drugs/ ResourcesForYou/Consumers/BuyingUsingMedicineSafely/ MedicationHealthFraud/ucm400595.htm.

# 37

# Scombrotoxinism: Protracted Illness following Misdiagnosis in the Emergency Department

**Ghan-Shyam Lohiya,**[1] **Sapna Lohiya,**[2] **Sunita Lohiya,**[3] **and Vijay Krishna**[4]

[1]*Occupational Medicine & Toxicology, Royal Medical Group, 1120 W. Warner Avenue, Santa Ana, CA 92707, USA*
[2]*University of Washington, Seattle, WA 98104, USA*
[3]*Royal Medical Group, 1120 W. Warner Avenue, Santa Ana, CA 92707, USA*
[4]*MidMichigan Medical Center, Midland, MI 48640, USA*

Correspondence should be addressed to Ghan-Shyam Lohiya; gslohiya@gmail.com

Academic Editor: Aristomenis K. Exadaktylos

*Background.* Scombrotoxinism is an acute toxin-induced illness caused primarily by bacterial synthesis of histamine in decomposed fish. *Case Report.* Immediately after taking 2-3 bites of cooked salmon, a clerical worker developed oral burning, urticaria, and asthma. In the emergency department, she was diagnosed with "allergies"; scombrotoxinism was never considered. She then developed wide-ranging symptoms (e.g., chronic fatigue, asthma, anxiety, multiple chemical sensitivity, and paresthesiae) and saw many specialists (in pulmonology, otorhinolaryngology, allergy, toxicology, neurology, psychology, and immunology). During the next 500+ days, she had extensive testing (allergy screens, brain MRI, electroencephalogram, electromyogram, nerve conduction velocity, heavy metal screen, and blood chemistry) with essentially normal results. She filed a workers' compensation claim since this injury occurred following a business meal. She was evaluated by a Qualified Medical Evaluator (GL) on day 504, who diagnosed scombrotoxinism. *Comment.* Scombrotoxinism should be considered in all patients presenting to the emergency department with "oral burning" or allergy symptoms following "fish consumption." Initial attention to such history would have led to a correct diagnosis and averted this patient's extended illness. Specialist referrals and tests should be ordered only if clinically indicated and not for diagnostic fishing expedition. Meticulous history is crucial in resolving clinical dilemmas.

## 1. Introduction

Scombrotoxinism is an acute self-limiting but potentially serious illness produced by consuming fish containing scombrotoxin, a mixture of histamine and related amines [1–5]. Under suboptimal refrigeration, contaminating anaerobic bacteria thrive in fish, and their carboxylase enzyme converts fish histidine into histamine. Ingestion produces immediate effects of histamine *toxicity* mimicking type-1 allergy. The affected fish need not look spoiled or malodorous. Scombrotoxin is heat-stable and therefore is not inactivated by cooking. Fish histamine concentration >50 ppm suggests decomposition. Scombrotoxinism responds well to antihistamines and corticosteroids [1–5]. We report a case of occupational scombrotoxinism where its correct diagnosis eluded recognition and led to a complex illness involving extensive medical care and disability. Real life lessons from this workers' compensation claim may help improve future case management.

## 2. Case Report

Immediately after taking 2-3 bites of cedar-plank-salmon during a business dinner, a clerk experienced "peppery burning in mouth, choking sensation, facial flushing, chest tightness, dizziness, and palpitations" (day 1). She had previously consumed salmon uneventfully many times. As first aid, she took 50 mg of oral diphenhydramine. Her weight was 93 Kg and height 172 cm; body mass index was 31 Kg/SqM (obese). She then received IV corticosteroids in an emergency room, followed by oral prednisone (50 mg daily, tapered 10 mg weekly to 10 mg daily maintenance dose). The diagnosis was an unspecified "allergic reaction." Although required, no report was made to the Health Department for this "foodborne and unusual" illness [6]. No toxicology or microbiologic test was performed on the fish.

Patient's symptoms persisted. On day 3, she was hospitalized and treated with IV corticosteroids, ranitidine, and cetirizine. She had moderate microcytic hypochromic anemia (hematocrit: 31.8%, normal 36–47%) probably from chronic menorrhagia. On day 4, she again required emergency room treatment.

For the next 4 months, patient experienced extreme fatigue, mostly remained in bed and saw several physicians. An otorhinolaryngologist diagnosed new asthma and prescribed beclomethasone and albuterol inhalers and allergen avoidance (HEPA air purifier, bedding covers). From day 28 onwards, a pulmonologist saw her monthly, recorded normal clinical examination and spirometry but continued the bronchodilators. A therapist diagnosed severe anxiety disorder from the allergic reaction, documented multiple symptoms (anxiety, excessive wariness, obsessions, compulsions, sleeplessness, and anticipatory fear of another reaction causing death or severe disability), and provided 40+ weekly psychotherapy treatments.

On day 191, a neurologist ordered five tests for patient's dizziness and paresthesiae. Brain MRI showed one hyperintense lesion perpendicular to the ventricular system (an unknown bright object) representing a nonspecific finding, lacunar infarct, or demyelinating disease. Electroencephalogram revealed intermittent nonspecific focal transient theta waves over the temporal lobes. Electromyogram and nerve conduction studies in both lower extremities were normal. Auditory evoked response test revealed normal hearing levels and brainstem activity. On day 219, the neurologist wrote "brain MRI and EEG changes are consequence rather than the cause of her problem," and prescribed gabapentin 200 mg daily. Repeat brain MRI 5 months later remained unchanged. Yet the neurologist recommended another MRI and cerebrospinal fluid testing.

Patient began developing dizziness and chest tightness following exposure to certain hair dyes, foods (potato chips), iron supplements, toiletries and cleaning chemicals. Monosodium glutamate sensitivity was suspected. The neurologist now advised hair analysis for "any stored neurotoxins." He also suspected "immune dysfunction." An immunologist found negative extractable-nuclear autoantibodies, negative antinuclear antibody, normal erythrocyte sedimentation rate, and normal serum thyroid stimulating hormone and immunoglobulins A, E, G, and M.

Since patient's illness occurred during the course of a business meal, she was eligible for workers' compensation benefits. To determine compensability (causation), patient was evaluated on days 133 and 193 by a defense allergist who diagnosed hypertension, anxiety, and nonoccupational allergies. He reported normal results for plasma norepinephrine, dopamine, vanillylmandelic acid (for pheochromocytoma), urine 5-hydroxyindoleacetic acid (for carcinoid tumor), serum tryptase (for mastocytosis), immunoglobulin E, serum chemistry panel, and blood mercury (patient: <3 mcg/L, acceptable: <6 mcg/L). Serum allergy testing for 49 allergens

and salmon revealed only dust mite allergy. Patient refused skin allergy testing.

A toxicology evaluator found normal levels of blood lead, arsenic, mercury, and cadmium. Repeat testing for 21 respiratory and ten food allergens was mildly positive for only dust mites. *Helicobacter pylori* antibody was absent. He diagnosed Multiple Chemical Sensitivity and phobia from the severe salmon-related reaction.

To help resolve medical disputes about causation, treatment, and permanent disability, patient was evaluated on day 504 by author GL for an independent State Panel Qualified Medical Evaluation (Occupational Medicine & Toxicology). He diagnosed scombrotoxinism based on a meticulous history and review of records.

## 3. Discussion

This was a classic case of scombrotoxinism. Patient developed oral burning, facial flushing, angioedema, and asthma immediately after salmon consumption. Although the diagnosis was never confirmed by determining the salmon's histamine content, *such incompleteness was inconsequential*. Extensive testing had ruled out all other competing diagnoses. In clinical practice, one may not achieve the level of diagnostic purity sought in research settings. Yet, this real life case offers unique and educationally useful insights to emergency physicians, toxicologists, and other specialists.

This case highlights the frequent underdiagnosis of scombrotoxinism. Despite this patient's tell-tale presentation, her physicians diagnosed "allergies." This probably occurred because allergies are common and scombrotoxinism is now rarer due to improved food handling. The emergency treatment of the patient was appropriate because symptoms in both allergies (type-1 hypersensitivity illness) and scombrotoxinism (toxic illness) are caused by histamine [4]. However in allergies the histamine source is *intrinsic (from mast cells and basophils)*, whereas in scombrotoxinism it is *extrinsic* (from decomposed fish). The diagnostic clue for scombrotoxinism is the "histamine-induced oral burning" and the history of fish consumption. The initial misdiagnosis occurred because the emergency physician did not recognize this link.

Scombrotoxin is synthesized by contaminating bacteria at room temperature. Therefore, fish, like any other food, should be handled carefully to avoid contamination and not be left in the "temperature danger zone" (21–40°C) for more than two hours. In this context, it is useful to remember the mnemonic "FAT-TOM" emphasizing the six pillars of food safety that need attention: Food, Acidity, Time, Temperature, Oxygen, Moisture [6]. Prompt notification of the local Health Department is essential to avert outbreaks from the same contaminated fish [7].

Patient had no toxicological permanent disability from this injury. Histamine has a very short half-life in extracellular fluid [8]. As a toxicological principle, a xenobiotic is deemed eliminated from blood after seven half-lives (<1% remainder). Thus patient's histamine-related symptoms ought to have resolved quickly, definitely within a week.

Missed diagnosis had significant adverse consequences in this case. This patient developed anxiety and required extended psychological treatment. She saw many specialists who screened her with numerous tests and diagnosed various unrelated conditions. Had patient learned at the outset that her illness was due to food poisoning caused by *that* particular salmon dish, she might not have developed this extended illness. Patient's ongoing symptoms probably represent an anxiety-panic disorder which requires a psychiatrist.

Illnesses from business meals are usually considered as "arising out of employment," and accepted for workers' compensation. California's Labor Code section 4600(a) specifies "Medical…treatment that is reasonably required to cure or relieve the injured worker from the effects of his or her injury shall be provided by the employer." Once a worker files a Workers' Compensation Claim, the employer must pay up to $10,000 for its treatment until the claim acceptance or denial [9]. Since patient's injury arose out of employment (the salmon consumption), the initial emergency treatment was the employer's responsibility. However, law does not require employers to diagnose and exclude all nonoccupational conditions that fall within the differential diagnosis. Patient's extensive testing and care after claim denial was unrelated to the injury.

Concern about mercury poisoning was unjustified. First, fish high on the food chain (swordfish, shark, king mackerel, and tilefish) may contain methyl mercury, but salmon is a low mercury fish (<0.09 ppm mercury) [10]. Second, there could not be sufficient mercury in 2-3 bites of salmon to produce mercurialism. Third, there would be a lag between mercury ingestion and symptom development. Finally, mercury toxicity does not produce immediate angioneurotic edema or asthma. Likewise, there was no indication for hair chemical analysis. Presence of a xenobiotic in hair may indicate exposure (both internal and external) but can neither indicate its source nor link it to an illness [11].

Ciguatera-toxinism was a competing diagnosis because of its fish origin and heat resistance. However it was unlikely because ciguatera toxin is tasteless, involves larger fish, has an 8-hour lag period, and produces vomiting and diarrhea [12]. Staphylococcal food poisoning was unlikely because patient did not experience vomiting, stomach cramps and diarrhea [13]. Assuming that the fish was adequately cooked, all potential fish-borne parasites (*Clonorchis sinensis*, *Anisakis*, and *Diphyllobothrium*) and bacteria (*Salmonella* and *Shigella*) would have been inactivated. Moreover, such infestations and infections have different specific clinical presentations, require an incubation period, and do not produce urticaria.

This case illustrates the need for physicians to base their opinions and recommendations on "evidence and science that is nationally recognized and peer reviewed" [14]. This patient was subjected to many tests without adequate justification. For example, the neurologist only cursorily noted "numbness" (without dermatomal or objective anomalies); yet he ordered nerve conduction velocity and electromyogram. Although the brain MRI revealed only a nonspecific change or mild leukoaraiosis which remained unchanged 5-months later, the neurologist still recommended repeat MRI and lumbar puncture, and then hair analysis and an immunologist. Patient was a nonsmoking office worker with no industrial chemical exposure; yet heavy metal levels were checked repeatedly. Likewise, there was no indication to test for environmental allergies, pheochromocytoma, mastocytosis, or carcinoid syndrome. Consequences of unnecessary testing for healthy patients are retesting, repeat venipuncture, unwarranted anxiety, waste, confusion, and false hope [15].

## Disclosure

This work was presented at the 64th Quarterly Coastal-Fairview Grand Rounds Conference in Costa Mesa, California.

## Conflict of Interests

The authors declare that there is no conflict of interests regarding the publication of this paper.

## Acknowledgments

Ghan-Shyam Lohiya, MD, evaluated this patient as a State Panel Qualified Medical Evaluator (Occupational Medicine and Toxicology). The workers' compensation insurer for the patient's employer paid Dr. Lohiya's fee according to California law.

## References

[1] C. K. Murray, G. Hobbs, and G. R. Gilbert, "Scombrotoxin and scombrotoxin-like poisoning from canned fish," *Journal of Hygiene*, vol. 88, no. 2, pp. 215–220, 1982.

[2] D. I. Ward, "'Mass allergy': acute scombroid poisoning in a deployed Australian Defence Force health facility," *Emergency Medicine Australasia*, vol. 23, no. 1, pp. 98–102, 2011.

[3] J. M. Hungerford, "Scombroid poisoning: a review," *Toxicon*, vol. 56, no. 2, pp. 231–243, 2010.

[4] N. K. Numbere, P. Featherstone, and H. L. Cooper, "Scombrotoxin poisoning: an important differential diagnosis for anaphylaxis," *Acute Medicine*, vol. 9, no. 2, pp. 80–81, 2010.

[5] Centers for Disease Control and Prevention (CDC), "Scombroid fish poisoning associated with tuna steaks—Louisiana and Tennessee, 2006," *Morbidity and Mortality Weekly Report*, vol. 56, no. 32, pp. 817–819, 2007.

[6] Iowa State University, "Food safety Lesson," 2015, http://www.extension.iastate.edu/foodsafety/Lesson/L4/L4p1.html.

[7] Illinois Department of Public Health, Illinois Reportable Diseases—Public Health Services, April 2015, http://www.idph.state.il.us/health/infect/ReportDiseasePoster.pdf.

[8] K. D. Stone, C. Prussin, and D. D. Metcalfe, "IgE, mast cells, basophils, and eosinophils," *Journal of Allergy and Clinical Immunology*, vol. 125, no. 2, pp. S73–S80, 2010.

[9] California Labor code section 4600-4614.1, 2015, http://law.onecle.com/california/labor/4600.html.

[10] Natural Resources Defense Council, "Consumer Guide to Mercury in Fish," 2015, http://www.nrdc.org/health/effects/mercury/guide.asp.

[11] Centers for Disease Control and Prevention (CDC), "Hair Analysis. Exploring the state of the science," http://www.atsdr.cdc.gov/HAC/hair_analysis/hairanalysis.pdf.

[12] C. Davis, "Ciguatera Fish Poisoning," 2015, http://www.emedicinehealth.com/wilderness_ciguatera_toxin/article_em.htm.

[13] Centers for Disease Control and Prevention (CDC), Staphylococcal food poisoning, 2015, http://www.cdc.gov/nczved/divisions/dfbmd/diseases/staphylococcal/.

[14] G.-S. Lohiya, P. Lohiya, V. Krishna, and S. Lohiya, "Death related to ibuprofen, valdecoxib, and medical errors: case report and medicolegal issues," *Journal of Occupational and Environmental Medicine*, vol. 55, no. 6, pp. 601–603, 2013.

[15] G.-S. Lohiya, L. Tan-Figueroa, and S. Lohiya, "Bloodborne pathogens exposure from occupational fingernail scratches," *Journal of the National Medical Association*, vol. 99, no. 11, pp. 1271–1275, 2007.

# 38

# Pitfalls in Suspected Acute Aortic Syndrome: Impact of Appropriate and If Required Repeated Imaging

## C. Meier,[1] M. Lichtenberg,[2] P. Lebiedz,[1] and F. Breuckmann[3]

[1]*Department of Cardiovascular Medicine, University Hospital Münster, 48149 Münster, Germany*
[2]*Department of Angiology, Arnsberg Medical Center, 59759 Arnsberg, Germany*
[3]*Department of Cardiology, Arnsberg Medical Center, 59759 Arnsberg, Germany*

Correspondence should be addressed to F. Breuckmann; f.breuckmann@klinikum-arnsberg.de

Academic Editor: Serdar Kula

The incidence of acute aortic syndrome is low, but the spontaneous course is often life-threatening. Adequate ECG-gated imaging is fundamental within the diagnostic workup. We here report a case of a 53-year-old man presenting with atypical chest pain, slight increase of D dimers at admission, and extended diameter of the ascending aorta accompanied by mild aortic regurgitation. Interpretation of an initial contrast-enhanced computed tomography was false negative due to inadequate gating and motion artifacts, thereby judging a tiny contrast signal in the left anterior quadrant of the ascending aorta as a pseudointimal flap. By hazard, cardiac magnetic resonance imaging demonstrated an ulcer-like lesion superior to the aortic root, leading to aortic surgery at the last moment. As sensitivity of imaging is not 100%, this example underlines that second imaging studies might be necessary if the first imaging is negative, but the clinical suspicion still remains high.

## 1. Introduction

The incidence of acute aortic dissection is estimated with 2,9–3,5/100.000 annual lives [1]. The pathogenesis starts with a laceration of the intima, in most cases accompanied by an off-peeling of the inner layer in the direction of the blood flow, so that a false lumen occurs [2]. As to the high mortality and low incidence, especially in type A aortic dissection, diagnosis and management require a fast and multidisciplinary approach, particularly with input from noninvasive imaging techniques in addition to clinical evaluation. Radiologic imaging technologies have improved in terms of detection accuracy in aortic diseases [3–6]. Several factors have an influence on accuracy, for example, scanning-technology, protocol standards, patient's anatomy, and especially the heart rate, producing motion artifacts. As referred to computed tomography (CT), for elimination of this artifact, the ECG-signal is detected synchronously to the acquisition of the CT data. Pictures are generated retrospectively, thereby minimizing artifacts by choosing the most convenient time frame. In contrast, the prospective triggering is an alternative to perform the examination. Using this method the radiation is applied in the expected ideal interval, enabling a reduction of radiation.

## 2. Case Presentation

A 53-year-old man presented to our emergency department with sudden onset of atypical chest pain and nonsignificant elevated ST-segments in the inferior leads. Baseline myocardial markers were negative and remained at the same level within the follow-up measurements. By contrast, D dimers at admission showed a slight increase (0.7 μg/mL, reference <0.5 μg/mL). Immediately performed transthoracic echocardiography demonstrated a preserved left ventricular global function without significant wall motion abnormalities and no signs of right ventricular strain, though an extended diameter of the ascending aorta of 52 mm was accompanied by a mild aortic regurgitation with hemodynamically noncompromising pericardial effusion. Thus, under the working diagnosis of an acute aortic syndrome, a contrast-enhanced CT using a triple rule out protocol

(a)

(b)

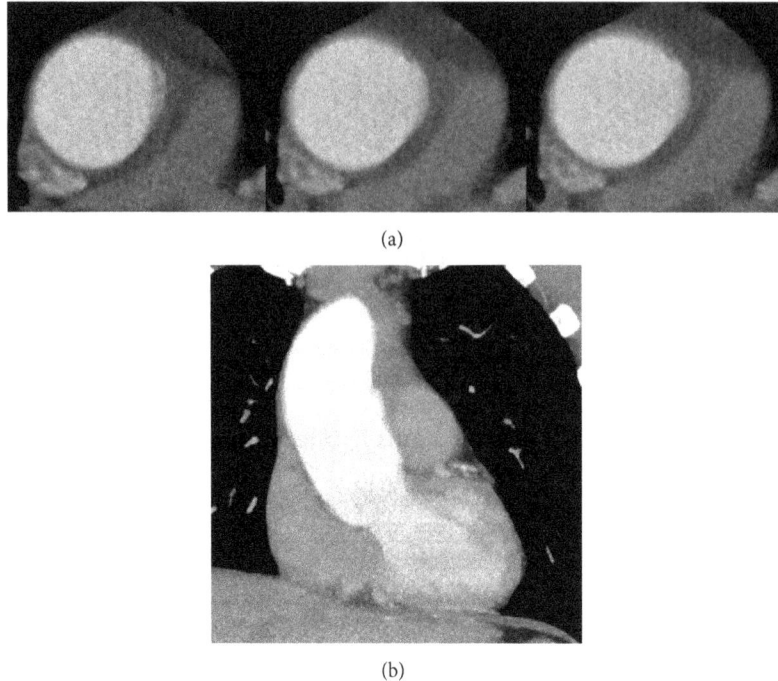

FIGURE 1: Double-oblique (a) and axial (b) reconstructions (spatial resolution $3 \times 0.5 \times 0.25$ mm) of the initial inadequate ECG-gated contrast-enhanced CT resulting from repeated premature ventricular contractions at the time of image acquisition. Consider the small contrast signal in the left anterior quadrant of the ascending aorta, misdiagnosed as a pseudointimal flap/motion artifact.

was initiated. Because of inadequate gating due to repeated premature ventricular contractions at the time of image acquisition despite administration of beta-blockers, finally a non-ECG-gated contrast-enhanced CT of the ascending aorta was completed in order to exclude aortic dissection. The CT showed an extended diameter of the ascending aorta with a maximum of 51 mm without hint for dissection membrane or false lumen. However, imaging of the aortic root as well as the supracoronary aorta was hampered by aortic motion artifacts, thereby judging a tiny contrast signal in the left anterior quadrant of the ascending aorta as a pseudointimal flap (Figures 1(a) and 1(b)).

In order to rule out a peri-/myocarditis as another possible explanation for the persistent clinical symptoms, we performed a cardiac magnet resonance imaging (CMR) shortly after initial presentation. Surprisingly, cine-CMR imaging demonstrated an ulcer-like lesion superior to the aortic root in the left anterior quadrant of the ascending aorta (Figure 2(a)) but no typical late enhancement pattern. A renewed and at this time adequately ECG-gated contrast-enhanced CT revealed a penetrating aortic ulcer exactly in the same location compared to the initially suspected area (Figures 2(b) and 2(c)), thereby showing a nearly similar accuracy as the preceding CMR.

The currently asymptomatic patient was directly admitted to our intensive care. Unfortunately, only a few minutes following the second CT the patient suffered a convulsive seizure with subsequent hemodynamic instability needing cardiopulmonary resuscitation for about 20 minutes until return of spontaneous circulation. The patient was brought immediately to the operation room for aortic surgery. At this time, the operative site demonstrated a supracoronary entry of an extensive classical type A aortic dissection reaching the aortic arch with an inversion of the intima flap that resulted in an occlusion of the supra-aortic limbs. A graft replacement of the ascending aorta under selective cerebral perfusion was done using a 30 mm artificial graft.

Despite the worsening scenario the patient recovered well without relevant neurological residuals until discharge and during subsequent outpatient follow-up consultations.

## 3. Discussion

Type A dissection has a 40–60% risk of death within the first 48 hours. However, not only acute type A dissection but all types of type A acute aortic syndrome require timely diagnosis and early surgery [7]. The classification by Svensson et al. takes account of the precursors of aortic dissection: classic dissection with a correct and a false lumen (class 1), intramural hematoma (class 2), localized dissection with dilatation (class 3), ulcer-like lesion and plaque rupture (class 4), and an iatrogenic or traumatic dissection (class 5) [8]. Urgent imaging of the aorta should be performed by transesophageal echocardiography, CT, or magnetic resonance imaging to identify or exclude thoracic aortic dissection. The selection of a specific imaging should be based on patient's condition as well as institutional capabilities [9]. A second imaging study should be performed if the first imaging is negative, but the clinical suspicion remains probable. As presented in our case, the initial clinical suspicion of acute

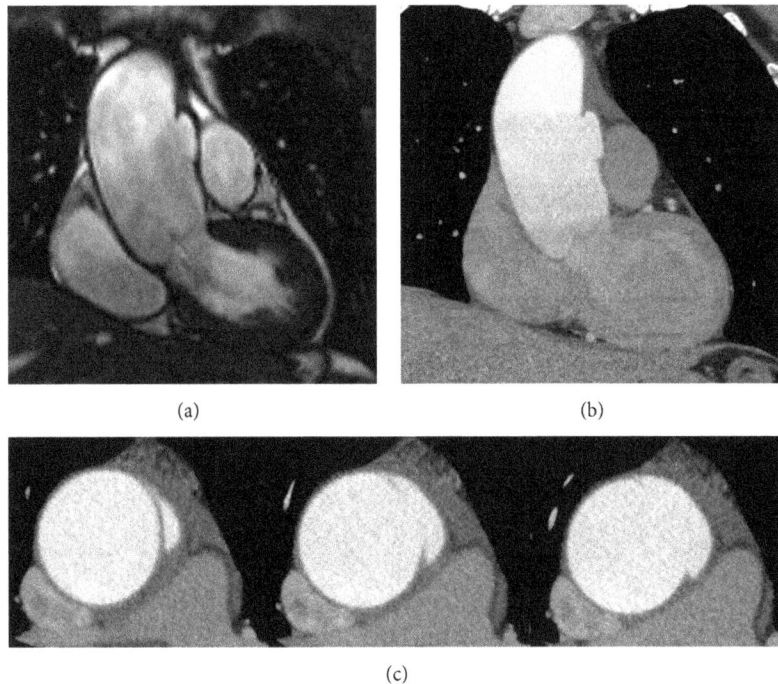

(a)

(b)

(c)

FIGURE 2: Corresponding double-oblique view of the cine-CMR demonstrating an ulcer-like lesion (acute aortic syndrome, class 4) superior to the aortic root in the even initially suspicious left anterior aortic quadrant (a) and nearly congruent double-oblique (b) and axial (c) reconstructions (spatial resolution $2 \times 0.5 \times 0.25$ mm) as compared to initial CT imaging, this time adequately prospectively ECG-gated. Note the precise demarcation and nearly similar accuracy compared to the preceding CMR of a penetrating aortic ulcer exactly in the same location compared to the initially suspected area.

aortic dissection was right and the interpretation of the presented symptoms was superior to the first CT scan. That points out that anamnesis and exploration should belong to the first important steps on the way to diagnosis. On the other hand, it emphasizes the importance of better correlating imaging data with the clinical picture, which might have led to a different interpretation of the initial CT scan.

Retrospectively, a localized dissection membrane or ulcer-like lesion should have been assumed, but diagnosis failed by insufficient imaging quality and missing of immediate reevaluation. This case should be a reminder that sensitivity of the first performed imaging and particularly CT scan is high but not 100%. Vice versa, the rate of false positive activation remains low and justifiable in such life-threatening disorder [10]. As a result, clinical knowledge about aortic diseases and right interpretation of the symptoms by the physician is fundamental and should in doubt lead to immediate therapy or a second imaging study.

## Conflict of Interests

The authors declare that there is no conflict of interests regarding the publication of this paper.

## References

[1] P. G. Hagan, C. A. Nienaber, E. M. Isselbacher et al., "The international registry of acute aortic dissection (IRAD): new insights into an old disease," *The Journal of the American Medical Association*, vol. 283, no. 7, pp. 897–903, 2000.

[2] M. Markl, A. Harloff, T. A. Bley et al., "Time-resolved 3D MR velocity mapping at 3T: improved navigator-gated assessment of vascular anatomy and blood flow," *Journal of Magnetic Resonance Imaging*, vol. 25, no. 4, pp. 824–831, 2007.

[3] A. D. Smith and P. Schoenhagen, "CT imaging for acute aortic syndrome," *Cleveland Clinic Journal of Medicine*, vol. 75, no. 1, pp. 7–24, 2008.

[4] R. R. Baliga, C. A. Nienaber, E. Bossone et al., "The role of imaging in aortic dissection and related syndromes," *JACC Cardiovascular Imaging*, vol. 7, no. 4, pp. 406–424, 2014.

[5] T. Shiga, Z. Wajima, C. C. Apfel, T. Inoue, and Y. Ohe, "Diagnostic accuracy of transesophageal echocardiography, helical computed tomography, and magnetic resonance imaging for suspected thoracic aortic dissection: systematic review and meta-analysis," *Archives of Internal Medicine*, vol. 166, no. 13, pp. 1350–1356, 2006.

[6] M. A. McMahon and C. A. Squirrell, "Multidetector ct of aortic dissection: a pictorial review," *Radiographics*, vol. 30, no. 2, pp. 445–460, 2010.

[7] E. Weigang, C. A. Nienaber, T. C. Rehders, H. Ince, C.-F. Vahl, and F. Beyersdorf, "Management of patients with aortic dissection," *Deutsches Ärzteblatt*, vol. 105, no. 38, pp. 639–645, 2008.

[8] L. G. Svensson, S. B. Labib, A. C. Eisenhauer, and J. R. Butterly, "Intimal tear without hematoma: an important variant of aortic dissection that can elude current imaging techniques," *Circulation*, vol. 99, no. 10, pp. 1331–1336, 1999.

[9] L. F. Hiratzka, G. L. Bakris, J. A. Beckman et al., "2010 ACCF/AHA/ AATS/ACR/ASA/SCA/SCAI/SIR/STS/SVM guidelines for the diagnosis and management of patients with thoracic aortic disease. A report of the American College of Cardiology Foundation/American Heart Association task force on practice guidelines, American Association for Thoracic Surgery, American College of Radiology, American Stroke Association, Society of Cardiovascular Anesthesiologists, Society for Cardiovascular Angiography and Interventions, Society of Interventional Radiology, Society of Thoracic Surgeons, and Society for Vascular Medicine," *Journal of the American College of Cardiology*, vol. 55, no. 14, pp. e27–e129, 2010.

[10] C. E. Raymond, B. Aggarwal, P. Schoenhagen et al., "Prevalence and factors associated with false positive suspicion of acute aortic syndrome: experience in a patient population transferred to a specialized aortic treatment center," *Cardiovascular Diagnosis and Therapy*, vol. 3, no. 4, pp. 196–204, 2013.

# 39

# A Broken Toothbrush in the Retropharyngeal Space in a Toddler of Sixteen Months

**Saileswar Goswami[1] and Choitali Goswami[2]**

[1]Department of Otolaryngology, Calcutta National Medical College, Kolkata, West Bengal 700014, India
[2]Department of General Emergency, Medical College, Kolkata, West Bengal 700073, India

Correspondence should be addressed to Saileswar Goswami; sgoswami1962@gmail.com

Academic Editor: Aristomenis K. Exadaktylos

A toddler of sixteen months fell while brushing his teeth and his mouth hit the ground. The toothbrush broke and one-third of it including the head got impacted in his throat. The attempt of his mother to remove it with her fingers further complicated the case and the toothbrush was ultimately lodged in the retropharyngeal space at the level from C1 to C5 vertebrae. It was strongly impacted due to the presence of the bristles. The broken end of the handle was just protruding into the nasopharynx and was very difficult to locate. The first attempt of its removal was unsuccessful. The toothbrush was removed safely in the second attempt without any complication.

## 1. Introduction

We frequently get patients with foreign bodies in the aerodigestive tract but a toothbrush is a very uncommon foreign body found there. Brushing of teeth is very safe when done properly but sometimes it can lead to life-threatening complications. As toddlers have a tendency to fall, they can easily get injured while left unsupervised during toothbrushing. In the present case, a child of sixteen months was the sufferer. The head of a broken toothbrush penetrated the posterior pharyngeal wall and entered the retropharyngeal space. The reason behind reporting this case is its rarity and the difficulty it posed in its management.

## 2. Case Presentation

In a remote village, a male child of one year and four months was playfully brushing his teeth in the late morning. He fell and his mouth hit the ground. The toothbrush broke and the head along with a part of the handle remained in his throat. His mother tried to remove it with her fingers but was unsuccessful. Her attempt resulted in further injury to the throat and the child started bleeding from his mouth. He was first taken to a paediatrician who advised his parents to take him to a tertiary care hospital.

At the time of admission in the ENT department of a rural medical college, he was unable to open his mouth completely or take foods and drinks. Blood stained saliva was coming out from his mouth. His oxygen saturation was 85% and he was having mild respiratory distress. His pulse was regular and was 110/min. Respiration was also regular and was 26/min. He was conscious but very restless and was not allowing examination of his throat.

X-ray of the neck revealed a faint radio-opaque foreign body in the prevertebral area extending from the level of C1 to C5 vertebrae (Figure 1). The airway was clearly in front of the foreign body. The shape of the foreign body and the dotted shadows in rows were in line with the head of a toothbrush with the bristles. The bristles were aligned in the coronal plane.

Treatment was started with antibiotics, analgesics, oxygen, and others. After his oxygen saturation was improved, further examination was carried out. The oral cavity was full of blood stained saliva. The mucosa of the oropharynx was edematous. There were multiple scattered superficial erosions in the mucosa of the oropharynx and the soft palate but there was no active bleeding.

The patient was taken to the operation theatre for removal of the toothbrush. He was operated under general anaesthesia with orotracheal intubation. The resident otolaryngologist,

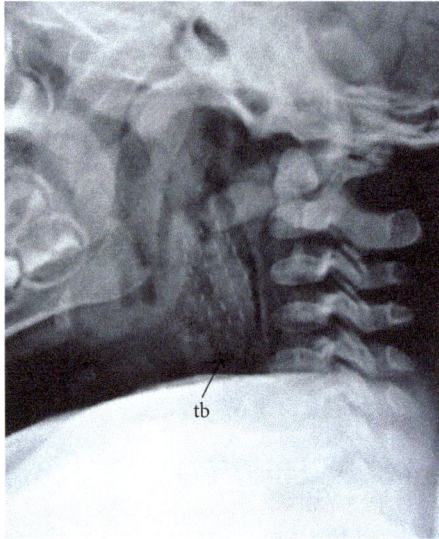

FIGURE 1: X-ray of the neck showing the head of the toothbrush (tb) with the bristles (dotted lines) in the retropharyngeal space extending from the level of C1 to C5 vertebrae.

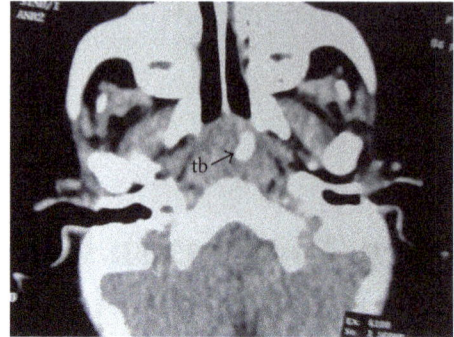

FIGURE 2: CT scan passing through the external auditory meatus, showing the handle of the toothbrush (tb) in the retropharyngeal space of the nasopharynx.

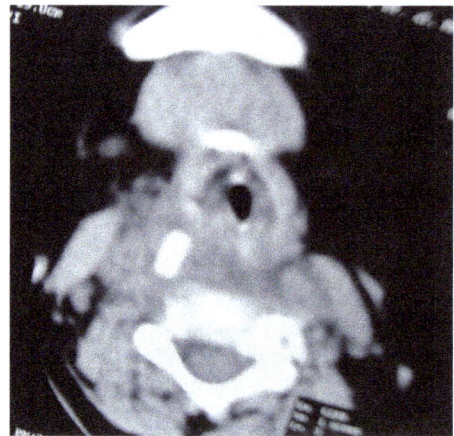

FIGURE 3: CT scan showing the lowermost part of the toothbrush in the retropharyngeal space of the hypopharynx.

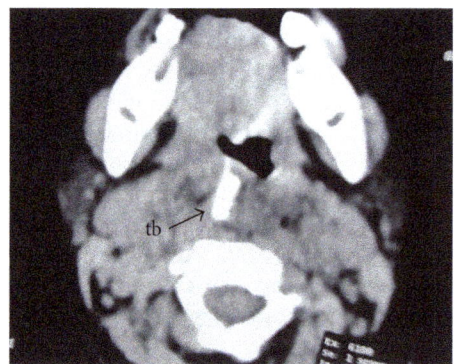

FIGURE 4: CT scan showing the toothbrush (tb) embedded in the retropharyngeal pace of the oropharynx.

who was on duty at that time, was unable to locate the toothbrush as there was edema of the pharyngeal mucosa and no part of the toothbrush was visible on the surface. The first attempt of its removal was unsuccessful.

Conservative treatment was continued with intravenous steroids, antibiotics, and others. CT scan was advised to know the precise location of the toothbrush and its relation to the nearby critical structures. CT scan was performed after two days because of financial constraints.

CT scan revealed the toothbrush embedded within the prevertebral soft tissue. It was lying obliquely across the midline, extending from the roof of the nasopharynx (Figure 2) to the level of the lower border of the C5 vertebra (Figure 3). The head was directed downwards and to the right, whereas the handle was directed upwards and to the left. The head and the neck were completely embedded within the prevertebral soft tissue (Figure 4). The broken end of the handle (Figure 2) was also embedded within the prevertebral soft tissue of the nasopharynx. However, a small part of the handle below the broken end was just coming out to the surface in the nasopharynx (Figure 5). The minimum distance between the carotid artery and the toothbrush was about 1.5 cm, which was at its upper end.

It was decided to wait for two more days for the edema to subside completely. The patient was operated for the second time on the fourth day of the injury. Under general anaesthesia, a Boyle Davis mouth gag was introduced. The oral cavity and the oropharynx were cleaned by suction. The oropharynx was searched thoroughly to locate the toothbrush but it was not found. Multiple scattered superficial injuries were seen over the mucosa of the oropharynx but no entry wound was found. There was a bulging over the posterior pharyngeal wall. On palpation, the toothbrush could be felt there.

A zero degree nasal endoscope was introduced through the left nostril. After cleaning by suction, a portion of the handle was found to be protruding from the posterior wall of the nasopharynx on the left side but both ends of the toothbrush were firmly embedded within the soft tissue.

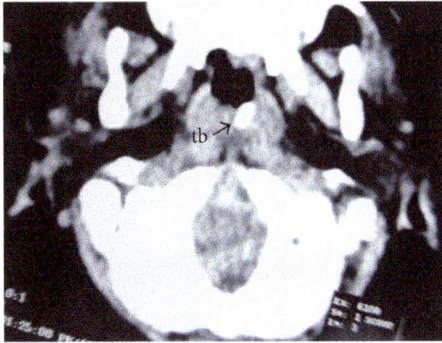

FIGURE 5: CT scan passing through the atlantooccipital joint, showing the handle of the toothbrush (tb) coming out to the surface from the retropharyngeal space of the nasopharynx.

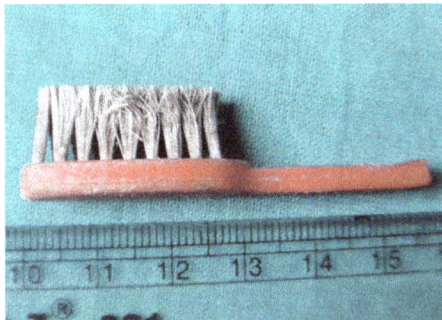

FIGURE 6: The toothbrush (5.8 cm × 1.5 cm) with sharp broken edge after removal.

It was not possible to remove the toothbrush through the nasal route. Two rubber catheters were used for velotraction. The soft palate was retracted anteriorly to expose the nasopharynx. The portion of the handle inside the lumen of the nasopharynx was visualised directly. It was impacted within the soft tissue. The upper entry point was widened first with the help of artery forceps and the broken end of the handle was gradually disimpacted. Then the lower point was widened in the same manner. The toothbrush was then removed by gently pulling as well as slightly rotating it in either direction to free it from the surrounding soft tissue. It was done slowly under direct vision taking care to avoid injury to the surrounding structures.

After removal of the toothbrush, the wound was carefully inspected. It was 5.8 cm long and 1.5 cm wide (Figure 6). The insignificant bleeding was controlled by applying pressure. The wounds were left as they were, to be healed on their own. Ryle's tube was introduced for feeding in the postoperative period.

The patient was kept on intravenous fluid on the day of operation. Ryle's tube feeding was started from the next day. The postoperative period was uneventful and the patient recovered quickly. Ryle's tube was removed after five days and oral feeding was started. The patient was discharged seven days after the operation.

## 3. Discussion

Impalement injury and implantation of a foreign body in the oral cavity are common in young children [1] but implantation of a toothbrush in the pharynx is not common. Oza et al. [1] reported a case of implantation of a broken toothbrush medial to the ramus of the mandible in a child following an injury with a cricket ball. Moran [2] reported a case of a toothbrush embedded in the buccal soft tissues. Sagar et al. [3] reported a case of life-threatening penetrating oropharyngeal trauma in a child by a toothbrush, which had penetrated the posterolateral part of the pharyngeal wall and reached the parapharyngeal space beyond the carotid sheath and pushed it laterally at the level of the second cervical vertebra.

There are few case reports of toothbrushes in the parapharyngeal space also. Burduk [4] and Aggarwal et al. [5] also reported cases of toothbrushes in the parapharyngeal space. However, toothbrush in the retropharyngeal space is an extreme rarity. Tanaka et al. [6] reported a case of a toothbrush in the retropharyngeal space embedded beside the carotid artery, which was removed by endoscopic surgical technique. In the present case, the toothbrush was embedded obliquely across the midline, extending from the roof of the nasopharynx to the level of the lower border of the C5 vertebra.

In most of the cases, injuries caused by an unimpacted toothbrush are minor and do not require much attention. However, penetrating injuries of the oral cavity and the pharynx, with or without impaction of foreign bodies, should not be taken lightly. They can lead to massive bleeding, retropharyngeal abscess, [7] mediastinitis, [8] carotid artery thrombosis, [9] jugular vein thrombosis, and cranial nerve involvement.

Attempt to remove a penetrating pharyngeal foreign body should be done after proper investigations, which are necessary to know its precise location and relation to the nearby critical structures. CT scan should be done routinely in all cases. Angiography may be necessary to exclude major vascular injury. MRI may be necessary in selected cases. In the present case, the first attempt was unsuccessful as CT scan was unavailable due to financial constraints.

Broad spectrum antibiotics including anaerobic coverage are very important to prevent sepsis. Tetanus prophylaxis is necessary in unimmunised patients. Anti-inflammatory agents like steroids may be necessary prior to surgical intervention to reduce the edema and increase the visibility of the impacted foreign body. If the wound is old and infected, it is better to leave it open [3]. Recent, uninfected, and clean wound may be sutured. Sutures may also be necessary in case of bleeding. If the foreign body is big and close to important neurovascular structures, an external exploration [5] may be preferred. Sagar et al. [3] removed a broken toothbrush from the parapharyngeal space close to the internal carotid artery, via the oral route. In the present case, the broken toothbrush was lodged obliquely in the retropharyngeal space, extending from the nasopharynx to the C5 vertebra. Although it was very difficult to approach, the toothbrush could be removed successfully via the oral route without any complications.

## Key Messages

Brushing of teeth should be done carefully. Children should always be supervised properly by their parents to prevent accidental impaction of a toothbrush. The injury may be further aggravated by the attempt of the parents to remove it. CT scan should be done routinely in all cases of penetrating pharyngeal foreign bodies. It should be removed by experienced surgeons. Proper imaging and prompt medical care are necessary to save the patient.

## Conflict of Interests

The authors declare that there is no conflict of interests regarding the publication of this paper.

## References

[1] N. Oza, K. Agrawal, and K. N. Panda, "An unusual mode of injury-implantation of a broken toothbrush medial to ramus: report of a case," *Journal of Dentistry for Children*, vol. 69, no. 2, pp. 193–195, 2002.

[2] A. J. Moran, "An unusual case of trauma: a toothbrush embedded in the buccal mucosa," *British Dental Journal*, vol. 185, no. 3, pp. 112–114, 1998.

[3] S. Sagar, N. Kumar, M. Singhal, S. Kumar, and A. Kumar, "A rare case of life-threatening penetrating oropharyngeal trauma caused by toothbrush in a child," *Journal of Indian Society of Pedodontics and Preventive Dentistry*, vol. 28, no. 2, pp. 134–136, 2010.

[4] P. K. Burduk, "Parapharyngeal space foreign body," *European Archives of Oto-Rhino-Laryngology*, vol. 263, no. 8, pp. 772–774, 2006.

[5] M. K. Aggarwal, G. B. Singh, R. Dhawan, and R. Kumar, "Rare case of a broken toothbrush as a parapharyngeal space foreign body," *Journal of Otolaryngology—Head and Neck Surgery*, vol. 38, no. 4, pp. E107–E109, 2009.

[6] T. Tanaka, M. Sudo, K. Iwai, S. Fujieda, and H. Saito, "Penetrating injury to the pharynx by a toothbrush in a pediatric patient: a case report," *Auris Nasus Larynx*, vol. 29, no. 4, pp. 387–389, 2002.

[7] Z. Luqman, M. A. M. Khan, and Z. Nazir, "Penetrating pharyngeal injuries in children: trivial trauma leading to devastating complications," *Pediatric Surgery International*, vol. 21, no. 6, pp. 432–435, 2005.

[8] M. F. López-Peláez, J. Roldán, and S. Mateo, "Cervical emphysema, pneumomediastinum, and pneumothorax following self-induced oral injury: report of four cases and review of the literature," *Chest*, vol. 120, no. 1, pp. 306–309, 2001.

[9] S. E. Pitner, "Carotid thrombosis due to intraoral trauma. An unusual complication of a common childhood accident," *The New England Journal of Medicine*, vol. 274, no. 14, pp. 764–767, 1966.

# 40

# A Rare Entity: Bilateral First Rib Fractures Accompanying Bilateral Scapular Fractures

**Gultekin Gulbahar,**[1] **Tevfik Kaplan,**[2] **Hasan Bozkurt Turker,**[3] **Ahmet Gokhan Gundogdu,**[4] **and Serdar Han**[2]

[1]*Division of Thoracic Surgery, Dr. Nafiz Korez Sincan State Hospital, Ankara, Turkey*
[2]*Department of Thoracic Surgery, Ufuk University School of Medicine, Ankara, Turkey*
[3]*Division of Orthopedics and Traumatology, Dr. Nafiz Korez Sincan State Hospital, Ankara, Turkey*
[4]*Division of Thoracic Surgery, Arnavutkoy State Hospital, Istanbul, Turkey*

Correspondence should be addressed to Tevfik Kaplan; tevfikkaplan@yahoo.com

Academic Editor: Vasileios Papadopoulos

First rib fractures are scarce due to their well-protected anatomic locations. Bilateral first rib fractures accompanying bilateral scapular fractures are very rare, although they may be together with scapular and clavicular fractures. According to our knowledge, no case of bilateral first rib fractures accompanying bilateral scapular fractures has been reported, so we herein discussed the diagnosis, treatment, and complications of bone fractures due to thoracic trauma in bias of this rare entity.

## 1. Introduction

Rib fractures commonly occur following blunt thoracic trauma and they are seen more frequently in the lower thoracic cage, where the ribs are relatively less protected. First rib fractures are scarce due to their well-protected anatomic locations. Generally, they occur following blunt traumas of high energy [1]. But indirect trauma, sudden contraction of the neck muscles, stress, and fatigue fractures may also give rise to this rare entity [2]. Close and cautious follow-up is necessary for early and late complications, because of the neighboring brachial plexus and the vascular structures. Similarly bilateral scapular fractures are rare and are related to high energy trauma [3]. While the treatment option for noncomplicated first rib fractures is conservative, some certain scapular fractures may necessitate surgical intervention. First rib fractures may be together with scapular or clavicular fractures but on the other hand the presence of these fractures together is very rare. Herein we report a case with bilateral first rib fracture accompanying bilateral scapular fracture treated nonsurgically.

## 2. Case

A seventy-seven-year-old female patient was admitted to the emergency department because of a motor vehicle accident. The patient was accepted to the trauma care unit. She was in good state of health, conscious with a Glasgow Coma Scale score of 15, and her hemodynamic state was stable. On physical examination, she had bilateral painful shoulder movements, bilateral tenderness of the lateral hemithoraces, tenderness on the back, and a 7 cm laceration of the scalp on the left parietal region. The hematological and biochemical blood analyses were consistent with the trauma. Bilateral first rib fractures were detected on chest X-ray (Figure 1(a)). Additionally computed axial tomography (CAT) of the chest revealed bilateral scapular fractures and bilateral limited pulmonary contusions in both hemithoraces (Figures 1(b), 1(c), and 1(d)). No neurovascular deficits were detected on the physical and radiologic examinations of the upper extremities. According to bone mineral densitometry the patient did not have osteoporosis. Conservative treatment was initiated in the intensive care unit. During the follow-up, the symptoms subsided and there was no complication.

(a)

(b)                                              (c)                                              (d)

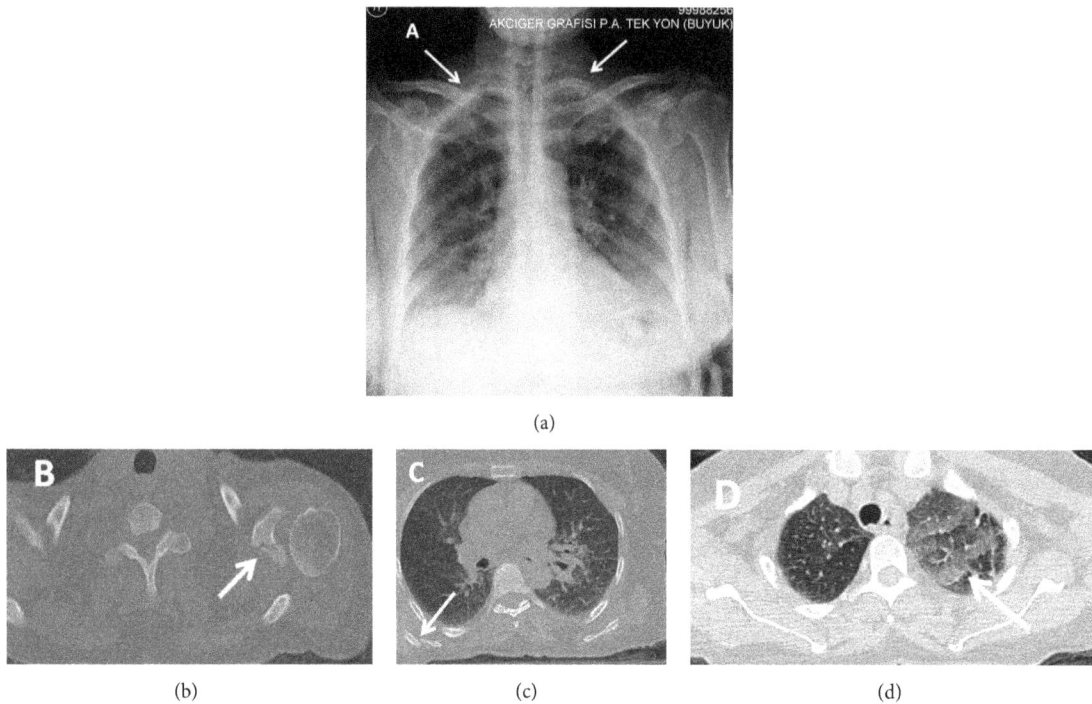

FIGURE 1: (a) Bilateral first rib fractures (white arrows). (b) Left scapular glenoid fracture (white arrow). (c) Right scapular body fracture (white arrow). (d) Pulmonary contusion (white arrow).

Thus, the patient was discharged with analgesics, bed rest, and bilateral body fixation for scapular fractures on the seventh day of the trauma.

## 3. Discussion

Fractures of the scapula and the first rib are quite rare [1–4]. The fractures of the first rib require injuries of high energy due to its profound location and good protection by the overlying soft tissue, clavicle, and scapula [3]. Similarly fractures of the scapula are scarce and constitute only about 1% of all fractures [4]. Although scapular and first rib fractures commonly occur with severe blunt trauma, first rib fractures can also be caused by sudden and powerful contraction of the muscles of the neck and stress fractures can also be seen [3, 5]. Scapular fractures can also develop due to muscle spasms, electrical shock, epileptic seizures, and metabolic imbalance [2].

In cases of high energy trauma caused first rib fractures, fatal complications of the neighboring structures such as subclavian vasculature, brachial plexus, and mediastinal contents. Early complications of the first rib fractures are pneumothorax, rupture of apex of lung, Horner's syndrome, injury of the brachial plexus, injury of the subclavian artery, pleurisy, trachea-esophageal fistula formation, aneurysm of the aortic arch, and abscess formation in the clavicular neighborhood [2]. Such complications are more common with unilateral fractures rather than bilateral ones. Thus, first rib fracture cases require immediate medical attention to evaluate the accompanying life-threatening injuries [1]. On

physical examination, pulse deficit of the upper extremity, blood pressure difference between the upper and lower extremities, edema of the extremity, and motor and sensory neurological deficits must be carefully sought and CAT, magnetic resonance imaging, and electromyography studies must be applied in case of suspicion. In cases without neurovascular injuries, the choice of treatment is analgesia, bed rest, and hot compression. Late complications of the first rib fracture cases are thoracic outlet syndrome and nonunion [2].

Since the scapular fractures are related to high energy traumas like the first rib fractures, multiple system traumas may accompany the situation [3]. So the patients with the scapular fractures must be examined thoroughly starting with the thoracic cage. In physical examination of the scapula, local tenderness, swelling, and painful shoulder movements may be observed. The deformation of the scapula may lead to hematoma formation and rotator cuff injury, which is characterized by the weakness in the movement of shoulder joint [5].

High quality X-ray and CAT are preferred for the diagnosis of scapular fracture [4]. Three-dimensional reconstructions of CAT images may be helpful in detecting the exact type of fracture but it may be insufficient in the diagnosis of nondisplaced fractures. Thus, it must be used along with CAT scan [6]. Such diagnostic procedures are also needed for deciding the modality of treatment. A displacement of greater than 5 millimeters of the glenoid fossa, greater than 10 mm displacement of the glenoid rim, disrupted superior shoulder suspensor complex, greater than 1 centimeter translation or greater than $40°$ angulations of the glenoid neck favor surgical treatment [4, 7, 8]. In scapular fracture cases which do not require surgery, bilateral shoulder joint immobilization is the treatment option [4].

In our case, the diagnosis was made through X-ray and CAT studies. Right-sided scapular body fracture and left-sided glenoid fracture were found to accompany bilateral rib fractures. No neurovascular or mediastinal complication was seen. Analgesics, hot compression, and bilateral shoulder joint immobilization were used for nonsurgical treatment. Immobilization was discontinued after three weeks. At the end of one-month follow-up, there was a significant decrease in the amount of pain.

## 4. Conclusion

Bilateral first rib fractures accompanying bilateral scapular fractures are quite rare and according to our knowledge our case is the single one in English medical literature. Although isolated bilateral scapular fracture and isolated bilateral first rib fractures may be related to indirect trauma, our case, which contains both entities, is related to high energy trauma. First rib fractures must be overinvestigated in the emergency department because of the probability of major vascular and neurological injuries that may accompany them.

## Conflict of Interests

The authors declared that there is no conflict of interests.

## References

[1] S. Chatterjee, R. Dey, P. Guha, R. Ray, and S. Sinha, "Isolated traumatic bilateral first rib fracture: a rare entity," *Tanaffos*, vol. 10, no. 4, pp. 60–63, 2011.

[2] R. Karuppal, C. M. Kumaran, A. Marthya, R. V. Raman, and S. Somasundaran, "Isolated bilateral first rib fracture associated with congenital cervical block vertebra—a case report," *Journal of Orthopaedics*, vol. 10, no. 3, pp. 149–151, 2013.

[3] M. Tuček, J. Bartoníček, P. Novotný, and M. Voldřich, "Bilateral scapular fractures in adults," *International Orthopaedics*, vol. 37, no. 4, pp. 659–665, 2013.

[4] S. C. Dwivedi and A. N. Varma, "Bilateral fracture of the first ribs," *Journal of Trauma*, vol. 23, no. 6, p. 538, 1983.

[5] B. Ejnisman, E. A. Figueiredo, B. B. Terra, G. C. Monteiro, A. C. Pochini, and C. V. Andreoli, "Exact moment of bilateral scapular fracture during skydiving captured on video," *BMJ Case Reports*, vol. 2011, Article ID bcr0920103351, 2011.

[6] B. M. Armitage, C. A. Wijdicks, I. S. Tarkin et al., "Mapping of scapular fractures with three-dimensional computed tomography," *The Journal of Bone and Joint Surgery—American Volume*, vol. 91, no. 9, pp. 2222–2228, 2009.

[7] A. van Noort, "Scapular fractures," in *Rockwood and Green's Fractures in Adults*, R. W. Bucholz, J. D. Heckman, and C. M. CourtBrown, Eds., pp. 1145–1164, Lippincott Williams & Wilkins, Philadelphia, Pa, USA, 7th edition, 2009.

[8] T. P. Goss, "Scapular fractures and dislocations: diagnosis and treatment," *Journal of the American Academy of Orthopaedic Surgeons*, vol. 3, no. 1, pp. 22–33, 1995.

# 41

# A Case of Palytoxin Poisoning in a Home Aquarium Enthusiast and His Family

**Christine Hall, David Levy, and Steven Sattler**

*Emergency Medicine Residency Program, Good Samaritan Hospital Medical Center, West Islip, NY 11795, USA*

Correspondence should be addressed to Christine Hall; crishalldo@gmail.com

Academic Editor: Michael Sand

Inhalational exposure to palytoxin is an extremely rare cause of respiratory distress. This little-known marine toxin has the potential to cause significant morbidity and mortality. Toxicity has been best documented in cases of ingestion but has also been seen in cases of dermal exposure and inhalation of vapors. Palytoxin has been found in several coral species, some of which are favored by home aquarium enthusiasts and are commercially available. We report a case of a family who were exposed to the aerosolized toxin following the cleaning of a coral in their home aquarium. It is important that clinicians be aware of this source of toxic exposure to provide necessary care to these patients.

## 1. Introduction

Palytoxin is a highly toxic substance and has been isolated from certain marine species including Zoantharia coral (Figure 1). This particular species is available to those who collect coral for home aquariums. In this case a 53-year-old male presented to the Emergency Department (ED) with dyspnea, starting shortly after cleaning his exotic coral species from his home aquarium which he identified as a Zoantharia species. A literature review identified only a limited number of cases of inhalational exposure attributable to palytoxin, although there is an abundance of self-reported exposures found on the Internet.

## 2. Case Report

A 53-year-old male presented to the ED with his wife and followed shortly by their daughter for evaluation of dyspnea which began approximately six hours prior to arrival. He had an associated nonproductive cough which had been worsening over that time period. He reported a subjective fever, chills, and myalgias. He had taken Robitussin and Aleve prior to arrival without relief. He stated that the symptoms began 1-2 hours following the cleaning of an exotic coral which he identified as a species of Zoantharia from his home aquarium. He had cleaned the coral using hot tap water in his basement sink. He identified the coral as a Zoantharia species of coral. He had not previously cleaned that particular coral and did not use any protective equipment while cleaning it. Both his wife and daughter were present in the home while he was cleaning the coral. His wife was in an adjoining basement room and his daughter was upstairs on the first floor of the home. Both presented to the ED with similar but less severe symptoms with the degree of severity commensurate with the distance from the location where the coral was being cleaned.

The patient's past medical history was significant only for hypothyroidism, hyperlipidemia, and psoriasis for which he was taking levothyroxine, rosuvastatin, and glucosamine chondroitin. Social history was significant for prior tobacco use, with a 20 pack-year history, with cessation one year prior to this encounter.

Vital signs included tachycardia at a rate of 112, a blood pressure of 155/83, respiratory rate of 18 with an oxygen saturation of 96% at room air, and a temperature of 102.6°F taken orally. On physical examination, bilateral expiratory wheezes with normal chest excursion were noted, with normal chest excursion. The patient had no evidence of respiratory distress. Cardiac examination revealed a regular tachycardia without murmurs, rubs, or gallops. The patient's wife's and daughter's examination revealed similar findings.

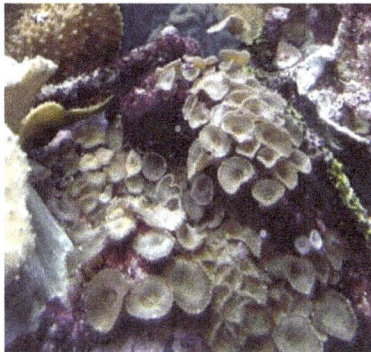

FIGURE 1: Coral similar to that encountered by the patient.

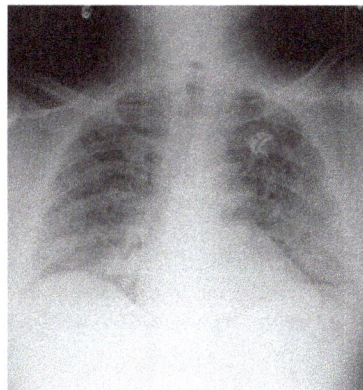

FIGURE 2: Chest X-ray from hospital day 3 showing worsening bibasilar opacities.

Acetaminophen was given for the fever with improvement of temperature to 100.8°F. Nebulized albuterol was given for the dyspnea and wheezing, with minimal improvement of symptoms. A portable chest X-ray was obtained and was normal. An EKG showed sinus tachycardia. Lab findings were significant for leukocytosis of 14,000, and an influenza swab was negative for influenza A and influenza B, and cardiac troponin I and brain natriuretic peptide (BNP) were normal.

The patient's condition continued to deteriorate requiring increasing supplemental oxygen to maintain his saturation above 90%. He received repeated doses of nebulized albuterol and oral acetaminophen with no change in condition. An arterial blood gas (ABG) was obtained while the patient was receiving four liters of oxygen by nasal cannula that was significant for a partial oxygen pressure ($pO_2$) of 65 mmHg. The New York City Poison Control Center was consulted and reported that certain toxic coral species have been found to cause pulmonary edema in cases of inhalational exposure when being handled out of water. As a result of the worsening clinical manifestations the patient was admitted to the intensive care unit with a diagnosis of respiratory distress from inhalational palytoxin exposure. During the course of the hospitalization the patient experienced a worsening cough, increased generalized weakness, and malaise. On the second inpatient day he developed hemoptysis. His $pO_2$ on ABG decreased further to 76 mmHg while on 85% $FiO_2$ via face mask. Serial chest X-rays demonstrated worsening bibasilar opacities (Figure 2). Lab work was significant for continued leukocytosis peaking at 22,000 on the third inpatient day. An echocardiogram was performed with no significant cardiac dysfunction identified. By day 4, the patient began to demonstrate mild clinical improvement with decreasing hemoptysis and improvement of generalized weakness. He continued to require supplemental oxygen by face mask throughout his hospitalization, with $O_2$ saturations dropping to the mid-80s with trials at room air.

After seven days of inpatient treatment the patient was discharged home with the diagnosis of acute toxic lung injury. At the time of discharge he required portable oxygen. He was also discharged with an albuterol metered dose inhaler and prednisone taper. The patient's wife and daughter were also hospitalized at the initial ED encounter but clinically improved after 24 hours and were discharged home in stable condition after symptomatic treatment and observation. The patient continued to require portable $O_2$ by nasal cannula and nebulized albuterol for 1 month following discharge, following which he made a complete recovery.

## 3. Discussion

Palytoxin is known to be a dangerous and often deadly toxin which can cause significant morbidity and mortality [1, 2]. Cases of human exposure have been documented from ingestion of contaminated seafood, dermal exposure, and inhalational exposure [3, 4]. This rare toxin which is most often found in soft corals and dinoflagellates has been definitively identified in zoanthid corals found both in the homes of collectors and for sale commercially [2].

Palytoxin is a marine polyether toxin which has effects on the cellular level. The toxin targets the sodium-potassium ATPase pumps inhibiting their function [4–6]. Human fatalities have been reported in cases of palytoxin ingestion [5]. In these cases mortality occurred primarily from myocardial damage and rhabdomyolysis resulting in renal failure [1].

One of the largest and earliest documented cases of inhalation exposures linked to palytoxin was reported during an *Ostreopsis ovata* bloom in the Mediterranean in 2006. It affected over 200 individuals in the local area. Exposure caused a spectrum of illness from mild symptoms such as rhinorrhea, cough, dyspnea, fever, and bronchospasm, to more severe illness in some of those exposed, requiring hospitalization and supportive care in approximately 10% of those reporting symptoms [2].

In recent literature, an increasing number of cases of home inhalational exposures have been reported [7–10]. The aerosolized toxin has affected entire families following exposure to Zoantharia coral in the home. To date, there have been no documented fatalities from inhalational exposure to palytoxin. These patients have frequently required hospitalization and supportive care for mild to severe respiratory reactions. The most commonly reported presenting symptoms are fever, cough, and dyspnea. Some patients additionally presented with chest pain and headache. Patients report a sudden onset of symptoms within minutes to hours after exposure to the coral species during cleaning or following attempted destruction of the coral with hot or boiling water. On presentation most patients were found to be febrile, tachycardic, and tachypneic, and in some cases wheezes were noted on physical examination. Lab findings of leukocytosis have been consistently reported in cases of inhalational exposure. Treatment in all of these cases was supportive, primarily with inhaled corticosteroids [7–10]. Most patients were discharged from the hospital following a short period of observation, although some patients with more severe respiratory symptoms required hospitalization [7].

Inhalational exposure to palytoxin is an extremely rare cause of respiratory distress. Although there is currently no definitive test to diagnose palytoxin exposure, a similar constellation of symptoms and laboratory findings have been described in previously reported inhalational exposures attributed to Zoantharia coral species. The presentation of this patient and his family and the synchronicity of symptomatic onset are highly indicative of a toxic inhalational exposure from the coral species in their home aquarium.

## Conflict of Interests

The authors declare that there is no conflict of interests regarding the publication of this paper.

## References

[1] J. R. Deeds and M. D. Schwartz, "Human risk associated with palytoxin exposure," *Toxicon*, vol. 56, no. 2, pp. 150–162, 2010.

[2] J. R. Deeds, S. M. Handy, K. D. White, and J. D. Reimer, "Palytoxin found in *Palythoa* sp. zoanthids (Anthozoa, Hexacorallia) sold in the home aquarium trade," *PLoS ONE*, vol. 6, no. 4, Article ID e18235, 2011.

[3] A. Tubaro, P. Durando, G. Del Favero et al., "Case definitions for human poisonings postulated to palytoxins exposure," *Toxicon*, vol. 57, no. 3, pp. 478–495, 2011.

[4] S. P. Nordt, J. Wu, S. Zahller, R. F. Clark, and F. L. Cantrell, "Palytoxin poisoning after dermal contact with zoanthid coral," *Journal of Emergency Medicine*, vol. 40, no. 4, pp. 397–399, 2011.

[5] P. Riobó and J. M. Franco, "Palytoxins: biological and chemical determination," *Toxicon*, vol. 57, no. 3, pp. 368–375, 2011.

[6] K. Hoffmann, M. Hermanns-Clausen, C. Buhl et al., "A case of palytoxin poisoning due to contact with zoanthid corals through a skin injury," *Toxicon*, vol. 51, no. 8, pp. 1535–1537, 2008.

[7] M. Bernasconi, D. Berger, M. Tamm, and D. Stolz, "Aquarism: an innocent leisure activity?" *Respiration*, vol. 84, no. 5, pp. 436–439, 2012.

[8] P. Sud, M. K. Su, H. A. Greller, N. Majlesi, and A. Gupta, "Case series: inhaled coral vapor—toxicity in a tank," *Journal of Medical Toxicology*, vol. 9, no. 3, pp. 282–286, 2013.

[9] L. Snoeks and J. Veenstra, "Family with fever after cleaning a sea aquarium," *Nederlands Tijdschrift voor Geneeskunde*, vol. 156, no. 12, Article ID A4200, 2012.

[10] N. Majlesi, M. K. Su, G. M. Chan, D. C. Lee, and H. A. Greller, "A case of inhalational exposure to palytoxin," *Clinical Toxicology*, vol. 46, article 637, 2008.

# 42

# Concurrent Spontaneous Sublingual and Intramural Small Bowel Hematoma due to Warfarin Use

**Gül Pamukçu Günaydın,[1] Hatice Duygu Çiftçi Sivri,[1] Serkan Sivri,[2] Yavuz Otal,[1] Ayhan Özhasenekler,[3] and Gülhan Kurtoğlu Çelik[1]**

[1]*Department of Emergency Medicine, Ankara Atatürk Training and Research Hospital, Çankaya, 06800 Ankara, Turkey*
[2]*Department of Cardiology, Ankara Atatürk Training and Research Hospital, Çankaya, 06800 Ankara, Turkey*
[3]*Department of Emergency Medicine, Faculty of Medicine, Yıldırım Beyazıt University, Çankaya, Ankara, Turkey*

Correspondence should be addressed to Gül Pamukçu Günaydın; gulpamukcu@gmail.com

Academic Editor: Kalpesh Jani

*Introduction.* We present a case of concurrent spontaneous sublingual and intramural small bowel hematoma due to warfarin anticoagulation. *Case.* A 71-year-old man presented to the emergency department complaining of a swollen, painful tongue. He was on warfarin therapy. Physical examination revealed sublingual hematoma. His international normalized ratio was 11.9. The computed tomography scan of the neck demonstrated sublingual hematoma. He was admitted to emergency department observation unit, monitored closely; anticoagulation was reversed with fresh frozen plasma and vitamin K. 26 hours after his arrival to the emergency department, his abdominal pain and melena started. His abdomen tomography demonstrated intestinal submucosal hemorrhage in the ileum. He was admitted to surgical floor, monitored closely, and discharged on day 4. *Conclusion.* Since the patient did not have airway compromise holding anticoagulant, reversing anticoagulation, close monitoring and observation were enough for management of both sublingual and spontaneous intramural small bowel hematoma.

## 1. Introduction

Sublingual hematoma is a rare and potentially life threatening complication of oral anticoagulation [1–3]. Spontaneous intramural small bowel hematoma (SISBH) due to oral anticoagulation is also rare but generally is not life threatening and may improve with medical treatment [4].

We present the case of concurrent spontaneous sublingual and intramural small bowel hematoma due to warfarin anticoagulation. To our knowledge, there is only one published case in Google scholar and none in PubMed that these two entities are seen together.

## 2. Case

A 71-year-old man presented to the emergency department complaining of a swollen, painful tongue and difficulty to speak that began a few hours ago. He did not have recent trauma, dental work, cough, or fever. He was on warfarin therapy, 5 mg/day for recurrent deep vein thrombosis for over a year.

His vital signs were within normal limits. Oral physical examination revealed 3 × 3 cm sized, red-purple, tense, and tender mass consistent with a sublingual hematoma (Figure 1). He was not in respiratory distress and did not have stridor. The submental triangle was swollen and ecchymotic (Figure 2).

Laboratory studies were significant for international normalized ratio (INR) of 11.9 (0.8–1.2), with a prothrombin time (PT) of 139.1 sec (8.8–14), and with partial thromboplastin time (PTT) of 108.7 sec (22–38). He said that his INR levels were not checked for over 6 months because he was living in a remote village that was 2 hours away from the nearest hospital that has the test. His hemoglobin was 14.2 g/dL, platelet count was 234 K/$\mu$L, and white blood cell count was 15.7 K/$\mu$L. His electrolytes, liver function tests, urea, and creatine levels were within normal limits. The computed tomography scan of the neck demonstrated sublingual hematoma.

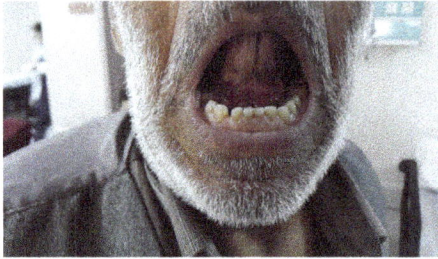

FIGURE 1: Sublingual hematoma.

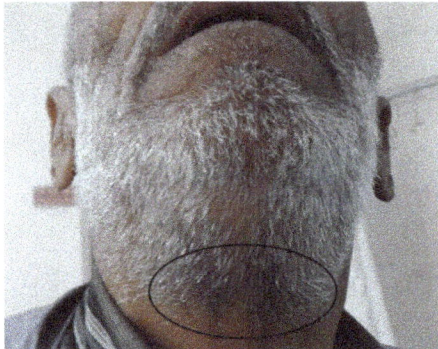

FIGURE 2: Submental ecchymosis.

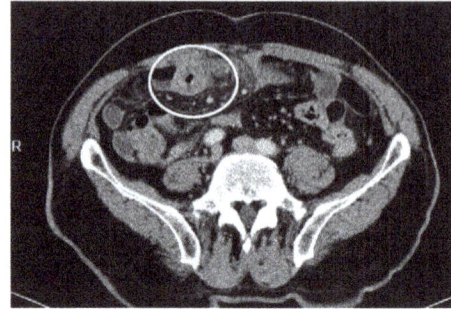

FIGURE 3: Intestinal submucosal hemorrhage.

The patient was evaluated by otolaryngologist. Flexible nasopharyngoscopy demonstrated that the hematoma was limited to the sublingual area. We stopped warfarin treatment and coagulopathy was reversed with 10 mg of IV vitamin K and 5 units of fresh frozen plasma. An INR measurement was 1.4 after 3 hours. He was given fentanyl for pain reduction.

26 hours after his arrival to the emergency department, his abdominal pain and melena started. Abdominal ultrasound revealed mural thickening in the intestinal wall. His abdomen tomography demonstrated intestinal submucosal hemorrhage in the ileum (Figure 3).

The patient was evaluated by general surgeon and was admitted. He was monitored closely and kept nothing by mouth. He was started on IV fluids and omeprazole. His hematocrit remained stable, and both sublingual and intestinal hemorrhage resolved slowly. He was started on oral diet on day 3 and discharged on day 4.

## 3. Discussion

Bleeding is the main complication of anticoagulation [5]. The incidence of hemorrhage is related to INR level [1]. Our patient had elevated INR level possibly due to not being regularly checked since he was living in village far away from the hospital.

Upper airway hematomas are rare. Retropharyngeal, submaxillary and epiglottic hematomas may be difficult to diagnose, but sublingual hematoma can be seen easily [2]. Computed tomography of the upper airway is needed to define the extent of hemorrhage [6, 7]. In our patient physical

exam revealed sublingual hematoma. CT was obtained to see the extent of hemorrhage.

Sublingual hematoma may be life threatening by causing airway obstruction. Some authors recommend that medical treatment combined with early prophylactic surgical airway should be standard of care but there is no consensus [8]. Surgical decompression of the hematoma is a treatment choice but it may cause edema, airway obstruction, and massive bleeding [9]. Awake fiber optic nasotracheal intubation is a good option for securing the airway; it can also show the extension of hemorrhage into other areas of upper airway [8]. Since the patient did not have airway compromise he was observed conservatively and we did not perform surgery or early intubation or surgical airway.

Medical treatment of overanticoagulation is withholding the drug, parenteral vitamin K and fresh frozen plasma or factor concentrates [1, 2, 10]. Some researchers recommend the use of antibiotics in the treatment of upper airway hematomas because it may be a result of localized infection and vasodilatation [1] but our patient did not have any symptoms of infection and antibiotics were not necessary. The use of systemic steroids is controversial and not of proven benefit in upper airway hematomas [1]; we did not use steroids.

The clinical presentation of SISBH depends on the location and extent of the hematoma. Acute abdominal pain and ileus symptoms in patient on anticoagulation treatment should raise suspicion. USG may show intramural bowel hematomas but its sensitivity is less than CT [11]. CT may show circumferential bowel wall thickening, intramural hyper density, luminal narrowing, and intestinal obstruction. In our patient the diagnosis was made with USG and CT was obtained to see the exact location and extent of hematoma.

Holding anticoagulant, reversing anticoagulation, close monitoring and observation will be enough in management of most SISBH cases [11]. Surgery should be reserved for cases with uncertain diagnosis or complications like intra-abdominal hemorrhage, perforation, peritonitis, and intestinal obstruction not responding to conservative treatment [12]. Our patient was monitored closely and reversal of anticoagulation was enough for successful treatment. Since melena was self-limited and it was not accompanied by hematemesis we think it may be due to the penetration of the intestinal hematoma that eventually healed by supportive treatment.

## Conflict of Interests

The authors have no conflict of interests to declare.

## Acknowledgments

The work should be attributed to Ankara Atatürk Training and Research Hospital, Department Of Emergency Medicine and Department Of Emergency Medicine, Faculty Of Medicine, Yıldırım Beyazıt University.

## References

[1] D. C. Bloom, T. Haegen, and M. A. Keefe, "Anticoagulation and spontaneous retropharyngeal hematoma," *Journal of Emergency Medicine*, vol. 24, no. 4, pp. 389–394, 2003.

[2] R. González-García, G. Schoendorff, M. F. Muñoz-Guerra, F. J. Rodríguez-Campo, L. Naval-Gías, and J. Sastre-Pérez, "Upper airway obstruction by sublingual hematoma: a complication of anticoagulation therapy with acenocoumarol," *American Journal of Otolaryngology—Head and Neck Medicine and Surgery*, vol. 27, no. 2, pp. 129–132, 2006.

[3] M. Buyuklu, E. M. Bakirci, E. Topal, and G. Ceyhun, "Spontaneous lingual and sublingual haematoma: a rare complication of warfarin use," *BMJ Case Reports*, 2014.

[4] F. Altintoprak, E. Dikicier, M. Akyüz et al., "A retrospective review of patients with non-traumatic spontaneous intramural hematoma," *Turkish Journal of Gastroenterology*, vol. 24, no. 5, pp. 392–399, 2013.

[5] S. Parvizi, S. Mackeith, and M. Draper, "A rare cause of upper airway obstruction: spontaneous synchronous sublingual and laryngeal haematomas," *BMJ Case Reports*, 2011.

[6] W. J. Frohna, R. C. Lowery Jr., and F. Pita, "Lingual and sublingual hematoma causing upper airway obstruction," *Journal of Emergency Medicine*, vol. 43, no. 6, pp. 1075–1076, 2012.

[7] R. E. Berthelsen, S. Tadbiri, and C. V. Rosenstock, "Spontaneous sublingual haematoma in a patient treated with warfarin," *Acta Anaesthesiologica Scandinavica*, vol. 57, no. 4, pp. 530–531, 2013.

[8] A. F. Cohen and S. P. Warman, "Upper airway obstruction secondary to warfarin-induced sublingual hematoma," *Archives of Otolaryngology—Head and Neck Surgery*, vol. 115, no. 6, pp. 718–720, 1989.

[9] E. Brotfain, L. Koyfman, S. Andrey et al., "Spontaneous sublingual hematoma: surgical or non-surgical management?" *International Journal of Case Reports and Images*, vol. 3, no. 1, pp. 1–4, 2012.

[10] E. Cashman, M. Shandilya, M. Amin, J. Hughes, and M. Walsh, "Warfarin-induced sublingual hematoma mimicking ludwig angina: conservative management of a potentially life-threatening condition," *Ear, Nose & Throat Journal*, vol. 90, no. 2, article E1, 2011.

[11] M. Moftah, R. Cahill, and S. Johnston, "Spontaneous sublingual and intramural small-bowel hematoma in a patient on oral anticoagulation," *Gastroenterology Insights*, vol. 4, no. 2, article e17, 2012.

[12] A. Abdel Samie, R. Sun, A. Huber, W. Höpfner, and L. Theilmann, "Spontaneous intramural small-bowel hematoma secondary to anticoagulant therapy: a case series," *Medizinische Klinik—Intensivmedizin und Notfallmedizin*, vol. 108, no. 2, pp. 144–148, 2013.

# 43

# Double Bolus Thrombolysis for Suspected Massive Pulmonary Embolism during Cardiac Arrest

**Gerard O'Connor,[1] Gareth Fitzpatrick,[2] Ayman El-Gammal,[2] and Peadar Gilligan[2]**

[1]*Department of Emergency Medicine, Mater Misericordiae University Hospital, Eccles Street, Dublin 7, Ireland*
[2]*Department of Emergency Medicine, Beaumont Hospital, Beaumont Road, Dublin 9, Ireland*

Correspondence should be addressed to Gerard O'Connor; geroconnor@me.com

Academic Editor: Kazuhito Imanaka

More than 70% of cardiac arrest cases are caused by acute myocardial infarction (AMI) or pulmonary embolism (PE). Although thrombolytic therapy is a recognised therapy for both AMI and PE, its indiscriminate use is not routinely recommended during cardiopulmonary resuscitation (CPR). We present a case describing the successful use of double dose thrombolysis during cardiac arrest caused by pulmonary embolism. Notwithstanding the relative lack of high-level evidence, this case suggests a scenario in which recombinant tissue Plasminogen Activator (rtPA) may be beneficial in cardiac arrest. In addition to the strong clinical suspicion of pulmonary embolism as the causative agent of the patient's cardiac arrest, the extremely low end-tidal $CO_2$ suggested a massive PE. The absence of dilatation of the right heart on subxiphoid ultrasound argued against the diagnosis of PE, but not conclusively so. In the context of the circulatory collapse induced by cardiac arrest, this aspect was relegated in terms of importance. The second dose of rtPA utilised in this case resulted in return of spontaneous circulation (ROSC) and did not result in haemorrhage or an adverse effect.

## 1. Introduction

Acute pulmonary embolism is a common disease with well-recognised morbidity and mortality [1–3]. It can present with variable, often nonspecific signs and symptoms, and this often leads to delayed diagnosis [4–6]. The TROICA study argued against the indiscriminate use of lysis in those in cardiac arrest [7]. Emergent thrombolysis is however being increasingly utilised for those with immediately life-threatening complications of pulmonary embolism [8–10].

In this regard, contemporary guidelines [11] suggest administration of thrombolysis for high-risk patients with pulmonary embolism (shock and/or hypotension present) and intermediate risk patients with pulmonary embolism where haemodynamic decompensation is present (as a result of evidence of both RV dysfunction—by echocardiography or CT angiography—and elevated cardiac biomarker levels in the circulation).

High level evidence in respect of thrombolysis of PE during cardiac arrest is lacking. While there are case reports and case series that describe successful resuscitation following administration of systemic thrombolytic therapy during cardiac arrest (from suspected PE) [12–16], there is also literature arguing against its use [17, 18]. This is in addition to the arguments that arise as a result of the publication bias of successful case reports and case series. Guidelines—including Class I recommendation from the European Society of Cardiology [11]—advocate proceeding with lysis in cardiac arrest associated with confirmed PE and also proceeding with lysis in cases of cardiac arrest associated with suspected PE [19, 20].

The most frequently used emergency thrombolysis dosing regimen for PE in cardiac arrest remains the prototypical 2003 British Thoracic Society regime of alteplase 50 mg intravenous (IV) bolus [21]. It is unclear on the optimum approach in those in which first-dose bolus systemic thrombolysis fails to achieve return of spontaneous circulation (ROSC). Options may involve a decision to administer a second bolus of thrombolysis, catheter directed thrombolysis, or other intervention. Extra-corporeal life support [22, 23] and surgical embolectomy [11, 20, 24–26] are treatment options in massive PE, although the decision on these options becomes even more complicated in those in cardiac arrest. This case of successful resuscitation following double dose thrombolysis should help to inform the decision making process for those facing a similar dilemma in the future.

## 2. Case

A 39 year-old gentleman presented to the Emergency Department with a two-day history of pleuritic chest pain, lethargy and associated symptoms of progressively increasing shortness of breath (now occurring with minimal exertion). This occurred on a background of more long-standing non-specific lethargy. There was a history of a recent long-haul flight from Nigeria to Ireland one week previously. At presentation, he exhibited a tachycardia of 116 beats per minute, blood pressure of 131/94 mmHg, and a respiratory rate of 22 breaths per minute.

An electrocardiogram revealed a sinus tachycardia with symmetrical T wave inversion in praecordial lead V3. Arterial blood gas analysis showed a $PaO_2$ of 7.5 kPa, $PaCO_2$ of 3.8 kPa, pH 7.47, and an oxygen saturation of 89%. A D-dimer assay performed at triage was significantly elevated at 10.5 mg/L. Given the working diagnosis of probable pulmonary embolus (high-risk pretest probability), therapeutic low-molecular-weight heparin (Enoxaparin 120 mg subcutaneously) was administered prior to emergent Computed Tomographic Pulmonary Angiography (CTPA).

Two hours later, while awaiting emergent CTPA, the patient collapsed and was found to be in cardiac arrest. Cardiopulmonary resuscitation was promptly initiated for pulseless electrical activity (PEA). Intubation with a cuffed oroendotracheal tube (COETT) was achieved without interruption of chest compressions. Despite primary confirmation of COETT placement, end-tidal $CO_2$ was not detected initially. Subxiphoid ultrasound—performed during brief interruption of chest compressions—did not reveal a dilated right side of heart. Despite this, given the overall clinical picture at this juncture, a presumptive diagnosis of massive or saddle pulmonary embolus was made.

Along with conventional ACLS adrenaline therapy, rtPA (alteplase) 50 mg was promptly administered. Despite continuing high quality chest compressions and a gradual rise in quantitative end-tidal $CO_2$, no cardiac output was detected after twenty minutes. A decision was taken to administer a second bolus of rtPA (alteplase) 50 mg. Ten minutes subsequent to this and following on-going advanced life support, return of spontaneous circulation (ROSC) was achieved with an initial non-invasive blood pressure of 144/50 mmHg.

Standard post-ROSC resuscitation care was instituted and this gentleman was admitted to the intensive care unit. A CTPA demonstrated multiple bilateral pulmonary emboli. He was continued on Enoxaparin and bridged to Warfarin once critical care stability was achieved. No major (or minor) bleeding was observed during this gentleman's hospital stay. The patient ultimately recovered to hospital discharge with a Glasgow Outcome Score of 4, secondary to watershed cerebellar infarcts.

## 3. Discussion

A number of trials and guidelines address the issue of thrombolysis during a massive pulmonary embolism and submassive pulmonary embolism. There are few specific guidelines which directly address the issue of thrombolysis during cardiac arrest in those with (suspected) massive pulmonary embolism [27], that is, fulminant cases.

The British Thoracic Society (BTS) recommends a bolus of 50 mg alteplase for massive PE [21] and states that this may be *"instituted on clinical grounds alone if cardiac arrest is imminent."* The American Heart Association seems to recommend a two-hour infusion of 100 mg of alteplase in those with haemodynamic compromise (though they do not explicitly address the issue of cardiac arrest) [28]. The 2014 European Society of Cardiology Guidelines [11] recommend a dose of 100 mg rtPA over 2 hours or 0.6 mg/kg over 15 minutes [29], though again they are not explicit regarding the approach in cardiac arrest. We felt that a prolonged infusion might not represent the best approach in the situation presented, given the understandable exigencies of cardiac arrest.

There are numerous case reports and case series describing survival post thrombolysis in cardiac arrest caused by PE. Er et al. [30] retrospectively studied 104 patients in whom thrombolysis was administered for presumptive PE cardiac arrest. ROSC was achieved in 40 patients with survival to hospital discharge in 19 patients. Both ROSC and survival to hospital discharge were associated with earlier initiation of thrombolysis. Patients in this trial were treated with bolus dose rtPA with an average dose of 80.5 ± 24 mg. Janata et al. [31] describe a retrospective review of cardiac arrest patients with the cause of arrest secondary to massive PE. Sixty-six patients were reviewed with 36 of these patients treated with rtPA. They administered rtPA as a bolus of 0.6–1.0 mg rtPA/kg body weight up to a maximum of 100 mg of rtPA. Return of spontaneous circulation showed a trend towards improvement in the rtPA group (67% versus 43%, $P = 0.06$) as well as survival to discharge (19% versus 7%, $P = 0.15$).

Once thrombolysis is initiated for a suspected PE in cardiac arrest, guidelines suggest that CPR should be continued for at least 60–90 minutes [13, 32–36].

Domino or double dose thrombolysis also appears in the literature. In the sentinel study by Böttiger et al. [37], 90 patients were assigned to intervention (thrombolysis) or control arms of treatment for cardiac arrest. Those in the intervention arm received a bolus of 5000 IU of heparin with 50 mg rtPA after 15 min of unsuccessful CPR, with a repeat bolus of heparin and rtPA 30 minutes later if ROSC was not achieved. While there is no breakdown on the numbers receiving double dose thrombolysis, in this early study on thrombolysis in cardiac arrest they noted statistically significant increases in ROSC and survival to hospital admission in the thrombolysis group. Kürkciyan et al. [38] describe intervening with regimens of 100 mg rtPA (either as a 50 mg double bolus or as a bolus dose of 15 mg, followed by continuous infusion of 85 mg over 90 minutes). In this intervention arm the two survivors to hospital discharge received double bolus doses. Similarly Fengler and Brady [39], in their suggested treatment algorithm, advocate a repeat bolus of alteplase 50 mg if ROSC is not achieved after 15 minutes after the first dose. In our case, we cannot discount that, despite achievement of ROSC after the second bolus, this success might be better explained by the haemodynamic improvements brought about by the first bolus [40].

There is general consensus that thrombolysis should be considered in cardiac arrest where pulmonary embolism is strongly suspected. The exact dosage and timing of fibrinolysis remain to be clarified [7, 19, 37, 41], though there does appear to be a trend towards improved survival in those in whom intervention is initiated at an earlier juncture. This is seen in the study by Er et al. [30] in which those patients who survived to hospital discharge benefitted from earlier initiation of lysis compared to all other patients ($11.0 \pm 1.3$ versus $22.5 \pm 0.9$ min; $P < 0.001$). The issue of risks and benefits in terms of haemorrhage remains a major consideration and while the principle of *primum non nocere* is more difficult to weigh in those in cardiac arrest, it should be remembered that the bleeding risks remain significant. Evidence would suggest that thrombolysis does not seem to be unduly associated with catastrophic haemorrhage in this critically ill patient group [31, 42, 43]; nevertheless there are still recognised major haemorrhage rates and intracranial haemorrhage rates of up to 10.4% [44] and 3.6% [45] in contemporary prospective trials.

Low end-tidal $CO_2$ ($ETCO_2$) is seen both in cardiac arrest [46–48] and in massive pulmonary embolism [49–55]. Increases in $ETCO_2$ are seen in recovery from both entities and have prognostic value in those in cardiac arrest in predicting the likelihood of ROSC [56]. The unrecordable levels seen at the outset of this case were assumed to result from the absolute no flow through the pulmonary circulation rather than the low flow that is seen in cardiac arrest.

Common echocardiographic findings in massive pulmonary embolism include that of an enlarged right ventricle [57] which may be associated with a flattened interventricular septum (D-sign of interventricular septal shift) and the "McConnell" sign [58, 59]. These tests were originally described in those with massive PE (and were originally performed with transthoracic approaches rather than with subxiphoid views) so their validity and applicability in terms of positive and negative predictive value for patients in cardiac arrest are unknown. Therefore, the absence of the echocardiographic features should not be used to rule out PE as a cause of cardiac arrest [60].

In conclusion, this particular case describes a clinical scenario in which double dose thrombolysis was successfully used. A similar strategy might be contemplated in the future by emergency physicians dealing with cardiac arrest caused by massive pulmonary embolism.

## Conflict of Interests

The authors declare that they have no conflict of interests regarding this paper.

## Authors' Contribution

All authors provided advice and guidance on the development and preparation of the paper.

## References

[1] S. B. Smith, J. B. Geske, J. M. Maguire, N. A. Zane, R. E. Carter, and T. I. Morgenthaler, "Early anticoagulation is associated with reduced mortality for acute pulmonary embolism," *Chest*, vol. 137, no. 6, pp. 1382–1390, 2010.

[2] J. L. Carson, M. A. Kelley, A. Duff et al., "The clinical course of pulmonary embolism," *The New England Journal of Medicine*, vol. 326, no. 19, pp. 1240–1245, 1992.

[3] V. F. Tapson, "Acute pulmonary embolism," *The New England Journal of Medicine*, vol. 358, no. 10, pp. 990–1052, 2008.

[4] P. D. Stein, A. Beemath, F. Matta et al., "Clinical characteristics of patients with acute pulmonary embolism: data from PIOPED II," *The American Journal of Medicine*, vol. 120, no. 10, pp. 871–879, 2007.

[5] P. D. Stein, F. Matta, M. H. Musani, and B. Diaczok, "Silent pulmonary embolism in patients with deep venous thrombosis: a systematic review," *American Journal of Medicine*, vol. 123, no. 5, pp. 426–431, 2010.

[6] PIOPED Investigators, "Value of the ventilation/perfusion scan in acute pulmonary embolism. Results of the Prospective Investigation of Pulmonary Embolism Diagnosis (PIOPED)," *The Journal of the American Medical Association*, vol. 263, no. 20, pp. 2753–2759, 1990.

[7] B. W. Böttiger, H.-R. Arntz, D. A. Chamberlain et al., "Thrombolysis during resuscitation for out-of-hospital cardiac arrest," *The New England Journal of Medicine*, vol. 359, no. 25, pp. 2651–2662, 2008.

[8] C. Jerjes-Sanchez, A. Ramírez-Rivera, M. de Lourdes García et al., "Streptokinase and heparin versus heparin alone in massive pulmonary embolism: a randomized controlled trial," *Journal of Thrombosis and Thrombolysis*, vol. 2, no. 3, pp. 227–229, 1995.

[9] B. Ly, H. Arnesen, H. Eie, and R. Hol, "A controlled clinical trial of streptokinase and heparin in the treatment of major pulmonary embolism," *Acta Medica Scandinavica*, vol. 203, no. 6, pp. 465–470, 1978.

[10] D. A. Tibbutt, J. A. Davies, J. A. Anderson et al., "Comparison by controlled clinical trial of streptokinase and heparin in treatment of life-threatening pulmonary embolism," *British Medical Journal*, vol. 1, no. 5904, pp. 343–347, 1974.

[11] S. V. Konstantinides and A. Torbicki, "2014 ESC guidelines on the diagnosis and management of acute pulmonary embolism," *European Heart Journal*, vol. 35, no. 43, pp. 3033–3073, 2014.

[12] M. R. Bailén, J. Á. R. Cuadra, and E. Aguayo De Hoyos, "Thrombolysis during cardiopulmonary resuscitation in fulminant pulmonary embolism: a review," *Critical Care Medicine*, vol. 29, no. 11, pp. 2211–2219, 2001.

[13] J.-P. Wu, D.-Y. Gu, S. Wang, Z.-J. Zhang, J.-C. Zhou, and R.-F. Zhang, "Good neurological recovery after rescue thrombolysis of presumed pulmonary embolism despite prior 100 minutes CPR," *Journal of Thoracic Disease*, vol. 6, no. 12, pp. E289–E293, 2014.

[14] B. W. Böttiger, H. Böhrer, A. Bach, J. Motsch, and E. Martin, "Bolus injection of thrombolytic agents during cardiopulmonary resuscitation for massive pulmonary embolism," *Resuscitation*, vol. 28, no. 1, pp. 45–54, 1994.

[15] T. Zhu, K. Pan, and Q. Shu, "Successful resuscitation with thrombolysis of a presumed fulminant pulmonary embolism during cardiac arrest," *The American Journal of Emergency Medicine*, vol. 31, no. 2, pp. 453.e1–453.e3, 2013.

[16] Q. Yin, X. Li, and C. Li, "Thrombolysis after initially unsuccessful cardiopulmonary resuscitation in presumed pulmonary

embolism," *The American Journal of Emergency Medicine*, vol. 33, no. 1, pp. 132.e1–132.e2, 2015.

[17] R. B. Abu-Laban, J. M. Christenson, G. D. Innes et al., "Tissue plasminogen activator in cardiac arrest with pulseless electrical activity," *The New England Journal of Medicine*, vol. 346, no. 20, pp. 1522–1528, 2002.

[18] N. Kucher, E. Rossi, M. De Rosa, and S. Z. Goldhaber, "Massive pulmonary embolism," *Circulation*, vol. 113, no. 4, pp. 577–582, 2006.

[19] E. J. Lavonas, I. R. Drennan, A. Gabrielli et al., "Part 10: special circumstances of resuscitation: 2015 American Heart Association guidelines update for cardiopulmonary resuscitation and emergency cardiovascular care," *Circulation*, vol. 132, no. 18, supplement 2, pp. S501–S518, 2015.

[20] A. Truhlar, C. D. Deakin, J. Soar et al., "European Resuscitation Council Guidelines for Resuscitation 2015: section 4. Cardiac arrest in special circumstances," *Resuscitation*, vol. 95, pp. 148–201, 2015.

[21] British Thoracic Society Standards of Care Committee Pulmonary Embolism Guideline Development G, "British Thoracic Society guidelines for the management of suspected acute pulmonary embolism," *Thorax*, vol. 58, no. 6, pp. 470–483, 2003.

[22] G. Maj, G. Melisurgo, M. De Bonis, and F. Pappalardo, "ECLS management in pulmonary embolism with cardiac arrest: which strategy is better?" *Resuscitation*, vol. 85, no. 10, pp. e175–e176, 2014.

[23] J. Swol, D. Buchwald, J. Strauch, and T. A. Schildhauer, "Extracorporeal life support (ECLS) for cardiopulmonary resuscitation (CPR) with pulmonary embolism in surgical patients—a case series," *Perfusion*, 2015.

[24] I. E. Konstantinov, P. Saxena, M. D. Koniuszko, J. Alvarez, and M. A. J. Newman, "Acute massive pulmonary embolism with cardiopulmonary resuscitation: management and results," *Texas Heart Institute Journal*, vol. 34, no. 1, pp. 41–46, 2007.

[25] H. C. Doerge, F. A. Schoendube, H. Loeser, M. Walter, and B. J. Messmer, "Pulmonary embolectomy: review of a 15-year experience and role in the age of thrombolytic therapy," *European Journal of Cardio-Thoracic Surgery*, vol. 10, no. 11, pp. 952–957, 1996.

[26] N. Meneveau, M.-F. Séronde, M.-C. Blonde et al., "Management of unsuccessful thrombolysis in acute massive pulmonary embolism," *Chest*, vol. 129, no. 4, pp. 1043–1050, 2006.

[27] K. P. Goran, "Thrombolysis during cardiopulmonary resuscitation should be addressed in guidelines for pulmonary embolism," *European Heart Journal*, vol. 29, no. 24, pp. 3066–3067, 2008.

[28] M. R. Jaff, M. S. McMurtry, S. L. Archer et al., "Management of massive and submassive pulmonary embolism, iliofemoral deep vein thrombosis, and chronic thromboembolic pulmonary hypertension: a scientific statement from the American Heart Association," *Circulation*, vol. 123, no. 16, pp. 1788–1830, 2011.

[29] S. V. Konstantinides, A. Torbicki, G. Agnelli et al., *2014 ESC Guidelines on the Diagnosis and Management of Acute Pulmonary Embolism-Web Addenda*, 2014, http://www.escardio.org/static_file/Escardio/Guidelines/publications/APEAcute PE_Web Addenda.pdf.

[30] F. Er, A. M. Nia, N. Gassanov, E. Caglayan, E. Erdmann, and U. C. Hoppe, "Impact of rescue-thrombolysis during cardiopulmonary resuscitation in patients with pulmonary embolism," *PLoS ONE*, vol. 4, no. 12, article e8323, 2009.

[31] K. Janata, M. Holzer, I. Kürkciyan et al., "Major bleeding complications in cardiopulmonary resuscitation: the place of thrombolytic therapy in cardiac arrest due to massive pulmonary embolism," *Resuscitation*, vol. 57, no. 1, pp. 49–55, 2003.

[32] B. W. Böttiger and E. Martin, "Thrombolytic therapy during cardiopulmonary resuscitation and the role of coagulation activation after cardiac arrest," *Current Opinion in Critical Care*, vol. 7, no. 3, pp. 176–183, 2001.

[33] F. Spöhr and B. W. Böttiger, "Safety of thrombolysis during cardiopulmonary resuscitation," *Drug Safety*, vol. 26, no. 6, pp. 367–379, 2003.

[34] C. Nobre, B. Thomas, L. Santos, and J. Tavares, "Prolonged chest compressions during cardiopulmonary resuscitation for in-hospital cardiac arrest due to acute pulmonary embolism," *Texas Heart Institute Journal*, vol. 42, no. 2, pp. 136–138, 2015.

[35] T. Hsin, F. W. Chun, and H. L. Tao, "Ultra-long cardiopulmonary resuscitation with thrombolytic therapy for a sudden cardiac arrest patient with pulmonary embolism," *American Journal of Emergency Medicine*, vol. 32, no. 11, pp. 1443.e3–1443.e4, 2014.

[36] D. K. Pedley and W. G. Morrison, "Role of thrombolytic agents in cardiac arrest," *Emergency Medicine Journal*, vol. 23, no. 10, pp. 747–752, 2006.

[37] B. W. Böttiger, C. Bode, S. Kern et al., "Efficacy and safety of thrombolytic therapy after initially unsuccessful cardiopulmonary resuscitation: a prospective clinical trial," *The Lancet*, vol. 357, no. 9268, pp. 1583–1585, 2001.

[38] I. Kürkciyan, G. Meron, F. Sterz et al., "Pulmonary embolism as a cause of cardiac arrest: presentation and outcome," *Archives of Internal Medicine*, vol. 160, no. 10, pp. 1529–1535, 2000.

[39] B. T. Fengler and W. J. Brady, "Fibrinolytic therapy in pulmonary embolism: an evidence-based treatment algorithm," *The American Journal of Emergency Medicine*, vol. 27, no. 1, pp. 84–95, 2009.

[40] H. Sors, G. Pacouret, R. Azarian, G. Meyer, B. Charbonnier, and G. Simonneau, "Hemodynamic effects of bolus vs 2-h infusion of alteplase in acute massive pulmonary embolism: a randomized controlled multicenter trial," *Chest*, vol. 106, no. 3, pp. 712–717, 1994.

[41] J. K. Logan, H. Pantle, P. Huiras, E. Bessman, and L. Bright, "Evidence-based diagnosis and thrombolytic treatment of cardiac arrest or periarrest due to suspected pulmonary embolism," *The American Journal of Emergency Medicine*, vol. 32, no. 7, pp. 789–796, 2014.

[42] K. H. Scholz, U. Tebbe, C. Herrmann et al., "Frequency of complications of cardiopulmonary resuscitation after thrombolysis during acute myocardial infarction," *The American Journal of Cardiology*, vol. 69, no. 8, pp. 724–728, 1992.

[43] M. Ruiz-Bailén, A. E. de Hoyos, M. Serrano-Córcoles, M. Díaz-Castellanos, J. Ramos-Cuadra, and A. Reina-Toral, "Efficacy of thrombolysis in patients with acute myocardial infarction requiring cardiopulmonary resuscitation," *Intensive Care Medicine*, vol. 27, no. 6, pp. 1050–1057, 2001.

[44] C. Wang, Z. Zhai, Y. Yang et al., "Efficacy and safety of low dose recombinant tissue-type plasminogen activator for the treatment of acute pulmonary thromboembolism: a randomized, multicenter, controlled trial," *Chest*, vol. 137, no. 2, pp. 254–262, 2010.

[45] C. Becattini, G. Agnelli, A. Salvi et al., "Bolus tenecteplase for right ventricle dysfunction in hemodynamically stable patients with pulmonary embolism," *Thrombosis Research*, vol. 125, no. 3, pp. e82–e86, 2010.

[46] J. L. Falk, E. C. Rackow, and M. H. Weil, "End-tidal carbon dioxide concentration during cardiopulmonary resuscitation,"

*The New England Journal of Medicine*, vol. 318, no. 10, pp. 607–611, 1988.

[47] A. R. Garnett, J. P. Ornato, E. R. Gonzalez, and E. B. Johnson, "End-tidal carbon dioxide monitoring during cardiopulmonary resuscitation," *Journal of the American Medical Association*, vol. 257, no. 4, pp. 512–515, 1987.

[48] K. R. Sheak, D. J. Wiebe, M. Leary et al., "Quantitative relationship between end-tidal carbon dioxide and CPR quality during both in-hospital and out-of-hospital cardiac arrest," *Resuscitation*, vol. 89, pp. 149–154, 2015.

[49] L. Hatle and R. Rokseth, "The arterial to end-expiratory carbon dioxide tension gradient in acute pulmonary embolism and other cardiopulmonary diseases," *Chest*, vol. 66, no. 4, pp. 352–357, 1974.

[50] R. Whitesell, C. Asiddao, D. Gollman, and J. Jablonski, "Relationship between arterial and peak expired carbon dioxide pressure during anesthesia and factors influencing the difference," *Anesthesia and Analgesia*, vol. 60, no. 7, pp. 508–512, 1981.

[51] C. Yosefy, E. Hay, Y. Nasri, E. Magen, and L. Reisin, "End tidal carbon dioxide as a predictor of the arterial $PCO_2$ in the emergency department setting," *Emergency Medicine Journal*, vol. 21, no. 5, pp. 557–559, 2004.

[52] U. K. H. Wiegand, V. Kurowski, E. Giannitsis, H. A. Katus, and H. Djonlagic, "Effectiveness of end-tidal carbon dioxide tension for monitoring of thrombolytic therapy in acute pulmonary embolism," *Critical Care Medicine*, vol. 28, no. 11, pp. 3588–3592, 2000.

[53] A. R. Hemnes, A. L. Newman, B. Rosenbaum et al., "Bedside end-tidal $CO_2$ tension as a screening tool to exclude pulmonary embolism," *European Respiratory Journal*, vol. 35, no. 4, pp. 735–741, 2010.

[54] M. Endoh, I. Yamanaka, and Y. Munetsugu, "Massive pulmonary thromboembolism during an orthopedic surgery in an obese patient," *Japanese Journal of Anesthesiology*, vol. 62, no. 10, pp. 1203–1206, 2013.

[55] I. Riaz and B. Jacob, "Pulmonary embolism in Bradford, UK: Role of end-tidal $CO_2$ as a screening tool," *Clinical Medicine, Journal of the Royal College of Physicians of London*, vol. 14, no. 2, pp. 128–133, 2014.

[56] O. Touma and M. Davies, "The prognostic value of end tidal carbon dioxide during cardiac arrest: a systematic review," *Resuscitation*, vol. 84, no. 11, pp. 1470–1479, 2013.

[57] P. MacCarthy, A. Worrall, G. McCarthy, and J. Davies, "The use of transthoracic echocardiography to guide thrombolytic therapy during cardiac arrest due to massive pulmonary embolism," *Emergency Medicine Journal*, vol. 19, no. 2, pp. 178–179, 2002.

[58] J. A. Lodato, R. P. Ward, and R. M. Lang, "Echocardiographic predictors of pulmonary embolism in patients referred for helical CT," *Echocardiography*, vol. 25, no. 6, pp. 584–590, 2008.

[59] M. V. McConnell, S. D. Solomon, M. E. Rayan, P. C. Come, S. Z. Goldhaber, and R. T. Lee, "Regional right ventricular dysfunction detected by echocardiography in acute pulmonary embolism," *American Journal of Cardiology*, vol. 78, no. 4, pp. 469–473, 1996.

[60] P.-M. Roy, I. Colombet, P. Durieux, G. Chatellier, H. Sors, and G. Meyer, "Systematic review and meta-analysis of strategies for the diagnosis of suspected pulmonary embolism," *British Medical Journal*, vol. 331, no. 7511, pp. 259–263, 2005.

# Colonic Foreign Body Retrieval Using a Modified TAMIS Technique with Standard Instruments and Trocars

**Shamir O. Cawich,**[1] **Fawwaz Mohammed,**[1] **Richard Spence,**[1] **Matthew Albert,**[2] **and Vijay Naraynsingh**[1]

[1]*Department of Clinical Surgical Sciences, University of the West Indies, St. Augustine Campus, St. Augustine, Trinidad and Tobago*
[2]*The Center for Colon and Rectal Surgery, 661 East Altamonte Drive, Altamonte Springs, FL 32701, USA*

Correspondence should be addressed to Shamir O. Cawich; socawich@hotmail.com

Academic Editor: Vasileios Papadopoulos

*Background.* Reports of retained colorectal foreign bodies (CFBs) are no longer considered uncommon. We present a case where a retained CFB was retrieved using a modified TAMIS technique using standard instruments and trocars. *Case Report.* A 52-year-old man presented with a CFB. We report our technique of extraction with standard laparoscopic instruments without specialized access platforms. *Conclusions.* This modified TAMIS technique is well suited for resource poor environments because it requires no specialized equipment, platforms, or additional skill sets compared to conventional laparoscopy.

## 1. Introduction

The earliest reports of patients presenting with retained colorectal foreign bodies (CFBs) date as far back as the 16th century [1]. Since that time, reports of retained CFBs have been increasing and it is no longer considered uncommon.

We present a case of a patient presenting with a retained CFB in which an unusual method of retrieval was used. We believe that this method is well suited for low cost environments.

## 2. Report of a Case

A 52-year-old man with no medical illnesses presented to the emergency room reporting constant pain in the gluteal region after he was allegedly abducted and beaten by a group of unknown individuals. No other useful history was volunteered.

On examination, vital signs were normal. There were no superficial lacerations or contusions in keeping with the history of an assault. Examinations of the abdomen, chest, nervous system, and musculoskeletal system were normal. There were no external injuries on examination of the gluteal

region but there was mild tenderness at the perianal region. Digital rectal examination revealed normal mucosa, an intact anal sphincter, and a normal prostate that was approximately 45 mls in volume. A plain radiograph of the pelvis was ordered as a part of the trauma series and revealed an unexpected finding: a cylindrical object with a tapered tip and radiolucent hollow base was present within the rectum (Figure 1).

With this unexpected finding, the history was revisited. Only then did the patient confess to his habit of inserting an object into the rectum for self-eroticism. The object used on this occasion was described as a metallic Cuban cigar sheath that had a tapered tip. Approximately 48 hours before, he grasped the rim of the cigar sheath with his thumb and index finger and inserted it into his rectum. However, on this occasion the cigar sheath ascended into the rectum and was not retrievable. Due to his embarrassment, he delayed presentation for 48 hours until he experienced vague rectal pain.

Although the foreign body appeared to be in the rectum on radiographs, it could not be palpated on digital rectal examination. The object was visualized on flexible sigmoidoscopy. By this time, it had ascended into the sigmoid colon

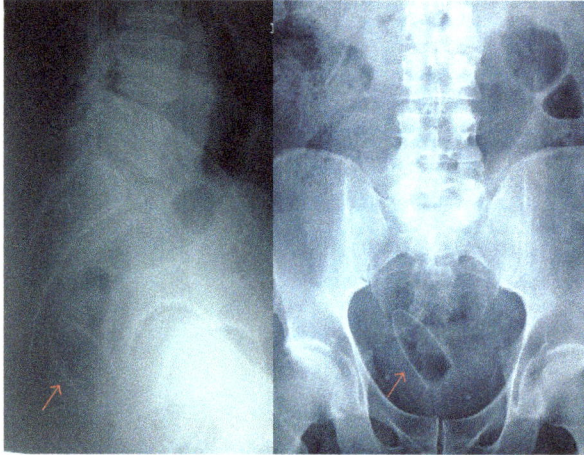

FIGURE 1: Plain radiographs of the pelvis outline a foreign body within the rectum (indicated by red arrow) that has a cylindrical shape and a tapered tip.

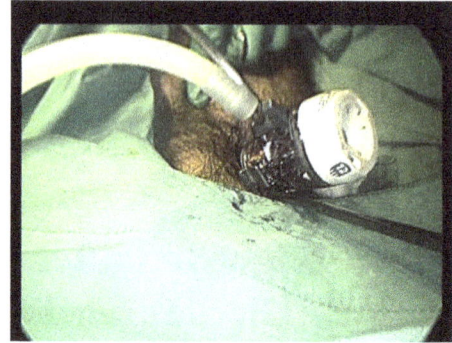

FIGURE 2: A photograph of the perineum. The patient is in lithotomy position and surgical drapes are applied. A 12 mm laparoscopic trocar is inserted into the anus and the trocar sleeve is fully advanced until the adjustable sleeve hub was pressed against the anus, creating a seal. A straight 35 mm laparoscopic grasper can be seen sliding beside the optical trocar into the anus. The seal is maintained by pressure from the anal sphincter.

but could not be retrieved since endoscopic tools could not grasp the smooth surface. An attempt to use the retroflexed scope to push the CFB distally for manual retrieval was not successful because the open end of the cigar sheath abutted the mucosa, creating a vacuum effect that kept it retained.

In order to retrieve the CFB, we secured consent for transabdominal retrieval using a laparoscopic approach. We considered retrieval by the transanal minimally invasive surgical (TAMIS) technique but we did not have specialized TAMIS platforms, instruments, or a SILS port available. Therefore, we considered inserting a laparoscope into the anus to visualize the CFB.

The patient was placed in lithotomy position and a 12 mm blunt-tip laparoscopic trocar (Endopath Excel, Ethicon, Somerville, NJ, USA) was inserted into the anus. The trocar sleeve was advanced fully until the adjustable sleeve hub was pressed against the anus, creating a seal (Figure 2). Two silk sutures were inserted into the gluteal skin at 3 and 9 o'clock and tied to the suture posts to secure the trocar. The resultant seal was sufficient to allow insufflation, enabling insertion of a standard 35 mm 0° laparoscope.

The cigar sheath was visualized in the sigmoid 30 cm proximal to the anus. It was oriented such that its base faced distally with the open rim firmly apposed to the sigmoid mucosa by vacuum effect (Figure 3). In an attempt to retrieve the CFB, two 35 mm straight laparoscopic graspers were slid beside the optical trocar into the anus (Figure 2). Apart from the optical trocar, no additional trocars were used. In order to prevent iatrogenic injury, we navigated the laparoscopic graspers into the sigmoid under laparoscopic vision (Figure 4). The instruments were sufficiently sturdy to allow the cigar sheath to be manipulated, overcoming the vacuum effect and dislodging it from the mucosa. This allowed the cigar case to be rotated within the colonic lumen so that the rim now faced the laparoscope (Figure 5). The laparoscopic graspers were used to grasp the rim of the cigar sheath and the CFB was extracted under vision (Figure 6).

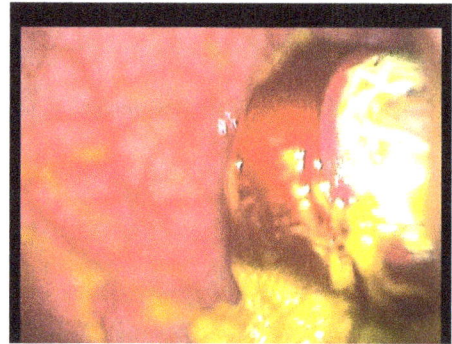

FIGURE 3: The cigar sheath is visualized in the sigmoid colon and is oriented such that the open base is firmly apposed to the sigmoid mucosa, creating a vacuum effect.

The patient recovered uneventfully and was spared laparotomy with the concomitant morbidity.

## 3. Discussion

In modern practice, CFBs are not uncommon although the true incidence remains unsettled because of inconsistent reporting. In our case, the patient initially refused to divulge the relevant history because he was embarrassed. This was not surprising since it has been established that many patients with CFB are deceptive historians [2, 3]. As many as 20% of patients will not divulge their history of CFB insertion at presentation [4] because the practice is still considered taboo. To overcome this barrier, clinicians should approach these patients in a candid manner in order to earn their trust during history taking.

An accurate history is important to ascertain the diagnosis because any delay increases the risk of complications, such as perforation or bleeding [3]. An accurate history is also important to plan the therapeutic approach. In retrospect, we could have predicted failure of endoscopic retrieval. Most

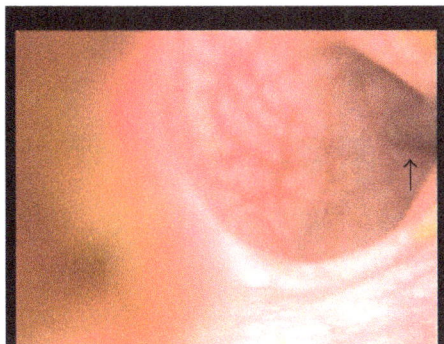

FIGURE 4: In order to retrieve the object, a straight 35 mm laparoscopic grasper was introduced into the lumen and advanced under laparoscopic vision (arrow) in order to avoid iatrogenic injury to the mucosa.

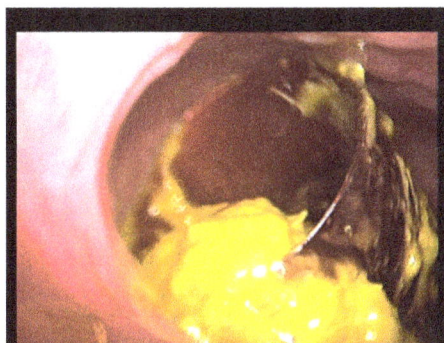

FIGURE 6: Laparoscopic graspers were used to grasp the rim of the cigar sheath and extract it under laparoscopic vision.

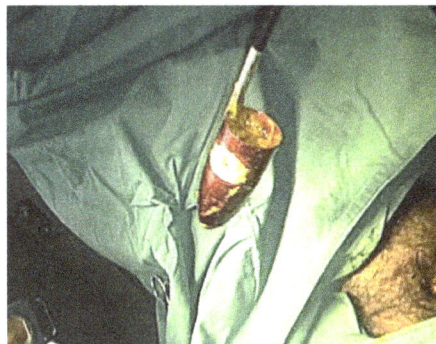

FIGURE 5: The instruments have been used to manipulate the cigar sheath and to overcome the vacuum effect. The dislodged cigar case has been rotated within the lumen so that the rim now faces the laparoscope.

reports of endoscopic retrieval involve encircling a part of the CFB with endoscopic polypectomy snares [3, 5–7]. However, there would have been no conceivable point to grasp a smooth, tapered cigar sheath with polypectomy snares.

Operative retrieval by either milking the CFB toward the anus [3, 8, 9] or by extracting via colostomy [10–12] has been described and is accepted therapeutic methods. However, they are both accompanied by attendant morbidity from laparotomy or laparoscopy. A transanal approach, when feasible, does not require a breach of the peritoneal cavity and therefore avoids potential formation of intraperitoneal collections, organ space infections, anastomotic leaks, and damage to surrounding viscera.

Transanal extraction has been documented to be successful in 60–75% of cases [3, 12–14]. In this case, transanal retrieval was not feasible because the CFB had ascended into the sigmoid colon. We were not surprised since there is free communication between the rectal and colonic lumina, with nothing to prevent retrograde migration of luminal contents. An alternative method that has been described to assist transanal extraction is to use a Foley catheter [3]. The catheter is advanced proximal to the CFB and then inflated. The inflated catheter is slowly withdrawn, pulling the CFB with it until it comes into grasp of the examining fingers.

This might have yielded success in our case, but it was not considered at the time.

We successfully utilized a modified TAMIS technique in this case. TAMIS was initially conceptualized to facilitate complete excision of upper rectal neoplasms that could not be extracted transanally [15]. This approach could theoretically spare patients the morbidity associated with anterior resections, including sexual dysfunction, urinary retention, and loss of the anal sphincter complex [15, 16]. In addition, it allows dissection under magnification leading to more accurate dissection and better hemostasis [15, 17].

There are several limitations, however, to widespread use of TAMIS including the requirement for specialized instruments, TAMIS access platforms, and a steep learning curve [15]. Some have also raised concern about post-TAMIS faecal incontinence with use of the TAMIS 40 mm rigid proctoscope [16]. Many of these concerns were overcome by using the SILS port (Covidien, Mansfield, MA, USA) to perform TAMIS [17, 18]. However, this is a limitation in a resource poor environment such as ours. In our setting, each SILS port costs US $470.21 from local distributors [19].

We believe that this modified TAMIS technique was better suited to a resource poor environment because there is no need for specialized instruments, TAMIS proctoscopes or SILS ports. The cost is contained because only standard laparoscopic instrumentation is used. It also provides a unique opportunity to repair any injuries using intraluminal laparoscopic suturing, requiring no additional skill sets compared to conventional laparoscopy. In this modified TAMIS technique, we used a single visual trocar and the working instruments were slid beside the trocar. This idea was inspired by the previously described direct transfascial puncture technique for single incision laparoscopy where instruments were slid along the working trocar without additional working ports [19]. However, sliding the instruments between the anal sphincter and the trocar did result in disruption of the air seal. Three manoeuvers were used to overcome this: we advanced the trocar fully into the rectum until the adjustable hub pressed against the anal sphincter, sutures were placed around the suture posts to maintain the seal, and the surgical assistant gently pressed the adjustable hub onto the anal sphincter during the procedure.

## 4. Conclusions

Patients with retained CFB are increasingly presenting to emergency rooms. Examination under anaesthesia and attempts at transanal extraction are important first line therapeutic steps. However, when these fail, a modified TAMIS technique can be considered using standard trocars and instruments. This is safe and cost effective and requires no specialized equipment or expertise to perform.

## Conflict of Interests

The authors declare that there is no conflict of interests regarding the publication of this paper.

## Authors' Contribution

All authors are responsible for concept and design of study, acquisition of data and analysis, and interpretation of data; drafting the paper and revising it critically for important intellectual content; and final approval of the version to be published. They contributed in concept, design, definition of intellectual content, literature search, clinical studies, experimental studies, data acquisition, data analysis, statistical analysis, paper preparation, paper editing, and paper review. Shamir O. Cawich should take responsibility for the integrity of the work as a whole from inception to published paper and should be designated as "guarantor."

## References

[1] G. M. Gould and W. Pyle, *Anomalies and Curiosities of Medicine*, W.B. Saunders, Philadelphia, Pa, USA, 1901.

[2] S. O. Cawich, R. Downes, A. C. Martin, N. R. Evans, D. I. G. Mitchell, and E. Williams, "Colonic perforation: a lethal consequence of cannabis body packing," *Journal of Forensic and Legal Medicine*, vol. 17, no. 5, pp. 269–271, 2010.

[3] K. G. Cologne and G. T. Ault, "Rectal foreign bodies: what is the current standard?" *Clinics in Colon and Rectal Surgery*, vol. 25, no. 4, pp. 214–218, 2012.

[4] M. A. Kurer, C. Davey, S. Khan, and S. Chintapatla, "Colorectal foreign bodies: a systematic review," *Colorectal Disease*, vol. 12, no. 9, pp. 851–861, 2010.

[5] J. E. Goldberg and S. R. Steele, "Rectal Foreign Bodies," *Surgical Clinics of North America*, vol. 90, no. 1, pp. 173–184, 2010.

[6] T. Pavlidis, G. Marakis, K. Psarras, A. Triantafyllou, T. Kontoulis, and A. Sakantamis, "The role of endoscopy for foreign bodies in the rectum," *The Internet Journal of Surgery*, vol. 8, no. 1, 2005.

[7] R. M. Singaporewalla, D. E. L. Tan, and T. K. Tan, "Use of endoscopic snare to extract a large rectosigmoid foreign body with review of literature," *Surgical Laparoscopy, Endoscopy and Percutaneous Techniques*, vol. 17, no. 2, pp. 145–148, 2007.

[8] G. Rispoli, C. Esposito, D. Monachese, and M. Armellino, "Removal of a foreign body from the distal colon using a combined laparoscopic and endoanal approach: report of a case," *Diseases of the Colon & Rectum*, vol. 43, no. 11, pp. 1632–1634, 2000.

[9] K. R. Berghoff and M. E. Franklin Jr., "Laparoscopic-assisted rectal foreign body removal: report of a case," *Diseases of the Colon and Rectum*, vol. 48, no. 10, pp. 1975–1977, 2005.

[10] M. D. Hellinger, "Anal trauma and foreign bodies," *Surgical Clinics of North America*, vol. 82, no. 6, pp. 1253–1260, 2002.

[11] D. L. Clarke, I. Buccimazza, F. A. Anderson, and S. R. Thomson, "Colorectal foreign bodies," *Colorectal Disease*, vol. 7, no. 1, pp. 98–103, 2005.

[12] J. P. Lake, R. Essani, P. Petrone, A. M. Kaiser, J. Asensio, and R. W. Beart Jr., "Management of retained colorectal foreign bodies: predictors of operative intervention," *Diseases of the Colon and Rectum*, vol. 47, no. 10, pp. 1694–1698, 2004.

[13] J. E. Barone, J. Yee, and T. F. Nealon Jr., "Management of foreign bodies and trauma of the rectum," *Surgery Gynecology and Obstetrics*, vol. 156, no. 4, pp. 453–457, 1983.

[14] J. S. Cohen and J. M. Sackier, "Management of colorectal foreign bodies," *Journal of the Royal College of Surgeons of Edinburgh*, vol. 41, no. 5, pp. 312–315, 1996.

[15] E. H. Aly, "SILS TEM: the new armamentarium in transanal endoscopic surgery," *Journal of Minimal Access Surgery*, vol. 10, no. 2, pp. 102–103, 2014.

[16] M. E. Allaix, F. Rebecchi, C. Giaccone, M. Mistrangelo, and M. Morino, "Long-term functional results and quality of life after transanal endoscopic microsurgery," *British Journal of Surgery*, vol. 98, no. 11, pp. 1635–1643, 2011.

[17] M. Ragupathi and E. M. Haas, "Transanal endoscopic video-assisted excision: application of single-port access," *Journal of the Society of Laparoendoscopic Surgeons*, vol. 15, no. 1, pp. 53–58, 2011.

[18] D. Dardamanis, D. Theodorou, G. Theodoropoulos et al., "Transanal polypectomy using single incision laparoscopic instruments," *World Journal of Gastrointestinal Surgery*, vol. 3, no. 4, pp. 56–58, 2011.

[19] S. O. Cawich, D. Thomas, D. Hassranah, and V. Naraynsingh, "Evolution of SILS cholecystectomy in the Caribbean: the direct transfascial puncture technique using conventional instruments without working ports," *Case Reports in Surgery*, vol. 2014, 4 pages, 2014.

# 45

# A Missed Case of Occult Bilateral Temporomandibular Dislocation Mistaken for Dystonia

**Evelyn Lee,[1] Jan Shoenberger,[2] and Jonathan Wagner[2]**

[1]LAC+USC Medical Center, 1200 North State Street 1060H, Los Angeles, CA 90033, USA
[2]LAC+USC Medical Center, Keck School of Medicine of USC, Los Angeles, CA, USA

Correspondence should be addressed to Evelyn Lee; evlee@dhs.lacounty.gov

Academic Editor: Aristomenis K. Exadaktylos

A 24-year-old male with a history of psychiatric disorder and no prior significant temporomandibular joint (TMJ) pathology presented to the emergency department for "lockjaw." Plain film X-rays of the mandible were read as unremarkable by an attending radiologist, leading to the initial diagnosis of medication-induced dystonic reaction. Following unsuccessful medical treatment a maxillofacial computed tomography (CT) was ordered. CT confirmed bilateral dislocation, illustrating the importance of clinical judgment, and limitations of certain radiographic images. The authors believe this case to be the first reported case in the medical literature of bilateral anterior TMJ dislocation with a false negative X-ray.

## 1. Case Presentation

A 24-year-old Hispanic male with a past medical history of an unknown psychiatric disorder was sent to the emergency department (ED) for "lockjaw" after opening his mouth widely while yawning. The patient was unable to close his mouth and complained of associated left jaw pain. He denied history of similar episodes, recent changes in his haloperidol dosing, history of trauma to the face, jaw clicking, dislocations, or other temporomandibular joint pathology.

On exam, the patient's mouth was symmetrically wide open with his lower mandible protruding forward. On palpation, there was mild tenderness to palpation of the left ramus and temporomandibular joint (TMJ) with no significant periauricular depressions. The patient was calm and able to communicate with mildly slurred speech. He was able to close his lips to form words and had minimal drooling, but the jaw remained open.

Common to many EDs, panoramic X-ray capabilities were not immediately available, and, therefore, plain film X-rays of the mandible were pursued. The mandible series, which includes anteroposterior, bilateral, and submental-vertex views, was read as an "unremarkable plain film of the mandible" (Figure 1) by an attending radiologist.

Upon consideration of the X-ray findings, the patient's calm demeanor, his ability to communicate relatively easily with little discomfort, and his history of psychotropic medication use, the presentation was thought to be consistent with a medication-induced dystonic reaction, rather than a dislocation. Intravenous diphenhydramine 25 mg, lorazepam 1 mg, and benztropine 1 mg were sequentially administered to the patient for presumed dystonia.

Following a period of observation, multiple reassessments, and a lack of response to the medications, the decision was made to pursue advanced imaging. Despite the normal X-ray read, a maxillofacial computed tomographic (CT) scan was ordered for further evaluation of the bony structures of the face, specifically looking for occult bilateral TMJ dislocation. The radiologist read of the CT stated that "the mandibular heads are dislocated anteriorly out of the TMJs bilaterally" (Figure 2).

The patient consented for reduction and was given midazolam 2 mg IV. Using the classic technique of placing the thumbs intraorally on the lower molars while applying steady pressure downward and posteriorly, the condylar heads were successfully reduced on the first attempt. An intraoral examination was not performed after the reduction, but the patient was able to easily open and close his jaw

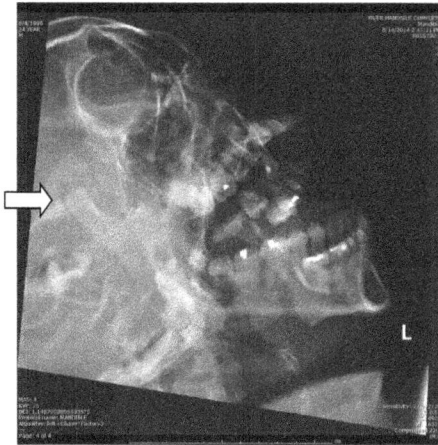

FIGURE 1: X-ray mandible series (left lateral view). The arrow is pointing to the condylar head.

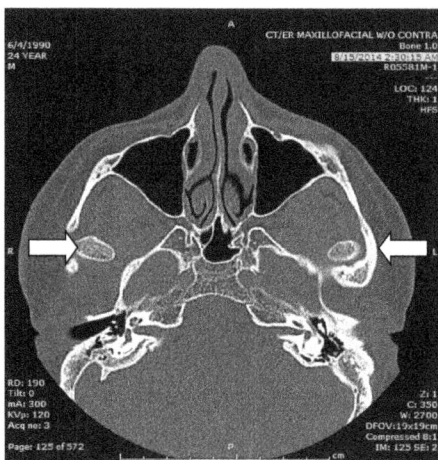

FIGURE 2: CT showing bilateral condylar heads (arrows) anterior to the glenoid fossa.

without difficulty, crepitus, or clicking. He also stated that his bite felt normal.

## 2. Discussion

Generally, atraumatic dislocations result from wide mouth opening (dental extraction, vomiting, laughing, oral sex, etc.) with yawning described as the most common associated mechanism [1–4]. Anterior head dislocations are most frequently seen, but the condylar heads can also slip inferiorly, medially, or posteriorly [2, 3]. Anterior TMJ dislocations occur when the mandibular condyle is displaced from the glenoid fossa anteriorly beyond the articular eminence and cannot be self-reduced [1, 5, 6]. Bilateral dislocations occur more often than unilateral dislocations [7, 8].

Typical clinical findings for mandible dislocation include the inability to close the mouth, visual or palpable depressions in the preauricular areas, prominent lower jaw or new onset prognathism, lateral chin deviation if unilaterally dislocated,

excessive drooling, difficulty speaking, and a general uncomfortable appearance [1, 3, 5].

The diagnosis of atraumatic mandibular dislocation frequently requires no imaging and should be obvious clinically in the majority of cases [3, 5, 9]. The decision to image is determined by practitioner preference and/or on a case-by-case basis, as no set guidelines for imaging exist. The American Academy of Oral and Maxillofacial Radiology suggests evaluating the entire clinical picture and determining whether imaging would assist with diagnosis given the risks of radiation exposure and cost [10, 11]. The general practice in the ED is to first start with plain film X-rays. The most important views are panoramic, transpharyngeal, transcranial, and submental-vertex views with recommendations for transcranial views [11, 12].

Currently, CT imaging is used more frequently than plain radiography in both traumatic and atraumatic mandibular dislocations, as it allows for evaluation of fractures, dislocations, and osseous changes [13, 14]. Magnetic resonance imaging (MRI) is rarely needed and is used primarily for diagnosing chronic changes and internal derangement of the TMJ [12, 15].

Internal derangement of the TMJ mainly involves the relationship of the mandibular condyle and the articular disc that sits between the condyle and the glenoid fossa. The articular disc helps with smooth joint movement. When displacement or derangement of the disc occurs, pain, clicking, popping, or joint locking can occur [15, 16]. When the articular disc displaces posteriorly, the mouth is locked in an open position, otherwise known as "open lock." The posteriorly displaced disc functions as a mechanical block that does not allow the condyle to return to the glenoid fossa and can appear clinically similar to a mandible dislocation [17]. Open lock is an uncommon finding and is rarely diagnosed in the emergency department. Therefore, if a mandibular dislocation is suspected, the appropriate next step is treatment with manual reduction [18]. In an outpatient setting, unenhanced MRIs or cone beam CTs (which use lower radiation to focus on the TMJ) are used to help evaluate and diagnose internal derangement of the TMJ. However, MRIs are the modality of choice in the evaluation of the articular disc [10, 14, 15]. Typically, treatment is nonsurgical and focused on patient education and counseling regarding behavior modification and anti-inflammatory medications. Serial muscle exercises that help to restore neuromuscular control, improve TMJ mobility, and decrease TMJ stress are recommended and may be useful in the treatment and prevention of future episodes of open lock [16].

In this case, the patient appeared comfortable and was speaking relatively clearly. He also was without major pain or anxiety. Due to the incongruence between the patient's clinical appearance and the described typical presentation of an acute bilateral mandible dislocation, in conjunction with the radiologist read of a negative mandible series, the coincidental nature of the patient's history of yawning with symptom onset was falsely assumed.

Although the final diagnosis of bilateral mandibular dislocation was slightly delayed from the initial X-rays to the final CT findings, the medications used to treat the suspected dystonic reaction likely aided in muscle relaxation and a simple and successful reduction in the emergency department.

## 3. Conclusion

While plain films of the mandible can provide a great deal of information, they may also mask the true underlying disorder [19]. Ultimately, it is important to keep an open mind when considering the differential diagnosis when the patient presentation does not correlate to the expected radiologic results. It is important to realize the limitations of certain radiographic images and the importance of clinical judgment. The authors believe that this is the first case of bilateral anterior TMJ dislocation with a false negative X-ray reported in the medical literature to date.

## Conflict of Interests

The authors declare that there is no conflict of interests regarding the publication of this paper.

## References

[1] C. W. Shorey and J. H. Campbell, "Dislocation of the temporomandibular joint," *Oral Surgery, Oral Medicine, Oral Pathology, Oral Radiology, and Endodontology*, vol. 89, no. 6, pp. 662–668, 2000.

[2] V. I. Ugboko, F. O. Oginni, S. O. Ajike, H. O. Olasoji, and E. T. Adebayo, "A survey of temporomandibular joint dislocation: aetiology, demographics, risk factors and management in 96 Nigerian cases," *International Journal of Oral and Maxillofacial Surgery*, vol. 34, no. 5, pp. 499–502, 2005.

[3] T. C. Chan, R. A. Harrigan, J. Ufberg, and G. M. Vilke, "Mandibular reduction," *Journal of Emergency Medicine*, vol. 34, no. 4, pp. 435–440, 2008.

[4] S. Pillai and M. R. Konia, "Unrecognized bilateral temporomandibular joint dislocation after general anesthesia with a delay in diagnosis and management: a case report," *Journal of Medical Case Reports*, vol. 7, article 243, 2013.

[5] N. H. Luyk and P. E. Larsen, "The diagnosis and treatment of the dislocated mandible," *The American Journal of Emergency Medicine*, vol. 7, no. 3, pp. 329–335, 1989.

[6] J. A. Marx, R. S. Hockberger, and R. M. Walls, "Oral medicine," in *Rosen's Emergency Medicine: Concepts and Clinical Practice*, pp. 895–908, Saunders, Philadelphia, Pa, USA, 8th edition, 2014.

[7] C. DelGross and A. J. Smally, "Spontaneous temporomandibular joint dislocation in an 80-year-old man," *Journal of Family Practice*, vol. 40, no. 4, pp. 395–398, 1995.

[8] B. O. Akinbami, "Evaluation of the mechanism and principles of management of temporomandibular joint dislocation. Systematic review of literature and a proposed new classification of temporomandibular joint dislocation," *Head and Face Medicine*, vol. 7, no. 1, article 10, 2011.

[9] T. Thangarajah, N. McCulloch, S. Thangarajah, and J. Stocker, "Bilateral temporomandibular joint dislocation in a 29-year-old man: a case report," *Journal of Medical Case Reports*, vol. 4, article 263, 2010.

[10] A. K. Bag, S. Gaddikeri, A. Singhal et al., "Imaging of the temporomandibular joint: an update," *World Journal of Radiology*, vol. 6, no. 8, pp. 567–582, 2014.

[11] S. L. Brooks, J. W. Brand, S. J. Gibbs et al., "Imaging of the temporomandibular joint: a position paper of the American Academy of Oral and Maxillofacial Radiology," *Oral Surgery, Oral Medicine, Oral Pathology, Oral Radiology, and Endodontics*, vol. 83, no. 5, pp. 609–618, 1997.

[12] J. B. Epstein, J. Caldwell, and G. Black, "The utility of panoramic imaging of the temporomandibular joint in patients with temporomandibular disorders," *Oral Surgery, Oral Medicine, Oral Pathology, Oral Radiology, and Endodontology*, vol. 92, no. 2, pp. 236–239, 2001.

[13] B. Schuknecht and K. Graetz, "Radiologic assessment of maxillofacial, mandibular, and skull base trauma," *European Radiology*, vol. 15, no. 3, pp. 560–568, 2005.

[14] E. L. Lewis, M. F. Dolwick, S. Abramowicz, and S. L. Reeder, "Contemporary imaging of the temporomandibular joint," *Dental Clinics of North America*, vol. 52, no. 4, pp. 875–890, 2008.

[15] R. de Leeuw, "Internal derangements of the temporomandibular joint," *Oral and Maxillofacial Surgery Clinics of North America*, vol. 20, no. 2, pp. 159–168, 2008.

[16] L. T. Hoglund and B. W. Scott, "Automobilization intervention and exercise for temporomandibular joint open lock," *Journal of Manual and Manipulative Therapy*, vol. 20, no. 4, pp. 182–191, 2012.

[17] S. Kai, H. Kai, E. Nakayama et al., "Clinical symptoms of open lock position of the condyle. Relation to anterior dislocation of the temporomandibular joint," *Oral Surgery, Oral Medicine, Oral Pathology*, vol. 74, no. 2, pp. 143–148, 1992.

[18] D. W. Nitzan, "Temporomandibular joint 'open lock' versus condylar dislocation: signs and symptoms, imaging, treatment, and pathogenesis," *Journal of Oral and Maxillofacial Surgery*, vol. 60, no. 5, pp. 506–511, 2002.

[19] R. W. Katzberg, Q. N. Anderson, J. V. Manzione, C. A. Helms, R. Tallents, and K. Hayakawa, "Dislocation of jaws," *Skeletal Radiology*, vol. 11, pp. 38–41, 1984.

# 46

# Assessment of Musculoskeletal Injuries from Domestic Violence in the Emergency Department

**Georgios F. Giannakopoulos[1] and Udo J. L. Reijnders[2]**

[1]Department of Trauma Surgery, VU University Medical Centre, P.O. Box 7057, 1007 MB Amsterdam, Netherlands
[2]Department of Forensic Medicine, Public Health Service, P.O. Box 2200, 1000 CE Amsterdam, Netherlands

Correspondence should be addressed to Georgios F. Giannakopoulos; gf.giannakopoulos@gmail.com

Academic Editor: Aristomenis K. Exadaktylos

Domestic violence is one of the most common causes of nonfatal injury in women, with musculoskeletal injuries representing the second most prevalent manifestation of this form of violence. It is therefore of great importance that healthcare providers such as emergency department (ED) physicians and surgeons are able to recognize and assess these kinds of injuries. In this case report, a woman is described visiting an ED with injuries caused by a fall. Thanks to the knowledge and attention of the ED physician, the real cause of the injury was discovered. What appeared to be an unsuspicious accident was actually the result of intimate partner violence.

## 1. Introduction

Domestic violence is a serious public health and medical problem that is prevalent in all classes of our population. In Netherlands each year over 200.000 women are victims of domestic violence in one form or another [1]. An estimated 12% of the acute injuries of women are caused by domestic violence [2]. More than half of these female victims who are treated for these injuries visit an emergency department (ED) [3]. Three-quarters of the attending physicians would not recognize these cases as abuse related [4].

## 2. Case Description

A 47-year-old woman visiting the ED is complaining of heavy pains in her left forearm. She claims to have fallen against a wardrobe. Examination by the attending ED physician reveals a purple-blue discoloration of the left forearm. He also notices a yellow discoloration around the left eye and forehead. This discoloration possibly dates from an earlier time. X-rays show a fracture of the forearm (both radius and ulna). When the physician expresses his doubts about the cause of the accident, the woman then admits being beaten and abused by her husband frequently. The fracture of her forearm was caused by a blow from a baseball bat and the "black eye" by a punch to the face at an earlier time. Further physical examination reveals extensive fingertip bruising caused by hefty grasping of the arms, back and buttocks, outline hematomas caused by beating with a round and cylindrically formed object (wooden spoon), and hematomas caused by beating with a looped cord.

## 3. Discussion

Previous studies have shown that musculoskeletal injuries represent the second most prevalent manifestation of intimate partner violence [5, 6]. It can be assumed that most ED physicians and (orthopedic) surgeons are treating victims of family violence, knowingly or unknowingly, in their practices [7–9].

In this case we observe a conscientious ED physician. Nevertheless even with visible exterior injuries physicians often overlook the possibility of abuse related causes. This is a serious matter because in Netherlands alone each year more than 80 women die as a direct consequence of domestic violence, whereas early recognition might have avoided the fatal outcome in most cases [1]. This situation has not been changed for the last decade [10, 11].

Reasons for not recognizing the abuse by physicians are often explained by lack of education and training, playing down the severity of the injury, fear of being mistaken, not wanting to be the policeman, not knowing the proper referral agencies, and lack of time. Bhandari et al. concluded from their study, in which 186 orthopedic surgeons participated by responding to a questionnaire, that discomfort with the issue and lack of education have led to misconceptions among Canadian orthopedic surgeons about intimate partner violence [5].

It is also commonly known that many women (>60%) are reluctant to speak of the violence because of shame and fear and do not dare speak of the true nature of their injuries [12, 13]. It is therefore the reason that the "fall from the stairs" or the "fall against the wardrobe" is often used as the reason for the injury [14]. More than half of these women would offer honest answers to the questions if the physician had only asked them directly. This is an important factor for opening the problem for discussion which stops the violence in 50% of the cases [15]. Another research has shown that in 72%–93% of the patients questioned by the physician over domestic violence where there was none in question those people reacted positively, expressing words of understanding, conscientious behavior, and agreeing it was advisable to subject victims to this line of questioning [16, 17].

When assessing injuries, one should always question whether the cause was accidental or intentional. Many accident injuries are caused by a fall, jolt, or jab. Preferential spots are the forehead, chin, knees and elbows, the inner side of hands and shins, and areas where bone structure exists low beneath the skin as in spinous processes and crista iliaca. Accidental injuries can also be caused by improper use of sharp utensils and machines. One-third of the injuries are to the more uncommon spots such as the eye, side of the face, throat and neck, upper arms and upper legs, mouth, outer side of the hand, back, hair on head, shoulder and chest, genitals, and buttocks [18]. Injuries and irregularities in these spots should be treated with more than the usual curiosity and necessary investigation. The physician should ask himself if the story matches with what is being observed. In regular abuse cases, one often observes contusions in various stages of healing (red, blue, green, yellow, and brown). They are often found in spots which are not easily accessible to the victim or there is question of various contusions of the same form.

But also with other injuries such as scrapes, tears, cuts, burns, injuries to the central nervous system, fractures, and bite wounds, one should consider the fact of it having been caused by someone else.

One must realize that for the outside world the only injuries that are visible are those not covered by clothing as in the face and the outer side of the hand. There might also be the injuries under the clothing that are not immediately visible. Research showed that 80% of the injuries were visible and 20% were hidden by clothing. But in 85% of the victims, there were injuries found in visible spots as well as those made invisible by clothing. This is because in 60% of the cases of victims of injuries the cause is usually the result of various forms of infliction to various parts of the body [18].

Physicians should familiarize themselves with recognizing the signs of injuries. When there is a question of abuse, the whole body should be inspected and it should be noted in the differential diagnosis. A high index of suspicion is necessary and the knowledge can be acquired by studying photo material of many forms of visible injuries [19]. Furthermore, it was demonstrated that after a brief training domestic violence was recognized four times more often than those who had not had the training [20].

If there is question of domestic violence, the ED physician can advise consultation with the GP. They can also make referrals to an advice and support center for domestic violence or a battered-women-house. Advising the victim to report the case to the police is also an option to be considered.

## 4. Conclusion

Knowledge and early recognition of inflicted injuries of domestic violence should be improved among healthcare providers such as (orthopedic) surgeons, ED physicians, and GPs. Domestic violence remains a difficult subject to discuss for the victim as well as the physician. Nevertheless, discussing the matter is the only way to make strides with this problem. This can help victims out of their isolation so they can be adequately helped and can also save lives for some. If physicians are not confident in critically examining injuries, they should ask professionals like forensic physicians for help. One must realize that ignoring the problem is even more harmful.

## Conflict of Interests

The authors declare that there is no conflict of interests regarding the publication of this paper.

## References

[1] L. van Gurp, *De veilige gemeente*, Stichting TransAct, Utrecht, The Netherlands, 2000.

[2] J. Abbott, R. Johnson, J. Koziol-McLain, and S. R. Lowenstein, "Domestic violence against women. Incidence and prevalence in an emergency department population," *The Journal of the American Medical Association*, vol. 273, no. 22, pp. 1763–1767, 1995.

[3] L. K. Hamberger, B. Ambuel, A. Marbella, and J. Donze, "Physician interaction with battered women: the women's respective," *Archives of Family Medicine*, vol. 7, no. 6, pp. 575–582, 1998.

[4] T. H. A. Compernolle, "Eerste hulp bij kindermishandeling en het Struisarts-syndroom," *Tijdschrift voor Kindergeneeskunde*, vol. 64, no. 4, pp. 168–179, 1996.

[5] M. Bhandari, S. Sprague, P. Tornetta III et al., "(Mis)perceptions about intimate partner violence in women presenting for orthopaedic care: a survey of Canadian orthopaedic surgeons," *The Journal of Bone & Joint Surgery Series A*, vol. 90, no. 7, pp. 1590–1597, 2008.

[6] M. Bhandari, S. Dosanjh, P. Tornetta III, and D. Matthews, "Violence against Women Health Research Collaborative. Musculoskeletal manifestations of physical abuse after intimate

partner violence," *The Journal of Trauma*, vol. 61, pp. 1473–1479, 2006.

[7]  D. A. Zillmer, D. K. Bynum Jr., M. S. Kocher, W. J. Robb III, and S. A. Koshy, "Family violence: tools for the orthopaedic surgeon," *Instructional Course Lectures*, vol. 52, pp. 791–802, 2003.

[8]  A. L. Chen and K. J. Koval, "Elder abuse: the role of the orthopaedic surgeon in diagnosis and management," *The Journal of the American Academy of Orthopaedic Surgeons*, vol. 10, no. 1, pp. 25–31, 2002.

[9]  M. E. Clarke and W. Pierson, "Management of elder abuse in the emergency department," *Emergency Medicine Clinics of North America*, vol. 17, no. 3, pp. 631–644, 1999.

[10]  U. J. L. Reijnders, M. C. van Baasbank, and G. van der Wal, "Diagnosis and interpretation of injuries: a study of Dutch general practitioners," *Journal of Clinical Forensic Medicine*, vol. 12, no. 6, pp. 291–295, 2005.

[11]  U. J. L. Reijnders, G. F. Giannakopoulos, and K. H. de Bruin, "Assessment of abuse-related injuries: a comparative study of forensic physicians, emergency room physicians, emergency room nurses and medical students," *Journal of Forensic and Legal Medicine*, vol. 15, no. 1, pp. 15–19, 2008.

[12]  B. Drijber, U. Reijnders, and M. Ceelen, "Female victims of domestic violence do not generally seek help from their GP," *Huisarts en Wetenschap*, vol. 52, no. 1, pp. 6–10, 2009.

[13]  N. K. Sugg and T. Inui, "Primary care physicians' response to domestic violence: opening pandora's box," *The Journal of the American Medical Association*, vol. 267, no. 23, pp. 3157–3160, 1992.

[14]  S. H. L. F. Wong, *The doctor and the woman 'who fell down the stairs'. Family doctor's role in recognising and responding to intimate partner abuse [Ph.D. thesis]*, Radboud Universiteit Nijmegen, Nijmegen, The Netherlands, 2006.

[15]  T. van Dijk, S. Flight, E. Oppenhuis, and B. Duesmann, *Huiselijk Geweld. Aard, Omvang en Hulpverlening*, Ministerie van Justitie, The Hague, The Netherlands, 1997.

[16]  U. J. L. Reijnders, B. C. Drijber, and T. Dorn, "Vragen naar huiselijk geweld," *Patiënt Care*, vol. 35, pp. 21–24, 2008.

[17]  K. M. Feldhaus, J. Koziol-McLain, H. L. Amsbury, I. M. Norton, S. R. Lowenstein, and J. T. Abbott, "Accuracy of 3 brief screening questions for detecting partner violence in the emergency department," *Journal of the American Medical Association*, vol. 277, no. 17, pp. 1357–1361, 1997.

[18]  U. J. L. Reijnders and M. Ceelen, "7208 Victims of domestic and public violence; an exploratory study based on the reports of assaulted individuals reporting to the police," *Journal of Forensic and Legal Medicine*, vol. 24, pp. 18–23, 2014.

[19]  U. J. L. Reijnders, C. Das, B. C. Drijber, and R. Lulf, *Herkenning van letsel door lichamelijk geweld*, Prelum Uitgevers, Houten, The Netherlands, 2008.

[20]  S. Lo Fo Wong, F. Wester, S. S. Mol, and T. L. Lagro-Janssen, "Increased awareness of intimate partner abuse after training: a randomized controlled trial," *British Journal of General Practice*, vol. 56, pp. 243–244, 2006.

47

# Acetabular Liner Dissociation following Total Hip Arthroplasty: A Rare but Serious Complication That May Be Easily Misinterpreted in the Emergency Department

**Christopher K. J. O'Neill, Richard J. Napier, Owen J. Diamond, Seamus O'Brien, and David E. Beverland**

*Primary Joint Unit, Musgrave Park Hospital, Stockmans Lane, Belfast BT9 7JB, UK*

Correspondence should be addressed to Christopher K. J. O'Neill; chrisoneill@doctors.org.uk

Academic Editor: Henry David

Acetabular liner dissociation is a rare complication of Total Hip Arthroplasty (THA) which requires urgent revision surgery. A case is presented in which the correct diagnosis was not appreciated on two separate Emergency Department attendances. The typical symptoms, signs, and radiological features are outlined and the importance of considering a rare complication following a commonly performed procedure is highlighted.

## 1. Introduction

Total Hip Arthroplasty (THA) remains one of the most frequently performed orthopaedic procedures performed worldwide [1–3]. Surgery involves implantation of both a femoral and acetabular component, with options for either cemented or uncemented fixation depending on Surgeon preference. The modern uncemented acetabular component is modular in design and provides several theoretical advantages. One of the primary attractions is the ability to implant alternative bearing surfaces with improved wear characteristics. The modular design also permits certain conservative revision options in the event of early infection, late polyethylene wear, or recurrent dislocation [4].

## 2. Case Presentation

An 83-year-old male was referred to Orthopaedic Outpatient Clinic by his General Practitioner (GP) for further assessment of a painful right THA.

The uncemented THA (Corail KLA12 stem, Pinnacle 100 Series 54 mm sell, 54/28 mm highly cross-linked polyethylene Marathon liner: DePuy, Warsaw, IN, USA) was performed five years previously for osteoarthritis. The patient had no other significant medical comorbidity. Body Mass Index was 27.4 kg/m$^2$ and activity level was relatively low demand.

Surgery was performed in the lateral decubitus position via a posterior approach, using the Transverse Acetabular Ligament (TAL) as a reference to control acetabular component orientation. Acetabular component radiological inclination (RI) and radiological anteversion (RA) were within the desired range (RI 45.1°, RA 10.7°).

The THA was a well-functioning implant until approximately 4 months prior to referral. At that time, the patient reported sudden onset of severe groin pain when getting into bed and attended the Emergency Department (ED) for assessment.

No significant limb length discrepancy or neurovascular deficit was documented. X-rays were interpreted as satisfactory, with no evidence of fracture or dislocation, and the patient was discharged.

The groin pain improved over a two-week period and the patient regained independent mobility. Both the patient and his wife described audible grinding and clicking from the hip when walking. The patient reattended the ED three months later with a further deterioration in groin pain and difficulty mobilizing. X-rays were again interpreted as satisfactory and the patient was discharged. Pain and grinding from the hip

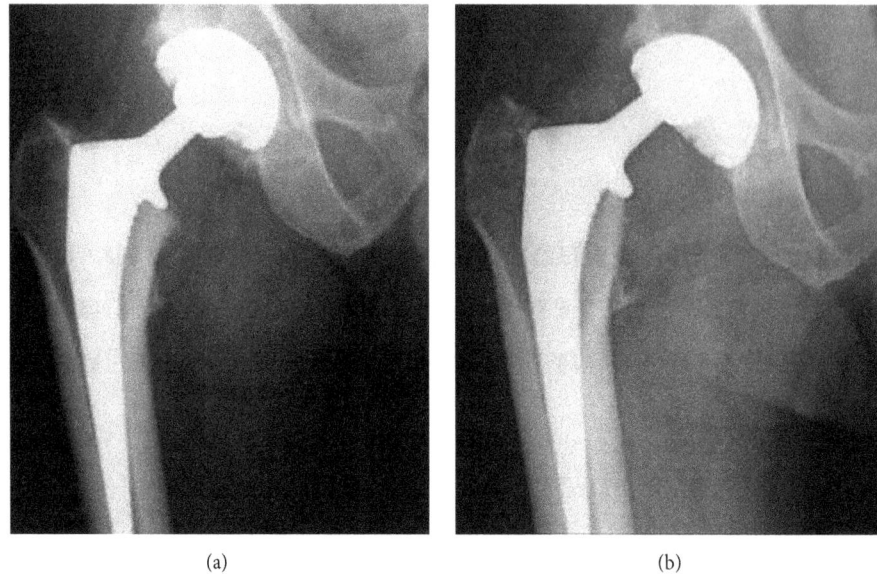

(a)                                                        (b)

FIGURE 1: (a) Previous AP Hip X-ray demonstrates satisfactory component positioning. (b) AP Hip X-ray from ED attendance demonstrates acetabular liner dissociation. Comparison to (a) shows grossly eccentric superior migration of the femoral head within the acetabular shell.

persisted and the patient was referred by his GP for an orthopaedic opinion.

On review of X-rays from both previous ED attendances, there was evidence of acetabular liner dissociation (Figures 1 and 2). The patient was scheduled for urgent acetabular revision surgery.

At time of revision surgery, there was evidence of soft tissue metallosis with significant damage to the surfaces of both the femoral head and acetabular shell. The polyethylene liner had completely dissociated from the shell and lay within the adjacent soft tissues. Though acetabular shell orientation was satisfactory, concern over integrity of the locking mechanism necessitated revision. A 58 mm Pinnacle Sector shell with screw augmentation, a 58/32 mm Marathon highly cross-linked polyethylene liner, and a 32 mm metal Articul/eze femoral head were implanted (DePuy, Warsaw, IN, USA).

Postoperative recovery was uneventful and progress at time of last review was satisfactory.

## 3. Discussion

Acetabular liner dissociation is a serious but rare complication following THA that is specific to the modern uncemented acetabular component. The most recent National Joint Registry (NJR) Report shows that over 76,000 primary THA procedures were performed in England, Wales, and Northern Ireland in 2013, with uncemented acetabular components implanted in 65.4% of cases. Review of ten-year NJR data suggests an acetabular liner dissociation incidence of approximately 0.04% [1].

The modern uncemented acetabular component is modular in design and consists of a metal shell which accepts a polyethylene or ceramic liner following insertion intraoperatively. Liner dissociation occurs due to failure of the locking

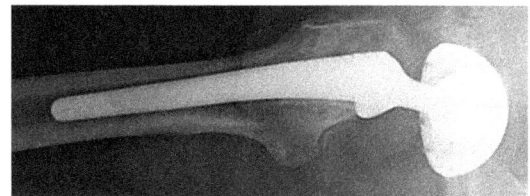

FIGURE 2: Lateral X-ray shows medial migration of the femoral head within the acetabular shell and excludes a dislocation as it confirms the prosthetic femoral head lies within the acetabular shell on a tangential view.

mechanism between the metal shell and liner (Figure 3). It appears to be more commonly associated with polyethylene liners due to a difference in ceramic liner locking mechanism design [5, 6].

The aetiology of locking mechanism failure is believed to be related to shell geometry design and liner material properties in the adverse environment of increased torque or component impingement [7–9].

In addition to a taper-lock mechanism, the Pinnacle shell design incorporates multiple Anti-Rotation Device (ARD) scallops which accept ARD tabs on the polyethylene liner in order to enhance stability (Figure 4(a)).

At time of acetabular component revision, multiple polyethylene liner ARD tabs were noted to have failed (Figure 4(b)).

Reports of both early and late liner dissociation are described in the literature and Joint Registries [1, 7–9]. It is likely that cases of early liner dissociation are more related to malseated components rather than true fatigue failure of the locking mechanism.

The senior author's routine practice includes checks to ensure correct liner seating and stability at time of initial

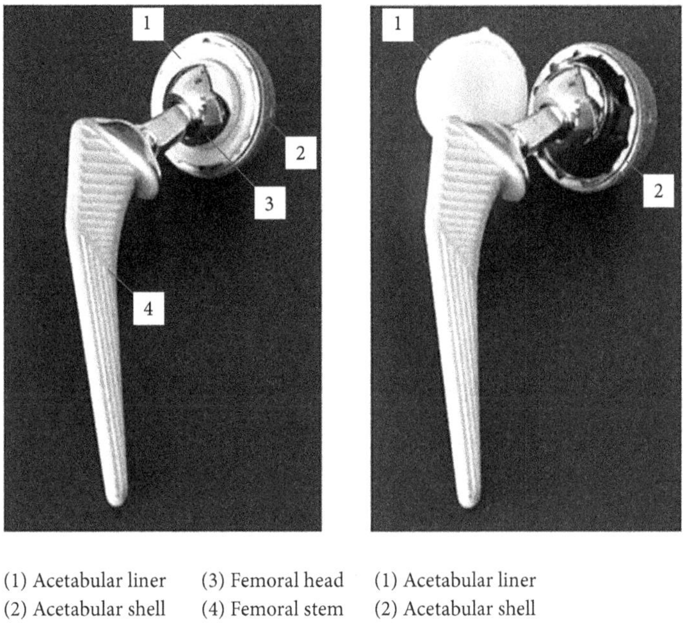

(1) Acetabular liner   (3) Femoral head     (1) Acetabular liner
(2) Acetabular shell   (4) Femoral stem    (2) Acetabular shell

(a)                                    (b)

FIGURE 3: (a) Normal THA implant appearance. The polyethylene liner is well seated within the acetabular shell. (b) Acetabular liner dissociation appearance. The polyethylene liner has clearly migrated from its original position in (a).

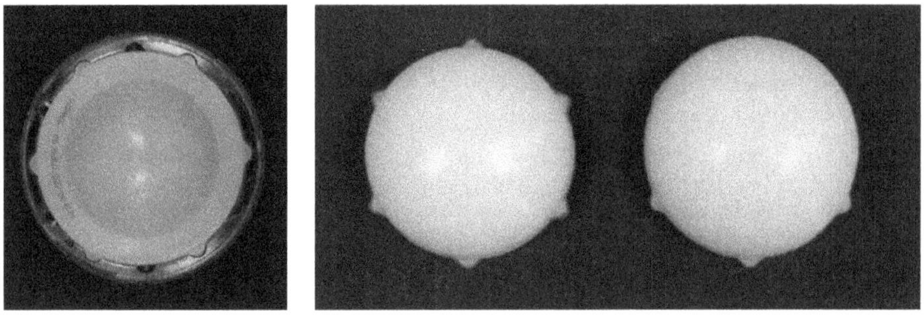

(a)                                    (b)

FIGURE 4: (a) Demonstrates shell Anti-Rotation Device (ARD) scallops which accept liner ARD tabs to enhance locking mechanism stability. (b) Normal appearance of polyethylene liner (6 ARD tabs highlighted in red) versus abnormal polyethylene liner in liner dissociation (failure of multiple ARD tabs).

implantation. Given the fact that the failure also occurred five years postoperatively, we believe the aetiology in this case was related to locking mechanism fatigue failure rather than initial component malseating.

Typical symptoms are of sudden onset of hip pain in a previously well-functioning prosthesis, followed by grinding or clicking with hip movements as the prosthetic femoral head articulates with the metal acetabular shell rather than the polyethylene liner [9, 10].

On examination, significant limb shortening or internal rotation as is commonly found with a posteriorly dislocated THA is unlikely. Audible grinding or clicking is reproduced with hip movements if pain permits.

AP Pelvic X-ray shows grossly eccentric superior migration of the femoral head within the acetabular shell [9]. Lateral X-ray shows medial migration of the femoral head within the acetabular shell and excludes a dislocation as it confirms the prosthetic femoral head lies within the acetabular shell on a tangential view. Comparison of previously normal X-rays on Picture Archived Communication Systems (PACS) can also be useful to aid the diagnosis if available (as shown in Table 1).

Appropriate management is orthopaedic referral for consideration of urgent acetabular component revision surgery.

Though acetabular liner dissociation is a rare complication following THA, increased awareness of the typical symptoms, signs, and radiological appearance will help avoid misdiagnosis.

A high index of clinical suspicion when assessing the painful THA is likely to improve patient outcomes and also reduce the risk of medical litigation.

TABLE 1: Findings suggestive of liner dissociation in the acutely painful THA.

| History | (i) Sudden onset of hip/groin pain in a previously well-functioning prosthesis<br>(ii) New "grinding/clicking" noise from affected hip<br>(iii) Difficulty fully weight bearing |
|---|---|
| Examination | (i) Audible "grinding/clicking" with passive hip movements<br>(ii) Lack of significant limb shortening/rotation |
| Investigations | *AP Hip X-ray*<br>Grossly eccentric superior migration of femoral head within acetabular shell<br>*Lateral Hip X-ray*<br>Medial migration of femoral head within acetabular shell. Excludes dislocation as confirms prosthetic femoral head lies within acetabular shell on a tangential view |

## Disclosure

Richard J. Napier, Owen J. Diamond, Seamus O'Brien, and David E. Beverland are coauthors.

## Conflict of Interests

The authors declare that there is no conflict of interests regarding the publication of this paper.

## References

[1] National Joint Registry for England, Wales and Northern Ireland, 11th Annual Report 2014, http://www.njrcentre.org.uk.

[2] Swedish Hip Arthroplasty Register, "Annual Report 2013," http://www.shpr.se/en/Publications/DocumentsReports.aspx.

[3] Australian Orthopaedic Association National Joint Replacement Registry, *Annual Report 2014*, 2014, https://aoanjrr.dmac .adelaide.edu.au/annual-reports-2014.

[4] C. C. Powers, K. B. Fricka, M. S. Austin, and C. A. Engh, "Five duraloc locking ring failures," *Journal of Arthroplasty*, vol. 25, no. 7, pp. 1170.e15–1170.e18, 2010.

[5] M. D. Ries, "Review of the evolution of the cementless acetabular cup," *Orthopedics*, vol. 31, no. 12, supplement 2, pp. 88–91, 2008.

[6] S. Tradonsky, P. D. Postak, A. I. Froimson, and A. S. Greenwald, "A comparison of the disassociation strength of modular acetabular components," *Clinical Orthopaedics and Related Research*, no. 296, pp. 154–160, 1993.

[7] M. D. Ries, D. K. Collis, and F. Lynch, "Separation of the polyethylene liner from acetabular cup metal backing: a report of three cases," *Clinical Orthopaedics and Related Research*, no. 282, pp. 164–176, 1992.

[8] J. Werle, S. Goodman, D. Schurman, and J. Lannin, "Polyethylene liner dissociation in Harris-Galante acetabular components: a report of 7 cases," *The Journal of Arthroplasty*, vol. 17, no. 1, pp. 78–81, 2002.

[9] A. Yun, E. N. Koli, J. Moreland et al., "Polyethylene liner dissociation is a complication of the DePuy pinnacle cup: a report of 23 cases," *Clinical Orthopaedics and Related Research*, 2015.

[10] C. F. Gray, R. E. Moore, and G.-C. Lee, "Spontaneous dissociation of offset, face-changing polyethylene liners from the acetabular shell: a report of four cases," *The Journal of Bone & Joint Surgery—American Volume*, vol. 94, no. 9, pp. 841–845, 2012.

# 48

# *P*-Chloroaniline Poisoning Causing Methemoglobinemia: A Case Report and Review of the Literature

**Anna Sarah Messmer, Christian Hans Nickel, and Dirk Bareiss**

*Department of Emergency Medicine, University Hospital Basel, Petersgraben 2, 4031 Basel, Switzerland*

Correspondence should be addressed to Anna Sarah Messmer; annamessmer@web.de

Academic Editor: Oludayo A. Sowande

*Background*. Methemoglobin (MetHb) most commonly results from exposure to an oxidizing chemical but may also arise from genetic, dietary, or even idiopathic etiologies. *P*-chloroaniline (PCA) was one of the first substances described in the context of acquired methemoglobinemia. *Case Report*. We report the case of a cyanotic chemistry worker who presented to our emergency department (ED) after working with PCA. His peripheral oxygen saturation ($SpO_2$) measured by pulse oximetry was at 81% and remained on that level despite oxygen administration (100% oxygenation via nonrebreather mask). His MetHb level was measured at 42.8% in arterial blood gas analysis. After treatment with intravenous methylene blue cyanosis resolved and the patient was discharged after 36 hours of observation. *Conclusion*. Acquired methemoglobinemia is a treatable condition, which may cause significant morbidity and mortality. The knowledge about the most common causes, fast diagnostic, and proper treatment is crucial.

## 1. Background

Methemoglobinemia is a treatable condition that may cause significant morbidity and mortality [1]. Various systems normally operate to keep methemoglobin (MetHb) at physiologic level, which is less than 1% of the total hemoglobin concentration [2]. Methemoglobinemia is a result of the oxidation of ferrous iron ($Fe^{2+}$) to ferric iron ($Fe^{3+}$) within the hemoglobin molecule.

This becomes important in the context of oxygen transport and delivery: the ferric state is unable to bind oxygen, and the remaining ferrous (reduced) hemoglobin has a higher affinity for oxygen molecules (allosteric effect), shifting the oxygen-hemoglobin dissociation curve to the left. Consequently, the release of oxygen to the tissues is limited [1–4]. As an example, a patient with a hemoglobin level of 10 g/dL who has 50% MetHb has only 5 g/dL functional hemoglobin able to bind oxygen and deliver it to tissues.

Most commonly, methemoglobinemia is acquired and a result of ingestion or skin exposure to an oxidizing agent such as certain medications or chemicals; see Table 1 [1, 2, 5, 6]. Aniline and its derivatives have been one of the first substances described to cause methemoglobinemia. Due to the awareness of its toxicity in industrial products, safety measures have been undertaken and acute aniline poisoning became rare in developed countries, reflected in case reports dated back to several decades [7, 8]. However, our case report shows that accidental aniline or *p*-chloroaniline (PCA) poisoning can nowadays still induce significant, life-threatening methemoglobinemia.

## 2. Case Report

A 56-year-old patient with known epilepsy in his past medical history presented to the emergency department (ED) with generalized cyanosis four hours after cleaning a floor in a chemical factory. He was using PCA in solid form, which was dissolved with methanol. While working, he was using a facemask and a full body protection suit, which, according to his team leader, might have been defective. Later, a work colleague noticed that his skin color turned blue. According to the local occupational health guidelines, the patient immediately changed his clothes and took a shower to decontaminate.

In the ED, he was mildly confused and giddy, but he did not suffer from dyspnea. His vital signs showed mild

TABLE 1: Substances that can cause MetHb[1].

| Drugs | | Chemical agents |
|---|---|---|
| Acetaminophen | Methylene blue | Acetanilide |
| Ammonium nitrate | Metoclopramide | Alloxan |
| Amyl nitrate | Nitrates/nitrites | Aminophenol |
| Anticonvulsants | Nitric oxide | Anilines |
|   Valproic acid | Nitrofurantoin | Automobile exhaust fumes |
|   Phenytoin | Nitroglycerine | Benzene |
| Antimalaria drugs | Nitroprusside | Bivalent copper |
|   Chloroquine | Nitrous oxide | Burning wood and plastic |
|   Quinacrine | Isobutyl nitrate | Chlorates |
|   Primaquine | Oral hypoglycemics | Chromates |
| Bismuth subnitrate | p-Aminosalicylic acid | Dimethyl sulfoxide |
| Dapsone | Phenacetin | Dinitrophenol |
| Flutamide | Phenazopyridine | Fumes |
| Hydroxylamine | Piperazine | Naphthalene |
| Local anesthetics | Rifampin | Nitrates |
|   Benzocaine | Riluzole | Nitrites |
|   Bupivacaine | Sulfadiazine | Nitrobenzene |
|   Lidocaine | | Nitroethane |
|   Prilocaine | | Nitrophenol |
|   EMLA* | | Paraquat |
| | | Propanil |
| | | Toluidine |
| | | Trinitrotoluene (TNT) |

This list is not complete. [1]References: see [6, 21, 25]. *Eutectic mixture of local anesthetics.

tachycardia with 107 beats per minute, blood pressure of 156/89 mmHg, and peripheral oxygen saturation (SpO$_2$) of 81% on a nonrebreather facemask (100% oxygenation). Arterial blood drawn immediately was of dark brown color and the blood gas analysis revealed a pH of 7.401, pO$_2$ of 8.33 kpa (62.5 mmHg), pCO$_2$ of 5.49 kpa (41.2 mmHg), and an arterial oxygen saturation (SaO$_2$) of 93.4%. The fraction MetHb measured in arterial blood by spectrophotometry was found to be elevated at 42.8%, while the fraction of oxyhemoglobin (O$_2$Hb) was 54.6%, and the fraction of reduced hemoglobin (HHb) was 3.9% (see Table 2).

The patient was treated immediately with 150 mg (2 mg/kg) intravenous methylene blue over 5 minutes. A sample of arterial blood gas obtained 30 minutes after treatment revealed a MetHb level of 12.3%; therefore, another dose of 150 mg of methylene blue was given. The patient's condition improved rapidly, the cyanosis resolved, and the patient was transferred to our intensive care unit for observation of possible rebound methemoglobinemia. Serial MetHb measurements showed a continued decrease to below 2%. The patient was discharged 36 hours later.

## 3. Discussion

In 1959, aniline poisoning has been first described in a case series of marking-ink poisoning causing methemoglobinemia in babies [7]. Later, more cases have been published, most often in correlation with dye or herbicides exposure [9–12]. PCA is a colorless or slightly amber colored crystalline solid with a mild aromatic odor. The chemical is soluble in water and in common organic solvents, such as methanol used in our case. The general public may be exposed to PCA from the use of PCA-based dyed or printed textiles, papers, cosmetics, and pharmaceutical products. It can be dermal (wearing of clothes, use of soaps, or mouthwashes), oral (small children sucking clothes and other materials and use of mouthwashes), or direct entry into the bloodstream (e.g., through breakdown products of chlorhexidine in spray antiseptics) [9, 13]. The mechanism of exposure in our case remains unclear. The team leader, who accompanied the patient to the ED, hypothesized a defective protection suit, whereas the PCA could have contaminated the skin.

Patients with methemoglobinemia typically present with skin discoloration ("chocolate cyanosis"), especially of the nails, lips, and ears, whereas the color is more often brown rather than blue. Even at low levels of MetHb, this discoloration can be striking [14].

The characteristic chocolate brown color of the blood is used as a simple bed side test to determine MetHb levels (visible at levels from 15% upwards) to guide treatment in settings of limited resources [15].

Acute methemoglobinemia should be suspected in patients with central cyanosis with low peripheral oxygen saturation not responding to high flow oxygen therapy [16].

TABLE 2: Arterial blood gas before and after administration of first dose of methylene blue 150 mg.

| | Before methylene blue | After methylene blue |
|---|---|---|
| $FiO_2$ (fraction of inspired oxygen) | 21% | 100% |
| pH | 7.401 | 7.378 |
| $pCO_2$ [kPa] | 5.59 | 5.01 |
| $pO_2$ [kPa] | 8.33 | 49.6 |
| $SaO_2$ [%] | 93.4 | 100 |
| $HCO_3$ [mmol/L] | 25.5 | 22.1 |
| Oximetry results | | |
| Hb (hemoglobin [g/L]) | 130 | 108 |
| $FO_2$Hb (fractional oxyglobin [%]) | 54.6 | 90.2 |
| FCOHb (fractional carboxyhemoglobin [%]) | 0 | 0 |
| FMetHb (fractional MetHb [%]) | 42.8 | 12.3 |
| Lactate [mmol/L] | 0.7 | 0.4 |

Arterial whole blood was analyzed on an ABL90 series blood gas analyzer, Radiometer Medical, Denmark. Arterial blood gas analyzers are based on electrochemistry and measure pH, $pCO_2$, and $pO_2$. Serum bicarbonate ($HCO_3$) and oxygen saturation ($SaO_2$) are calculated values (using the Henderson-Hasselbalch equation for serum bicarbonate and the standard oxygen-hemoglobin saturation curve for oxygen saturation).

The reason is that pulse oximetry may be inaccurate for monitoring oxygen saturation in the presence of methemoglobinemia since conventional pulse oximeters measure ultraviolet absorption at only two wavelengths (940 and 660 nm) to differentiate oxyhemoglobin from deoxyhemoglobin. To determine the oxygen saturation, the oximeter calculates the ratio of absorbance at the 2 wavelengths. A ratio of absorbance (660 nm/940 nm) of 0.43 corresponds to 100%, whereas a ratio of 1.0 corresponds to a saturation of 85%. MetHb absorbs light equally at both 940 and 660 nm. In the presence of 100% MetHb the ratio of absorbance of light at 660 nm over 940 nm is about 1.0. Therefore, at higher MetHb levels, $SaO_2$ tends toward 85% regardless of the true percentage of oxyhemoglobin [2, 17]. In our case, the peripheral oxygen saturation was 81%.

Another interesting phenomenon is demonstrated in our case report: the oxygen saturation shown in the arterial blood gas analysis ($SaO_2$) may be falsely elevated in patients with methemoglobinemia. The value is calculated based on the patients' $pO_2$. The latter refers to dissolved gas and not to oxygen molecules bound to hemoglobin. Subjects with MHb may have normal $pO_2$ levels despite life-threatening MHb [2].

Additionally, if an oxygen saturation gap >5% exists between the calculated arterial saturation ($SaO_2$) in the blood gas analysis and the reading from the pulse oximeter ($SpO_2$) abnormal hemoglobin (e.g., methemoglobinemia) should be suspected [1, 18]. In our case, the gap was 12.4%.

Regardless of etiology, the severity of symptoms depends on the MetHb levels, reported as a percentage of total hemoglobin. Cyanosis caused by MetHb becomes clinically apparent at a MetHb level of about 15% of total hemoglobin. At levels between 30 and 50%, as observed in our patient, dyspnea, headache, weakness and fatigue, dizziness, and sometimes syncope are described. Levels above 70% may cause death [2, 14]. Anemia, acidosis, respiratory compromise, and cardiac disease may make patients more symptomatic than expected for a given MetHb level.

The most effective and widely used antidotal therapy is methylene blue, which was first described in 1933 in aniline dye poisoning [19, 20].

Treatment should be guided by the severity of the disorder and blood levels of MetHb represent a secondary parameter in the definition of the treatment. However, several authors suggest that methylene blue should be considered with MetHb above 30%, regardless of the presence of symptoms [14, 20, 21]. Symptomatic patients or patients with preexisting conditions that interfere with tissue oxygenation should be treated at levels between 10% and 30%. Standard dose of the intravenous administration is 1 to 2 mg/kg given as a 1% solution over 5 minutes [4]. In our case, the MetHb concentration after 30 min was still elevated at 12.3%, and the patient seemed to still be clinically unwell. We were concerned about the patient's state and the fact that he may develop a possible rebound methemoglobinemia. Therefore, we have applied a second dose of methylene blue.

Notably, "desaturation" on the pulse oximeter after methylene blue administration, as seen in our patient, has been well documented and is known to be a result of interference by methylene blue on light absorbance [22]. This interference complicates the assessment of the patient's ability to oxygenate properly and may lead to administration of repeated doses of methylene blue. The patient's clinical status will provide the most useful information about their ability to oxygenate. According to the literature, a repeated dose may be necessary in severe cases of MetHb levels over 60% or if the patient's condition does not improve [20]. The maximal dose should not exceed 7 mg/kg, since methylene blue at high doses may also precipitate MetHb formation [14, 20].

Methylene blue should be used with caution in individuals with severe renal insufficiency and in young patients with G6PD deficiency. This group of patients can develop hemolytic anemia characterized by formation of Heinz bodies without any reduction in MetHb levels [14, 20, 23]. Alternative therapies include exchange transfusion, hyperbaric oxygen, and ascorbic acid [24].

Excretion of PCA in humans occurs primarily via the urine, with PCA and its conjugates appearing as early as 30 min after exposure. Excretion takes place mainly during the first 24 h and is almost complete within 72 h. Nephrotoxic and hepatotoxic potential of PCA has only been described in animal studies [13].

## 4. Conclusion

Our case shows a rare cause of methemoglobinemia. However, methemoglobinemia can be a complication of commonly used or prescribed medication in the ED, that is, nitroglycerin, local anesthetics such as lidocaine, or metoclopramide. Methemoglobinemia should be suspected in a patient presenting with cyanosis not responsive to oxygen administration. The administration of methylene blue should be considered as antidotal therapy for MetHb concentrations over 30%.

## List of Abbreviations

MetHb:  Methemoglobin
PCA:      $p$-Chloroaniline
ED:        Emergency department
$SpO_2$:   Peripheral oxygen saturation
$SaO_2$:   Arterial oxygen saturation
$pO_2$:    Partial pressure of oxygen
$pCO_2$:  Partial pressure of carbon dioxide.

## Consent

Written informed consent was obtained from the patient for publication of this case report and any accompanying images. A copy of the written consent is available for review.

## Conflict of Interests

The authors have declared that no competing interests exist.

## References

[1] R. Ash-Bernal, R. Wise, and S. M. Wright, "Acquired methemoglobinemia: a retrospective series of 138 cases at 2 teaching hospitals," *Medicine*, vol. 83, no. 5, pp. 265–273, 2004.

[2] R. O. Wright, W. J. Lewander, and A. D. Woolf, "Methemoglobinemia: etiology, pharmacology, and clinical management," *Annals of Emergency Medicine*, vol. 34, no. 5, pp. 646–656, 1999.

[3] S. M. Bradberry, "Occupational methaemoglobinaemia. Mechanisms of production, features, diagnosis and management including the use of methylene blue," *Toxicological Reviews*, vol. 22, no. 1, pp. 13–27, 2003.

[4] L. S. Nelson, N. A. Lewin, M. A. Howland, R. S. Hoffman, and L. R. Goldfrank, *Goldfrank's Toxicoloic Emergencies*, McGraw-Hill, New York, NY, USA, 2011.

[5] J. B. Sullivan and G. R. Krieger, "Clinical hematotoxicology," in *Clinical Environmental Health and Toxic Exposures*, chapter 28, Lippincott Williams & Wilkins, Philadelphia, Pa, USA, 2nd edition, 2001.

[6] D. M. Roberts, R. Heilmair, N. A. Buckley et al., "Clinical outcomes and kinetics of propanil following acute self-poisoning: a prospective case series," *BMC Clinical Pharmacology*, vol. 9, article 3, 2009.

[7] D. E. Ramsay and C. Harvey, "Marking-ink poisoning: an outbreak of methemoglobin cyanosis in newborn babies," *The Lancet*, vol. 273, no. 7079, pp. 910–912, 1959.

[8] B. S. Kulkarni, V. N. Acharya, R. M. Khanna, S. Nath, R. P. Mankodi, and P. Raghavan, "Methemoglobinemia due to nitroaniline intoxication. Review of the literature with a report of 9 cases," *Journal of Postgraduate Medicine*, vol. 15, no. 4, pp. 192–200, 1969.

[9] A. F. Pizon, A. R. Schwartz, L. M. Shum et al., "Toxicology laboratory analysis and human exposure to p-chloroaniline," *Clinical Toxicology*, vol. 47, no. 2, pp. 132–136, 2009.

[10] A. Bazylewicz, T. Kłopotowski, M. Kicka, Ł. Miśkiewicz, and S. Picheta, "Acute poisoning due to chemical substances inducing methemoglobinemia—two cases report," *Przegląd lekarski*, vol. 67, no. 8, pp. 636–639, 2010.

[11] B. E. Watt, A. T. Proudfoot, S. M. Bradberry, and J. A. Vale, "Poisoning due to urea herbicides," *Toxicological Reviews*, vol. 24, no. 3, pp. 161–166, 2005.

[12] R. Thier, J. Lewalter, S. Selinski, and H. M. Bolt, "Biological monitoring in workers in a nitrobenzene reduction plant: haemoglobin versus serum albumin adducts," *International Archives of Occupational and Environmental Health*, vol. 74, no. 7, pp. 483–488, 2001.

[13] A. K. J. Boehncke, G. Könnecker, C. Poehlenz-Michel et al., "Concise International Chemical Assessment," Document 48: 4-Chloroaniline 2003.

[14] K. R. Olsen, "Poisoning and drug overdose," in *Methylene Blue by Fabian Garza*, pp. 902–904, McGraw-Hill, New York, NY, USA, 5th edition, 2007.

[15] F. Shihana, D. M. Dissanayake, N. A. Buckley, and A. H. Dawson, "A simple quantitative bedside test to determine methemoglobin," *Annals of Emergency Medicine*, vol. 55, no. 2, pp. 184–189, 2010.

[16] S. BheemReddy, F. Messineo, and D. Roychoudhury, "Methemoglobinemia following transesophageal echocardiography: a case report and review," *Echocardiography*, vol. 23, no. 4, pp. 319–321, 2006.

[17] S. J. Barker, K. K. Tremper, and J. Hyatt, "Effects of methemoglobinemia on pulse oximetry and mixed venous oximetry," *Anesthesiology*, vol. 70, no. 1, pp. 112–117, 1989.

[18] J. Akhtar, B. D. Johnston, and E. P. Krenzelok, "Mind the gap," *The Journal of Emergency Medicine*, vol. 33, no. 2, pp. 131–132, 2007.

[19] C. F. Williams, "Methylene blue as an antidote for aniline dye poisoning," *Journal of Laboratory and Clinical Medicine*, vol. 1, pp. 166–171, 1933.

[20] J. Clifton II and J. B. Leikin, "Methylene blue," *The American Journal of Therapeutics*, vol. 10, no. 4, pp. 289–291, 2003.

[21] T. S. do Nascimento, R. O. L. Pereira, H. L. D. de Mello, and J. Costa, "Methemoglobinemia: from diagnosis to treatment," *Revista Brasileira de Anestesiologia*, vol. 58, no. 6, pp. 651–664, 2008.

[22] M. R. Kessler, T. Eide, B. Humayun, and P. J. Poppers, "Spurious pulse oximeter desaturation with methylene blue injection," *Anesthesiology*, vol. 65, no. 4, pp. 435–436, 1986.

[23] P. Sikka, V. K. Bindra, S. Kapoor, V. Jain, and K. K. Saxena, "Blue cures blue but be cautious," *Journal of Pharmacy and Bioallied Sciences*, vol. 3, no. 4, pp. 543–545, 2011.

[24] P. Boran, G. Tokuc, and Z. Yegin, "Methemoglobinemia due to application of prilocaine during circumcision and the effect of ascorbic acid," *Journal of Pediatric Urology*, vol. 4, no. 6, pp. 475–476, 2008.

[25] R. B. Abu-Laban, P. J. Zed, R. A. Purssell, and K. G. Evans, "Severe methemoglobinemia from topical anesthetic spray: case report, discussion and qualitative systematic review," *Canadian Journal of Emergency Medicine*, vol. 3, no. 1, pp. 51–56, 2001.

# 49

# An Unusual Presentation of a Massive Pulmonary Embolism with Misleading Investigation Results Treated with Tenecteplase

**David Migneault,[1] Zachary Levine,[2] and François de Champlain[2]**

[1]Department of Emergency Medicine, Vancouver General Hospital, University of British Columbia, Room 3300 910, West 10th Avenue, Vancouver, BC, Canada V5Z 1M9

[2]Emergency Department, Montreal General Hospital, McGill University Health Centre, 1650 Cedar Avenue, Room B2.117, Montreal, QC, Canada H3G 1A4

Correspondence should be addressed to David Migneault; dmemubc@interchange.ubc.ca

Academic Editor: Ching H. Loh

*Background.* There is no foolproof strategy to identify a pulmonary embolism (PE) in the emergency department, and atypical presentations are common. Negative test results may mislead physicians away from the diagnosis of PE. *Objectives.* The current report aims to raise awareness of an unusual presentation of massive PE and its diagnosis and management, in the face of limited evidence in the scientific literature. *Case Reports.* We report the case of a patient with a negative D-Dimer and a negative Computed Tomography contrast angiography of the chest who was diagnosed twenty-seven hours later with a massive PE, as suggested by a bedside echocardiography. The patient was successfully treated with tenecteplase (TNK). *Conclusions/Summary.* Pulmonary embolism frequently presents atypically and is often a diagnostic challenge. There is limited literature about the treatment of massive PE. Further research on bedside echocardiography for diagnosing PE in unstable patients is warranted. In addition, further study into new thrombolytic agents like tenecteplase in the context of massive and submassive PE is warranted.

## 1. Introduction

There is no foolproof strategy to identify cases of pulmonary embolism (PE) in the emergency department (ED). One in every 500 to 1000 ED patients who present to the ED has a PE, and atypical presentations are common [1]. No matter how aggressively one pursues the diagnosis and work-up, it is believed that about 1-2% of patients with PE will be missed. We report the case of a patient with a negative D-Dimer and a negative Computed Tomography contrast angiography (CTA) of the chest who was diagnosed with a massive PE as suggested by a bedside echocardiography and who was subsequently treated successfully with tenecteplase (TNK).

## 2. Case Report

*2.1. Day 1.* A 63-year-old woman known for erythema nodosum, cholelithiasis, hypertension, and remote breast reduction surgery presented to the ED with a two-day history of constant right upper quadrant (RUQ) "tearing/sharp" pain radiating to the back which was worsened with breathing and movement. The pain was accompanied by occasional nausea and anorexia which had begun two weeks earlier. The patient had never experienced similar pain before and denied associated vomiting, chest pain, dyspnea, or fever.

On examination, her vital signs were as follows: temperature 36.5°C, heart rate (HR) 100 beats/min, respiratory rate (RR) 20 breaths/min, oxygen saturation (O2Sat) of 97% on room air, and blood pressure (BP) 145/100 mmHg. The cardiopulmonary examination was normal. The abdominal examination was remarkable only for mild RUQ tenderness without guarding or rebound and negative Murphy's sign. Normal bowel sounds were present and no costovertebral angle tenderness was noted.

Laboratory work-up (CBC, electrolytes, lipase, amylase, LFTs, troponin, and D-Dimer (The assay used for the D-Dimer at our institution is the STA-Liatest D-DI and a result below 0.5 $\mu$g/ml is considered normal or negative.)) was all normal except for a total hyperbilirubinemia of 45 $\mu$mol/L. The ECG showed few premature atrial contractions with no other significant abnormalities. In order to rule out the diagnosis of acute cholecystitis versus referred pain from T-spine compression fracture, an abdominal ultrasound, chest X-ray (CXR), and thoracic spine X-ray were requested as well as a general surgery consult. The CXR showed blunting of the left costophrenic angle and bibasilar atelectatic changes. The spine X-ray showed only degenerative changes. Analgesia with IV morphine was provided.

The patient was reevaluated ninety minutes later and found to have increased right sided posterior thoracic pain with deep breathing and worsening abdominal pain. The vital signs and the rest of the physical examination remained unchanged. The diagnosis of PE was entertained and a spiral CT scan of the chest with IV contrast using a PE protocol and an infused CT of the abdomen were requested. The CTA of the chest read by the radiology attending staff showed no evidence of clots in the central, segmental, or proximal subsegmental pulmonary arteries. The study was slightly limited by the fact that the left lower lobe segmental pulmonary arteries were not well visualized. Both lower lobes and the lingula were remarkable for subsegmental atelectasis. The CT abdomen was unremarkable overall, showing approximately 15 subcentimetric gallbladder stones with no complication or biliary tree dilatation seen.

*2.2. Day 2.* The next morning, the patient was reassessed and her condition judged to be stable. The abdominal ultrasound was performed and showed the same findings as the abdominal CT, that is, gallstones with no sign of an acute process. Repeat laboratory work-up (CBC, electrolytes, and liver profile) showed only an elevated total bilirubin (45 $\mu$mol/L) and an alanine aminotransferase (ALT) of 34. Internal medicine was consulted and they suggested the possibility of early herpes zoster versus background chronic abdominal pain which could be investigated as an outpatient. They specified that there was no evidence of PE, vascular, soft tissue, or rib/bone abnormalities.

*2.3. Day 3.* At 1:35 a.m. the next morning, the patient was found to be confused, moaning, and trembling, with cold extremities. She denied chest pain. Her vital signs were as follows: RR 28/min, O2Sat 88% on room air, BP 92/70 mmHg, HR 141/min, and temperature 36.5°C. The O2Sat increased to 90% on a nonrebreather mask. A venous blood gas was obtained and a femoral line was established. An ECG was done and showed sinus tachycardia with no ST-T changes. The oxygen saturation decreased progressively and the patient developed cyanosis and pallor.

The decision was made to intubate the patient, the intensive care unit (ICU) was consulted, and some blood work, including a repeat D-Dimer, was ordered. A bedside cardiac ultrasound was performed by an attending emergency physician. It demonstrated a dilated, hypokinetic right ventricle as well as increased right sided pressures as demonstrated by inferior vena cava (IVC) distention greater than 20 mm with no inspiratory collapse (Figure 1).

The D-Dimer came back positive at >4.0 $\mu$g/mL. A massive PE was suspected and since it was not possible to obtain

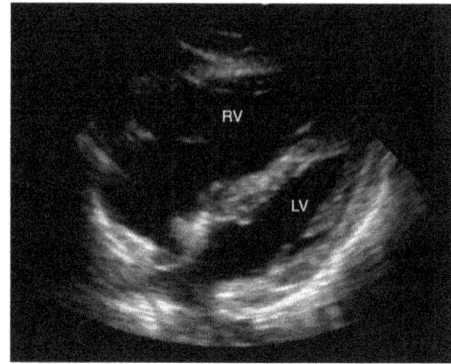

FIGURE 1: Cardiac ultrasound, subxiphoid view showing a dilated right ventricle (RV).

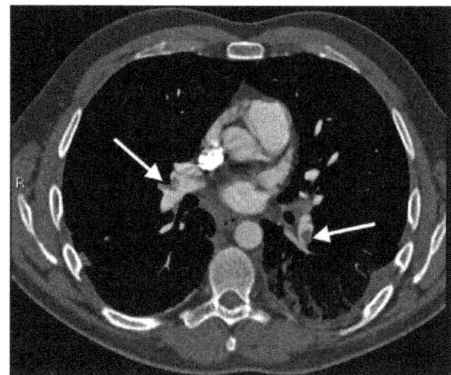

FIGURE 2: CT pulmonary angiography (CTPA) showing a bilateral pulmonary embolisms with clots in branch arteries.

a transesophageal echocardiogram (TEE) as a confirmatory test at that time of the night and the patient was too unstable for a repeat CTA of the chest, a decision was made to attempt thrombolysis using tenecteplase (TNK). A dose of 35 mg (7000 U) (0.5 mg/kg (100 U/kg)) was used in conjunction with 5000 U of unfractionated heparin. The patient was then transferred to the ICU. A repeat CTA of the chest was performed and showed bilateral extensive pulmonary embolus (Figure 2).

## 3. Discussion

This case highlights several controversies related to the diagnosis and treatment of a PE in the ED. Herein, we review the diagnostic accuracy of the D-Dimer and CTA of the chest, the use of bedside echocardiography, and the off-label use of tenecteplase for the treatment of PE.

*3.1. Diagnostic Modalities for PE.* Our patient was initially evaluated as low risk for PE. Based on Wells et al., her pretest probability for PE was approximately 3.4% [2]. The literature shows a great variability in the sensitivity and specificity of the D-Dimer. Brown et al. report 93% and 74%, respectively [3]. With a negative D-Dimer, we can infer a posttest probability of approximately 0.33%. The initial decision not to order a CTA was therefore justified. As mentioned earlier, the imaging was later ordered and found to be negative for PE. Again, there is variability in the literature on the sensitivity and specificity of the CTA of the chest. As per PIOPED II, they are 83% and 96%, respectively [4]. Based on those values, we can calculate a reassuring combined negative D-Dimer and CTA of the chest posttest probability of 0.06% for low risk patients.

Another approach which has been proven to be safe and effective is to combine the CTA of the chest with bilateral lower extremity Doppler ultrasonography (US) for all patients with moderate to high pretest probability of PE [5]. Notably, the lower extremity US was not done on this patient in the ED. Hence, it is impossible to know if a positive result would have been found on the initial presentation, prompting earlier therapy. Our case report also raises the question of the relative benefit of adding CT venography to the chest CTA protocol as it is done routinely in some institutions. This combination yields an absolute increase in detection of venothromboembolism (VTE) of 2-3%. This is similar to the additional yield of lower extremity US with CTA chest but at the expense of increased radiation exposure [4, 6–8].

In our case, the finding that triggered treatment was the evidence of a dilated, hypokinetic right ventricle and the increased right sided pressures as demonstrated by the inferior vena cava (IVC) distention on bedside echocardiography. It is important to note that this bedside echocardiogram was performed while the patient was intubated where evaluation of the IVC distention is less specific for the evaluation of elevated right sided pressures. The literature is very limited on the use of a bedside echocardiogram performed by an emergency physician in the diagnosis of PE. Its utilization seems most useful in the situation in which a massive PE is suspected in the periarrest situation, especially when a bedside TEE is not available in a timely manner. In such a situation, the bedside ultrasound can help the physician to narrow the differential diagnosis and to consider further investigations and/or immediate definitive treatment [9].

*3.2. Thrombolysis for PE.* Indications for thrombolysis for PE are controversial and are poorly defined. The risk-benefit analysis suggests that it is of greatest value in the subset of patients with proven PE who are likely to die or to develop circulatory shock or recurrence [10]. In the absence of an evidence based definition, it is generally accepted that a massive PE is defined by a systolic blood pressure less than 90 mm Hg for more than 15 minutes. In the absence of contraindications, patients with proven massive PE probably benefit from thrombolysis. When to administer a fibrinolytic agent to a patient with profound shock remains controversial when the decision is based solely on clinical suspicion of PE derived from information obtained at the bedside (i.e., empirical fibrinolysis in absence of pulmonary vascular imaging).

Administration of alteplase to patients with PE results in more rapid symptomatic improvement than standard antithrombotic therapy alone and causes more rapid normalization of right ventricular function [11, 12]. Tenecteplase is a recombinant plasminogen-activating enzyme that differs from alteplase by its longer half-life, resistance to plasminogen activator inhibitor-1, and increased fibrin specificity, which results in less fibrinogenolysis and less coagulopathy [12]. Its efficacy and safety have not yet been verified by a well-designed randomized clinical trial. However, a literature review reveals 16 case reports where tenecteplase was used as "off-label" to treat PE. Since no standard dose has been determined, the perceived consensus is to use the recommended dose for thrombolytic therapy for acute myocardial infarction [13–28].

A recently published study examining the indications for fibrinolysis in the treatment of submassive pulmonary embolism evaluated the efficacy and safety of single IV bolus of tenecteplase in addition to heparin as compared to heparin alone for normotensive patients with acute PE who have echocardiographic and laboratory evidence of right ventricular dysfunction. Hemodynamically unstable patients were being excluded. Nevertheless, they concluded that fibrinolytic therapy prevented hemodynamic decompensation but increased the risk of major hemorrhage and stroke. A more recent meta-analysis similarly concluded that thrombolytic therapy was associated with lower rates of all-cause mortality and increased risks of major bleeding and ICH. These results are likely not applicable to our unstable patient [29, 30].

## 4. Conclusion

Pulmonary embolism in the context of a negative D-Dimer and a negative CT chest, although uncommon, does occur, and emergency physicians should be aware of this possibility. Bedside echocardiography can help the emergency physician support the diagnosis of PE in hemodynamically unstable patients. Tenecteplase is a treatment option to consider in such patients with suspected PE, as reported in this case and in other published case reports. Further research on the diagnosis and treatment of massive and submassive PE is clearly warranted.

## Conflict of Interests

The authors declare that there is no conflict of interests regarding the publication of this paper.

## References

[1] R. H. White, "The epidemiology of venous thromboembolism," *Circulation*, vol. 107, no. 23, supplement 1, pp. I4–I8, 2003.

[2] P. S. Wells, J. S. Ginsberg, D. R. Anderson et al., "Use of a clinical model for safe management of patients with suspected pulmonary embolism," *Annals of Internal Medicine*, vol. 129, no. 12, pp. 997–1005, 1998.

[3] M. D. Brown, S. J. Vance, and J. A. Kline, "An emergency department guideline for the diagnosis of pulmonary embolism: an outcome study," *Academic Emergency Medicine*, vol. 12, no. 1, pp. 20–25, 2005.

[4] P. D. Stein, S. E. Fowler, L. R. Goodman et al., "Multidetector computed tomography for acute pulmonary embolism,"

*The New England Journal of Medicine*, vol. 354, no. 22, pp. 2317–2327, 2006.

[5] D. R. Anderson, M. J. Kovacs, C. Dennie et al., "Use of spiral computed tomography contrast angiography and ultrasonography to exclude the diagnosis of pulmonary embolism in the emergency department," *Journal of Emergency Medicine*, vol. 29, no. 4, pp. 399–404, 2005.

[6] M. D. Cham, D. F. Yankelevitz, and C. I. Henschke, "Thromboembolic disease detection at indirect CT venography versus CT pulmonary angiography," *Radiology*, vol. 234, no. 2, pp. 591–594, 2005.

[7] P. B. Richman, J. Wood, D. M. Kasper et al., "Contribution of indirect computed tomography venography to computed tomography angiography of the chest for the diagnosis of thromboembolic disease in two United States emergency departments," *Journal of Thrombosis and Haemostasis*, vol. 1, no. 4, pp. 652–657, 2003.

[8] K. E. Lim, Y. Y. Hsu, W. C. Hsu, and C. C. Huang, "Combined computed tomography venography and pulmonary angiography for the diagnosis PE and DVT in the ED," *The American Journal of Emergency Medicine*, vol. 22, no. 4, pp. 301–306, 2004.

[9] J. Wright, R. Jarman, J. Connolly, and P. Dissmann, "Echocardiography in the emergency department," *Emergency Medicine Journal*, vol. 26, no. 2, pp. 82–86, 2009.

[10] G. Agnelli, C. Becattini, and T. Kirschstein, "Thrombolysis vs heparin in the treatment of pulmonary embolism: a clinical outcome-based meta-analysis," *Archives of Internal Medicine*, vol. 162, no. 22, pp. 2537–2541, 2002.

[11] S. Konstantinides, A. Geibel, G. Heusel, F. Heinrich, and W. Kasper, "Heparin plus alteplase compared with heparin alone in patients with submassive pulmonary embolism," *The New England Journal of Medicine*, vol. 347, no. 15, pp. 1143–1150, 2002.

[12] S. Z. Goldhaber, W. D. Haire, M. L. Feldstein et al., "Alteplase versus heparin in acute pulmonary embolism: randomised trial assessing right-ventricular function and pulmonary perfusion," *The Lancet*, vol. 341, no. 8844, pp. 507–511, 1993.

[13] N. D. Brunetti, R. Ieva, M. Correale et al., "Massive pulmonary embolism immediately diagnosed by transthoracic echocardiography and treated with tenecteplase fibrinolysis," *Journal of Thrombosis and Thrombolysis*, vol. 28, no. 2, pp. 238–241, 2009.

[14] C. Becattini, G. Agnelli, A. Salvi et al., "Bolus tenecteplase for right ventricle dysfunction in hemodynamically stable patients with pulmonary embolism," *Thrombosis Research*, vol. 125, no. 3, pp. e82–e86, 2010.

[15] F. Lapostolle, J. Levasseur, N. Dardel, and F. Adnet, "Cardiac arrest after air travel successfully treated by presumptive fibrinolysis," *Resuscitation*, vol. 80, no. 5, p. 606, 2009.

[16] S. Fasullo, S. Paterna, and P. Di Pasquale, "An unusual presentation of massive pulmonary embolism mimicking septal acute myocardial infarction treated with tenecteplase," *Journal of Thrombosis and Thrombolysis*, vol. 27, no. 2, pp. 215–219, 2009.

[17] A. Hovland, H. Bjørnstad, R. F. Hallstensen et al., "Massive pulmonary embolism with cardiac arrest treated with continuous thrombolysis and concomitant hypothermia," *Emergency Medicine Journal*, vol. 25, no. 5, pp. 310–311, 2008.

[18] J. M. van Opstal, S. C. Bekkers, and A. P. M. Gorgels, "A dancing thrombus in the right atrium going hand-in-hand with the electrocardiogram," *European Journal of Echocardiography*, vol. 9, no. 1, pp. 80–81, 2008.

[19] D. V. F. Hefer, A. Munir, and H. Khouli, "Low-dose tenecteplase during cardiopulmonary resuscitation due to massive pulmonary embolism: a case report and review of previously reported cases," *Blood Coagulation & Fibrinolysis*, vol. 18, no. 7, pp. 691–694, 2007.

[20] H. Isma'eel, A. Taher, S. Alam, and M. S. Arnaout, "Massive pulmonary embolism in a Lebanese patient doubly heterozygous for MTHFR and Factor V Leiden presenting with syncope and treated with tenecteplase," *Journal of Thrombosis and Thrombolysis*, vol. 21, no. 2, pp. 179–184, 2006.

[21] C. Melzer, C. Richter, P. Rogalla et al., "Tenecteplase for the treatment of massive and submassive pulmonary embolism," *Journal of Thrombosis and Thrombolysis*, vol. 18, no. 1, pp. 47–50, 2004.

[22] B. D. Adams, J. Y. Kim, and W. O. Jackson, "Tenecteplase and return of spontaneous circulation after refractory cardiopulmonary arrest," *Southern Medical Journal*, vol. 97, no. 10, pp. 1015–1017, 2004.

[23] I. G. Livaditis, M. Paraschos, and K. Dimopoulos, "Massive pulmonary embolism with ST elevation in leads V1-V3 and successful thrombolysis with tenecteplase," *Heart*, vol. 90, no. 7, article e41, 2004.

[24] D. Clément, R. Loyant, and T. Labet, "Tenecteplase and massive pulmonary embolus," *Annales Francaises d'Anesthesie et de Reanimation*, vol. 23, no. 4, pp. 440–441, 2004.

[25] D. Caldicott, S. Parasivam, J. Harding, N. Edwards, and F. Bochner, "Tenecteplase for massive pulmonary embolus," *Resuscitation*, vol. 55, no. 2, pp. 211–213, 2002.

[26] D. Y. Sze, M. B. Lewis Carey, and M. K. Razavi, "Treatment of massive pulmonary embolus with catheter-directed tenecteplase," *Journal of Vascular and Interventional Radiology*, vol. 12, no. 12, pp. 1456–1457, 2001.

[27] W. Abdulla and U. Netter, "Case report. Successful use of tenecteplase in massive pulmonary embolism with cardiopulmonary resuscitation immediately following tracheostomy," *Acta Anaesthesiologica Belgica*, vol. 56, no. 2, pp. 179–182, 2005.

[28] G. Allocca, V. Dall'Aglio, and G. L. Nicolosi, "Massive pulmonary embolism in ambiguous presentation in a 90-year-old patient treated with fibrinolysis: clinical case and clinico-echocardiographic considerations," *Italian Heart Journal Supplement*, vol. 6, no. 6, pp. 390–393, 2005.

[29] G. Meyer, "The PEITHO study: for a clarification of the indications for the fibrinolytic treatment of pulmonary embolism," *Revue de Pneumologie Clinique*, vol. 64, no. 6, pp. 326–327, 2008.

[30] S. Chatterjee, A. Chakraborty, I. Weinberg et al., "Thrombolysis for pulmonary embolism and risk of all-cause mortality, major bleeding, and intracranial hemorrhage: a meta-analysis," *The Journal of the American Medical Association*, vol. 311, no. 23, pp. 2414–2421, 2014.

# 50

# Not Just Painless Bleeding: Meckel's Diverticulum as a Cause of Small Bowel Obstruction in Children—Two Cases and a Review of the Literature

**Khalida Itriyeva,[1] Matthew Harris,[2] Joshua Rocker,[2] and Robert Gochman[2]**

[1]Department of Pediatrics, Cohen Children's Medical Center of New York, 269-01 76th Avenue, New Hyde Park, NY 11040, USA
[2]Pediatric Emergency Medicine, Cohen Children's Medical Center of New York, 269-01 76th Avenue, New Hyde Park, NY 11040, USA

Correspondence should be addressed to Matthew Harris; mharris13@nshs.edu

Academic Editor: Vasileios Papadopoulos

Physicians are educated with the classical teaching that symptomatic patients with Meckel's diverticulum (MD) most often present with painless rectal bleeding. However, a review of the literature reveals that young patients with MD will most commonly present with signs of intestinal obstruction, an etiology not frequency considered in patients presenting to the emergency department with obstruction. We present two cases of intestinal obstruction diagnosed in our emergency department, with Meckel's diverticulum being the etiology.

## 1. Case 1

An 18-month-old male with a past medical history significant for constipation and reflux presented to our pediatric emergency department with an approximately 5-hour history of lethargy, intermittent crying, and abdominal pain. The parents denied fever, vomiting, or abdominal distension but reported a decrease in oral intake and urine output. He had not stooled that day and had no prior surgical history.

Upon arrival to the emergency department (ED), the patient was afebrile with a rectal temperature of 98.2°F, heart rate of 129 bpm, blood pressure of 115/71, respiratory rate of 28, and oxygen saturation of 100% on room air. On physical exam, he was notably lethargic and pale, with sunken eyes and dry mucus membranes. He had periods of wakefulness, during which he appeared uncomfortable. He was intermittently tachycardic. The abdominal exam was notable for decreased bowel sounds and moderate distension with diffuse tenderness to palpation.

Intravenous access was obtained and the patient was given a 20 mL/kg normal saline bolus. Laboratory studies drawn were notable for a leukocytosis of 26,000 with a neutrophilic predominance and thrombocytosis. The chemistry obtained was grossly normal.

Intussusception was high on our differential diagnosis. Multiple-view abdominal plain films and an ultrasound of the abdomen were requested.

The supine abdominal plain film (Figure 1) revealed a moderately dilated loop of bowel in the mid-abdomen, a paucity of air in the right colon, and a large amount of stool. The abdominal ultrasound revealed marked bowel wall thickening in the right hemiabdomen with free fluid present both in the abdomen and in the pelvis. There was no evidence of appendicitis or intussusception.

The patient received a second 20 mL/kg saline bolus for persistent tachycardia and a pediatric fleet enema which did not produce significant stool. The patient developed worsening abdominal tenderness and bilious emesis and appeared obtunded, increasing our concern for an acute obstructive process. Intravenous piperacillin-tazobactam was empirically administered to the patient, given that a third 20 mL/kg normal saline bolus was administered, and a nasogastric tube was placed. A pediatric surgery consult was obtained and a noncontrast CT scan of the abdomen and pelvis was performed. The CT scan revealed a distal small bowel obstruction with evidence of ischemia and significant ascites.

A diagnostic laparoscopy and subsequent exploratory laparotomy revealed a congenital band extending from

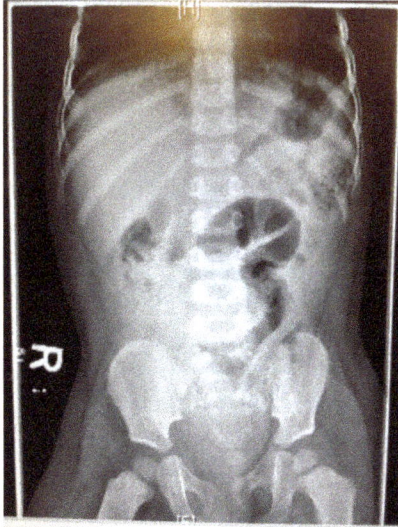

FIGURE 1: Supine abdominal plain film.

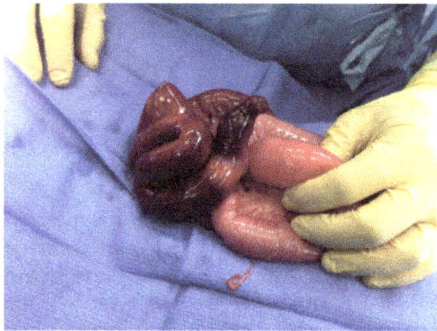

FIGURE 2: Intraoperative photograph showing portion of ischemic bowel.

Meckel's diverticulum to the root of the mesentery, with thickened loops of dilated and ischemic bowel strangulated within this space (Figure 2). Significant ascites was also noted. A resection of the terminal ileum and cecum was performed, with subsequent primary ileocolic anastomosis. Forty-five cm of the distal ileum was found to be ischemic and subsequently resected. The postoperative period was unremarkable and the patient made a full recovery.

## 2. Case 2

A 3-month-old full-term male with no prior medical history was referred to our pediatric emergency department after presenting to an outside institution with voluminous emesis and dehydration. Abdominal plain films were suspicious for malrotation (Figure 3). There had been no recent fever or URI symptoms, nor any diarrhea or rash.

On presentation to our pediatric ED, the patient was afebrile, with a pulse of 123 bpm, blood pressure 103/57 mmHg, respiratory rate of 26, and oxygen saturation of 100% on room air. On physical exam, the patient was alert, active, and playful and in no acute distress. He had dry lips,

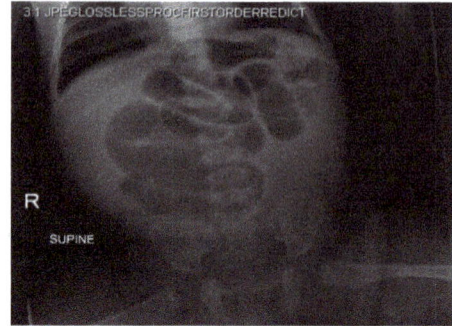

FIGURE 3: Supine abdominal plain film.

but his skin was warm and with brisk capillary refill. His abdomen was soft, nontender, and nondistended and without hepatosplenomegaly. He had a normal testicular and inguinal exam.

An abdominal ultrasound revealed multiple air filled loops of bowel within the mid-abdomen, with no evidence of intussusception. An upper GI series and barium enema were subsequently performed, revealing an abnormal position of the duodenum without the expected course of contrast to the left upper quadrant, suggesting the possibility of malrotation without volvulus.

Pediatric surgery was consulted, and the patient was taken to the operating room for diagnostic laparoscopy. Surgical evaluation revealed Meckel's diverticulum with a congenital band, causing an extra-luminal obstruction of the adjacent bowel—the cause of his vomiting. Ironically, the patient did also have a malrotation, without volvulus or obstruction from the Ladd's bands that were present; however this abnormal anatomy was not the cause of the patient's symptoms.

The congenital band and Meckel's diverticulum were resected to resolve the obstruction, without loss of bowel. Ladd's procedure was also performed to correct the malrotation. Final pathology report revealed Meckel's diverticulum without perforation lined by small intestinal and gastric antral mucosa showing active inflammation and reactive changes, with a nodule of pancreatic tissue in its wall.

## 3. Discussion

The differential diagnosis for a child with vomiting is broad and ranges from relatively benign conditions such as gastroenteritis to life-threatening causes such as volvulus. While the physical exam, laboratory studies, and imaging can often elucidate the cause of vomiting, it is sometimes incumbent upon the pediatric emergency medicine physician to recognize a surgical abdomen that requires an intraoperative evaluation for formal diagnosis and intervention.

Meckel's diverticulum (MD) is the most common congenital anomaly of the gastrointestinal tract, with an incidence of 2–4% in the general population [1]. Meckel's diverticulum is a persistence of the vestigial vitelline duct and is comprised of the three layers of the intestinal wall: mucosa, submucosa, and muscularis. While it may contain jejunal, duodenal, and even pancreatic tissue, it classically contains heterotopic gastric tissue. Most patients with MD are asymptomatic. Children are more likely to be symptomatic at presentation than adults. Twenty-five to fifty percent of all symptomatic Meckel's patients present before the age of 10. The incidence in males is twice that of females [2]. MD is most commonly found in the distal ileum, within 2 feet of the ileocecal valve, and, on gross resection, is approximately two inches in length. (The oft quoted "rule of 2's" is defined as follows: 2% incidence, 2 feet from the ileocecal junction, 2 inches in length, and 2 : 1 incidence in males over females.)

Most children with Meckel's diverticulum are asymptomatic. Complications of Meckel's diverticulum are seen more frequently in those who present at a younger age and in male patients [3, 4]. The classical description of painless bleeding is more commonly seen in adult patients, whereas in children, especially those younger than four years of age, the presentation is more likely to be that of an obstruction, as was the case with the patients in our case series. One large study of over 1400 patients, including 58 pediatric patients, found that obstruction was the most common presenting sign (40%) in children [3]. In their 2006 review of the literature, Sagar and colleagues found this number to be closer to 50% [1].

The etiologies of obstruction in children with symptomatic Meckel's diverticula include intussusception, volvulus, Littre's hernia, omphalomesenteric band, and diverticulitis [1–4]. Pediatric patients presenting with obstruction may exhibit irritability, paroxysmal abdominal pain, abdominal distension, nausea, vomiting, and anorexia.

Classically, one should suspect Meckel's diverticulum in children who present with painless lower gastrointestinal bleeding without evidence of infectious gastroenteritis or inflammatory bowel disease. MD may also be suspected in children with recurrent intussusception, as it may serve as a lead point. MD is also in the differential for right lower quadrant pain, especially in those patients with a previous appendectomy [2].

There are classically three diagnostic modalities in the evaluation of a patient with suspected Meckel's diverticulum. Meckel's scan is a nuclear medicine study that uses technetium 99m pertechnetate, which detects gastric mucosa, to identify ectopic gastric mucosa [2, 5]. Its sensitivity is much higher in pediatrics (85–90%) than in the adult population (60%) [5]. Mesenteric angiography may be helpful in identifying MD when a patient presents with active gastrointestinal bleeding. With this imaging modality, an anomalous superior mesenteric artery branch feeding the diverticulum may be visualized [2, 6]. Active contrast extravasation may also be seen in patients with persistent bleeding [2]. Finally, abdominal exploration in the operating room may lead to a finding of Meckel's diverticulum.

Our patients presented with evolving obstructive processes. To be clear, in the setting of a suspected obstructive process, the aforementioned imaging modalities are superfluous. Upright and decubitus abdominal radiographs to assess the patient for the presence of air-fluid levels, with computer aided tomography of the abdomen and pelvis with oral and intravenous contrast, may be necessary to identify the obstruction.

For the pediatric patient who presents with evidence of an obstructive process, there are a number of important aspects of management that should be addressed early. Intravenous access should be obtained immediately, and aggressive fluid resuscitation should be considered. A nasogastric tube should be placed for continuous suction and the patient made NPO. Any electrolyte abnormalities should be corrected, and a surgical consult should be obtained promptly. One can consider the empiric use of antibiotics with broad Gram-negative and anaerobic coverage, and some studies suggest the use of proton pump inhibitors [2]. Perhaps most importantly, urgent consultation with a pediatric surgeon can expedite both diagnosis and management.

The first patient in our series became progressively lethargic and obtunded. This is likely due to the release of inflammatory mediators as part of a SIRS response to strangulated tissue, as was evident by his tachycardia, tachypnea, and leukocytosis [7]. Previous studies have established that patients with a systemic inflammatory response in the setting of a suspected small bowel obstruction are more likely to have strangulated bowel [8].

In addition to Meckel's diverticulum, the second patient in our series was noted to have malrotation. The association between malrotation and other congenital gastrointestinal anomalies has been well reported. In one study, Meckel's diverticulum was the 2nd most common anomaly found with malrotation, behind duodenal atresia [9].

Both of our patients required resection of MD and associated bands to relieve their respective obstructive processes.

Meckel's diverticulum is occasionally found incidentally during abdominal surgery. Resection of incidental MD is generally not recommended, although this is an area of controversy and there may be exceptions [2, 3, 10]. One study suggested resection of asymptomatic Meckel's diverticula when they fulfilled one or more of the following four criteria: patient age younger than 50 years, male sex, diverticulum length greater than 2 cm, and ectopic or abnormal features within the diverticulum, as these were all associated with symptomatic diverticula in the study [3]. Resection is also recommended in all children under the age of 8 years, as they are more at risk of complications of MD [11]. In those patients who meet operative requirements, surgeons may choose either a simple diverticulectomy or small bowel resection with primary anastomosis [2]. Surgical complications and perioperative morbidity and mortality are very low [2, 10].

Younger children with Meckel's diverticulum are more likely to be symptomatic than older children. While the classical association of MD with painless rectal bleeding is still taught, obstruction is the more common presenting symptom in pediatric patients. Our case series identified two patients with different clinical presentations of obstruction, both of whom were found to have complications of MD. Small bowel obstruction is relatively uncommon in pediatrics, and our cases highlight the importance of early recognition and management to minimize morbidity and mortality. We strongly recommend early, urgent consultation with a pediatric surgeon in setting of suspected small bowel obstruction.

## Conflict of Interests

The authors declare that there is no conflict of interests regarding the publication of this paper.

## References

[1] J. Sagar, V. Kumar, and D. K. Shah, "Meckel's diverticulum: a systematic review," *Journal of the Royal Society of Medicine*, vol. 99, no. 10, pp. 501–505, 2006.

[2] P. Javid and E. M. Pauli, *Meckel's Diverticulum*, edited by: T. W. Post, UpToDate, Waltham, Mass, USA, 2014.

[3] J. J. Park, B. G. Wolff, M. K. Tollefson, E. E. Walsh, and D. R. Larson, "Meckel diverticulum: the Mayo Clinic experience with 1476 patients (1950–2002)," *Annals of Surgery*, vol. 241, no. 3, pp. 529–533, 2005.

[4] J. H. Rho, J. S. Kim, S. Y. Kim et al., "Clinical features of symptomatic Meckel's diverticulum in children: comparison of scintigraphic and non-scintigraphic diagnosis," *Pediatric Gastroenterology, Hepatology and Nutrition*, vol. 16, no. 1, pp. 41–48, 2013.

[5] S. Lin, P. V. Suhocki, K. A. Ludwig, and M. A. Shetzline, "Gastrointestinal bleeding in adult patients with Meckel's diverticulum: the role of technetium 99 m pertechnetate scan," *Southern Medical Journal*, vol. 95, no. 11, pp. 1338–1341, 2002.

[6] W. D. Routh, R. B. Lawdahl, E. Lund, J. H. Garcia, and F. S. Keller, "Meckel's diverticula: angiographic diagnosis in patients with non-acute hemorrhage and negative scintigraphy," *Pediatric Radiology*, vol. 20, no. 3, pp. 152–156, 1990.

[7] J. Pavare, I. Grope, and D. Gardovska, "Prevalence of systemic inflammatory response syndrome (SIRS) in hospitalized children: a point prevalence study," *BMC Pediatrics*, vol. 9, article 25, 2009.

[8] H. Tsumura, T. Ichikawa, E. Hiyama, Y. Murakami, and T. Sueda, "Systemic inflammatory response syndrome (SIRS) as a predictor of strangulated small bowel obstruction," *Hepato-Gastroenterology*, vol. 51, no. 59, pp. 1393–1396, 2004.

[9] E. G. Ford, M. O. Senac Jr., M. S. Srikanth, and J. J. Weitzman, "Malrotation of the intestine in children," *Annals of Surgery*, vol. 215, no. 2, pp. 172–178, 1992.

[10] A. Zani, S. Eaton, C. M. Rees, and A. Pierro, "Incidentally detected meckel diverticulum: to resect or not to resect?" *Annals of Surgery*, vol. 247, no. 2, pp. 276–281, 2008.

[11] A. Önen, M. K. Ciğdem, H. Öztürk, S. Otçu, and A. I. Dokucu, "When to resect and when not to resect an asymptomatic Meckel's diverticulum: an ongoing challenge," *Pediatric Surgery International*, vol. 19, no. 1-2, pp. 57–61, 2003.

# 51

# Development of ST Elevation Myocardial Infarction and Atrial Fibrillation after an Electrical Injury

**Erdal Gursul,[1] Serdar Bayata,[2] Ercan Aksit,[1] and Basak Ugurlu[1]**

[1]Biga State Hospital, Kibris Sehitleri Street, Biga, 17200 Canakkale, Turkey
[2]Katip Celebi University Ataturk Training and Research Hospital, Izmir, Turkey

Correspondence should be addressed to Erdal Gursul; erdalgrsul@yahoo.com.tr

Academic Editor: Aristomenis K. Exadaktylos

Electrical energy is a type of energy that is commonly used in daily life. Ventricular premature beats, ventricular tachycardia, ventricular fibrillation, atrial tachycardia, atrial fibrillation, bundle branch blocks, and AV block are arrhythmic complications that are encountered in case of electric shocks. Myocardial infarction is one of the rarely seen complications of electric shocks yet it has fatal outcomes. Coronary arteries were detected to be normal in most of the patients who had myocardial infarction following an electric shock. So, etiology of myocardial infarction is thought to be unrelated to coronary atherosclerosis in these cases. Coronary artery vasospasm is thought to be the primary etiological cause. In our case report, we presented a patient who developed ST elevation MI with atrial fibrillation after an electric shock.

## 1. Introduction

Electrical energy is the commonly used energy type in daily life. However, electric shocks can lead to a wide range of clinical conditions from skin burns to fatal arrhythmic complications. Cardiac effects of electric shock include accelerated hypertension, arrhythmia, acute myocardial infarction (MI), and cardiac rupture [1–3]. Ventricular premature beats, ventricular tachycardia, ventricular fibrillation, atrial tachycardia, atrial fibrillation (AF), bundle branch blocks, and AV block can be seen as the arrhythmic complications of electric shock [3, 4]. MI is one of the rarely seen complications which may lead to fatal outcomes. In most of the cases, patients who had myocardial infarction after electric shock have been reported to have normal coronary arteries. Particularly in case of ST elevation MI, etiology is considered to be vasospasm occurring after electric shock [5].

In our case report, we presented a patient who developed ST elevation MI with atrial fibrillation after an electric shock.

## 2. Case

A 50-year-old male patient admitted to the emergency because of an electric shock which occurred 15 minutes before (alternative current, 50 Hz, 220 V). The patient indicated that as soon as he touched the wall plug to switch on light, he was shocked from his right hand and found himself lying on the floor of his home. He stated that he had lost his consciousness with the shock and after recovery he had found out he had a tightening chest pain radiating to his left arm. His pain had continued increasingly. Arterial blood pressure ratio was measured as 140/80 mmHg on examination of the patient. Pulse was arrhythmic and tachycardic. No lesion was observed regarding the electric shock entry and exit points. Sinus tachycardia, increase in the amplitude of the T-wave at inferior derivations, and ventricular premature beats were monitored in the performed ECG (Figure 1).

After establishing a vascular access, routine blood tests were performed and the patient was monitored by connecting to a defibrillator. Nearly after ten minutes, atrial fibrillation developed with a sharpened chest pain. In the performed ECG, ST segment elevation in inferior derivations and ST segment depression in V1–V3 derivations were observed (Figure 2). In order to maintain the ventricular rate under control, intravenous beta-blocker was applied to the patient whose blood pressure was stable. Due to continuous ST segment elevation, ASA 300 mg and clopidogrel 600 mg were

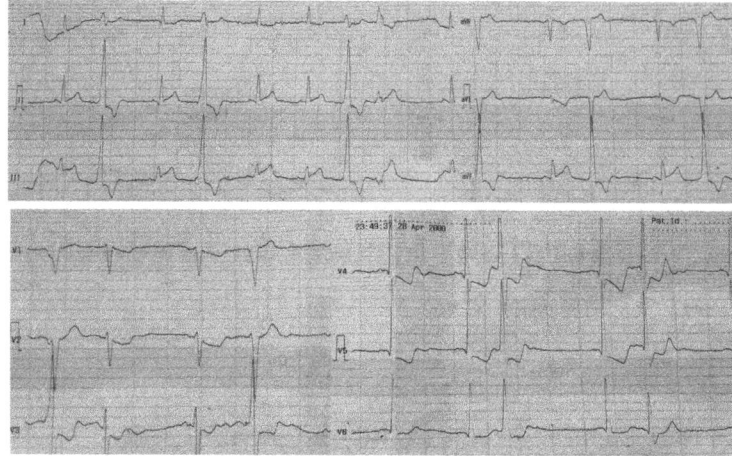

FIGURE 1: This electrocardiogram demonstrates ventricular premature beats and increased amplitude of the T-wave in inferior derivations.

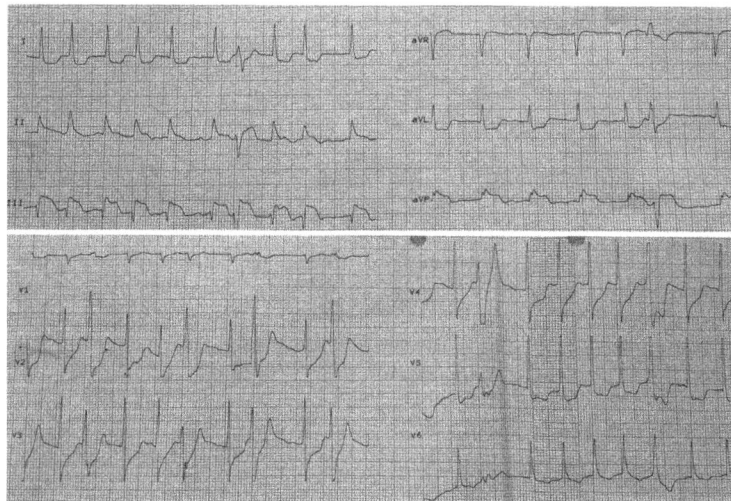

FIGURE 2: At this electrocardiogram, ST segment elevation in inferior derivations and ST segment depression in V1–V3 are seen with the rhythm of atrial fibrillation.

given and enoxaparin 0.6 cc was applied subcutaneously. In an effort to exclude a potential Type 1 myocardial infarction, the patient was immediately transferred to a center where primary angioplasty could be performed in 120 minutes. Before coronary angiography in the hospital where he transferred, the patient's chest pain disappeared, ST segment descended to isoelectric line, and the patient returned to sinus rhythm approximately 100 minutes after the detection of symptom. In the performed coronary angiography, normal coronary arteries were determined and dominancy of right coronary artery was observed. The patient was thought to have right coronary arterial vasospasm (Type 2 MI) which was probably triggered by electric shock. A moderate increase in troponin and CK-MB levels was seen in the monitorization of the patient. In echocardiographic examination, EF was estimated as 58% and segmental motion defect was not detected. The patient was discharged with full recovery after four-day-long observation in the hospital.

## 3. Discussion

Electric shock can cause adverse outcomes on human body. Various clinical conditions from simple burn lesions to fatal arrhythmias could be observed in case of electric shocks. In a recently conducted study, electric shock was found to be only 2.2% of the injuries admitted to emergency service; however, it was reported to be 42.9% of the fatal injuries [6]. It is indicated that cardiac pathologies are more frequently encountered when direction of electric current passes through the heart in injuries related to electric shock [7]. Electric shock may lead not only to arrhythmia, but also to myocardial infarction, accelerated hypertension, and myocardial rupture of heart [3, 4]. Pathophysiology of arrhythmia due to electric current has not been fully enlightened yet. Necrotic areas created by current and alterations in cardiac sodium/potassium pump activity are considered to be primary responsible mechanisms [7, 8].

Butler and Gant investigated 182 electric shock incidents over 20 years and they reported only 2 AF cases [2]. Arrowsmith et al. detected 3 ectopic beats and 1 AF (exposed to high voltage) among 145 cases they evaluated regarding cardiac complications over 5 years. In this study, it is emphasized that cardiac complications occurred more frequently if loss of consciousness was seen after electric shock [9]. In our case, loss of consciousness was also developed and cardiac complications were experienced as it is mentioned in literature.

Coronary arteries were detected to be normal in most of the patients who had MI following an electric shock. So, etiology of myocardial infarction is thought to be unrelated to coronary atherosclerosis in these cases. Coronary arterial vasospasm [5], direct thermal effect on myocardium [5], arrhythmia induced hypotension [10], depredation of coronary artery during cardiopulmonary resuscitation [11], and hypoxia due to cardiopulmonary arrest [12] are thought to be primary etiological causes of electric shock induced MI. Development of ST-elevated MI due to electric shock is a rarely encountered situation [13]. It is stated in the literature that right coronary artery lays closer to the chest wall on its course and it is more sensitive to electrical current, so ST elevation in inferior derivations is more frequently observed after electric shock [14]. Al et al. determined normal coronary arteries after electric shock induced inferior MI and they reported that the patient's ECG findings were recovered after 6 hours [15]. Celebi et al. also presented an electric shock induced inferior MI patient with normal coronary arteries. They reported that minimal ST elevation was continued at inferior derivations even after 1 year of shock [16]. In our case, right coronary arterial vasospasm was probably developed after electrical current exposure through right hand. Recovery of ECG findings within 100 minutes after the electric shock and detection of normal coronary arteries in performed angiography also support the idea of vasospasm.

In our case, association of electric shock induced ST elevation at inferior derivations and AF was observed. The AF developed during monitorization can be due to either direct arrhythmic effect of the electric shock or ischemic myocardium. AF disappeared soon after normalization of ST segment. This makes us consider the ischemic etiology on foreground.

Since the primary cause is vasospasm, fibrinolytic therapy should not be considered as the first option for electric shock induced ST elevation MI treatment. Electric shock induced multiple traumas and/or hematomas may also cause contraindication for fibrinolytic treatment. According to all of these, in such cases first treatment option should be percutaneous coronary angioplasty [15, 16].

## 4. Conclusion

Electric shock injuries can result in serious situations such as arrhythmia and myocardial infarction. Arterial vasospasm should be considered as one of the etiologies of ST-elevated MI developed after an electric shock.

## Conflict of Interests

The authors declare that there is no conflict of interests regarding the publication of this paper.

## References

[1] F. C. DiVincenti, J. A. Moncrief, and B. A. Pruitt Jr., "Electrical injuries: a review of 65 cases.," *Journal of Trauma*, vol. 9, no. 6, pp. 497–507, 1969.

[2] E. D. Butler and T. D. Gant, "Electrical injuries, with special reference to the upper extremities. A review of 182 cases," *The American Journal of Surgery*, vol. 134, no. 1, pp. 95–101, 1977.

[3] L. Solem, R. P. Fischer, and R. G. Strate, "The natural history of electrical injury," *The Journal of Trauma*, vol. 17, no. 7, pp. 487–492, 1977.

[4] G. S. Wander, R. K. Bansal, I. S. Anand, S. Arora, S. B. Khurana, and L. S. Chawla, "Atrial fibrillation following electrical injury," *Japanese Heart Journal*, vol. 33, no. 1, pp. 131–134, 1992.

[5] N. Xenopoulos, A. Movahed, P. Hudson, and W. C. Reeves, "Myocardial injury in electrocution," *The American Heart Journal*, vol. 122, no. 5, pp. 1481–1484, 1991.

[6] S. Özkan, Ş. Kiliç, P. Durukan et al., "Occupational injuries admitted to the emergency department," *Ulusal Travma ve Acil Cerrahi Dergisi*, vol. 16, no. 3, pp. 241–247, 2010.

[7] H. Boggild, L. Freund, and J. P. Bagger, "Persistent atrial fibrillation following electrical injury," *Occupational Medicine*, vol. 45, no. 1, pp. 49–50, 1995.

[8] P. J. Jensen, P. E. Thomsen, J. P. Bagger, A. Nørgaard, and U. Baandrup, "Electrical injury causing ventricular arrhythmias," *British Heart Journal*, vol. 57, no. 3, pp. 279–283, 1987.

[9] J. Arrowsmith, R. P. Usgaocar, and W. A. Dickson, "Electrical injury and the frequency of cardiac complications," *Burns*, vol. 23, no. 7-8, pp. 576–578, 1997.

[10] C. L. Oltman, C. B. Clark, N. L. Kane et al., "Coronary vascular dysfunction associated with direct current shock injury," *Basic Research in Cardiology*, vol. 98, no. 6, pp. 406–415, 2003.

[11] P. B. Oliva and J. C. Breckinridge, "Acute myocardial infarction with normal and near normal coronary arteries. Documentation with coronary arteriography within 12 1/2 hours of the onset of symptoms in two cases (three episodes)," *The American Journal of Cardiology*, vol. 40, no. 6, pp. 1000–1007, 1977.

[12] A. C. Koumbourlis, "Electrical injuries," *Critical Care Medicine*, vol. 30, no. 11, pp. S424–S430, 2002.

[13] N. C. Chandra, C. O. Siu, and A. M. Munster, "Clinical predictors of myocardial damage after high voltage electrical injury," *Critical Care Medicine*, vol. 18, no. 3, pp. 293–297, 1990.

[14] T. N. James, L. Riddick, and J. H. Embry, "Cardiac abnormalities demonstrated postmortem in four cases of accidental electrocution and their potential significance relative to nonfatal electrical injuries of the heart," *The American Heart Journal*, vol. 120, no. 1, pp. 143–157, 1990.

[15] B. Al, P. Yarbil, H. O. Özer, S. Aslan, C. Yıldırım, and V. Davutoğlu, "A rare complication of electric shock: myocardial infarction," *Journal of Academic Emergency Medicine: Case Reports*, vol. 3, no. 1, pp. 4–8, 2012.

[16] A. Celebi, O. Gulel, H. Cicekcioglu, S. Gokaslan, G. Kututcularoglu, and V. Ulusoy, "Myocardial infarction after an electric shock: a rare complication," *Cardiology Journal*, vol. 16, no. 4, pp. 362–364, 2009.

# 52

# Necrotizing Fasciitis Secondary to a Primary Suture for Anoperineal Trauma by Motorcycle Accident in a Healthy Adult

**Susumu Saigusa,**[1,2] **Masaki Ohi,**[1,2] **Hiroki Imaoka,**[1,2] **Ryo Uratani,**[1,2]
**Minako Kobayashi,**[1,2] **and Yasuhiro Inoue**[1,2]

[1]*Department of Surgery, Wakaba Hospital, 28-13 Minami-Chuo, Tsu, Mie 514-0832, Japan*
[2]*Department of Gastrointestinal and Pediatric Surgery, Mie University Graduate School of Medicine, 2-174 Edobashi, Tsu, Mie 514-8507, Japan*

Correspondence should be addressed to Susumu Saigusa; saigusa@wakabahsp.jp

Academic Editor: Vasileios Papadopoulos

A 41-year-old man experienced a swollen scrotum three days after a motorcycle accident and presented to our hospital. He had had a primary suture repair for anoperineal trauma in an outside hospital at the time of the injury. He presented to us with general fatigue, low grade fevers, and perineal pain. Abdominal computed tomography showed subcutaneous emphysema from the scrotum to the left chest. The sutured wound had foul-smelling discharge and white exudate. We made the diagnosis of necrotizing fasciitis and immediately opened the sutured wound and performed initial debridement and lavage with copious irrigation. We continued antibiotics and lavage of the wound until the infection was controlled. Fortunately, the necrotizing fasciitis did not worsen and he was discharged after 15 days. Our experience indicates that anoperineal injuries should not be closed without careful and intensive follow-up due to the potential of developing necrotizing fasciitis.

## 1. Introduction

Necrotizing fasciitis (NF) is an uncommon, rapidly progressive soft tissue infection involving necrosis of subcutaneous tissues with an alarmingly high mortality rate. Appropriate diagnosis and prompt treatment are extremely important [1–4]. However, early recognition of NF is difficult clinically because there may only be minor skin changes such as local pain upon palpation and erythema in the early phases. Although there is no age or gender predilection, higher rates of NF are seen in obese, diabetic, and immunocompromised patients, as well as in alcoholics and patients with peripheral vascular disease. However, NF can also occur in young, otherwise healthy patients with none of these predisposing factors [1, 3, 5]. We report a case of necrotizing fasciitis after primary suture repair for an anoperineal injury by motorcycle accident with a favorable clinical outcome in a healthy adult.

## 2. Case Presentation

A 41-year-old Brazilian man with scrotal swelling presented to our hospital, thinking that perhaps he had a recurrence of an inguinal hernia which had been repaired at our hospital three years prior. Upon evaluation at our hospital, we discovered that at an outside hospital he had undergone primary suture repair of anoperineal trauma 3 days prior, secondary to a motorcycle accident. Cefalexin (300 mg/day) and a nonsteroidal anti-inflammatory drug were prescribed by the doctors at that initial presentation, and he was scheduled to return there five days after the repair for follow-up. At our hospital, he presented with general fatigue, low grade fevers, perineal pain, and crepitus from the left chest to the flank.

Abdominal computed tomography (CT) showed that there was subcutaneous emphysema from the scrotum to the left chest (Figure 1), multiple fractures of bilateral ribs, a right pleural effusion, multiple transverse process fractures, fracture of the fourth lumber vertebral body, and a retroperitoneal hematoma; he had no recurrence of a right inguinal hernia. Neither pelvic fracture nor urethral injury was observed. Upon examination of the anoperineal area, the sutured and contused/lacerated wound had foul-smelling discharge and white exudate. Digital examination demonstrated reduced anal sphincter tone. Magnetic resonance

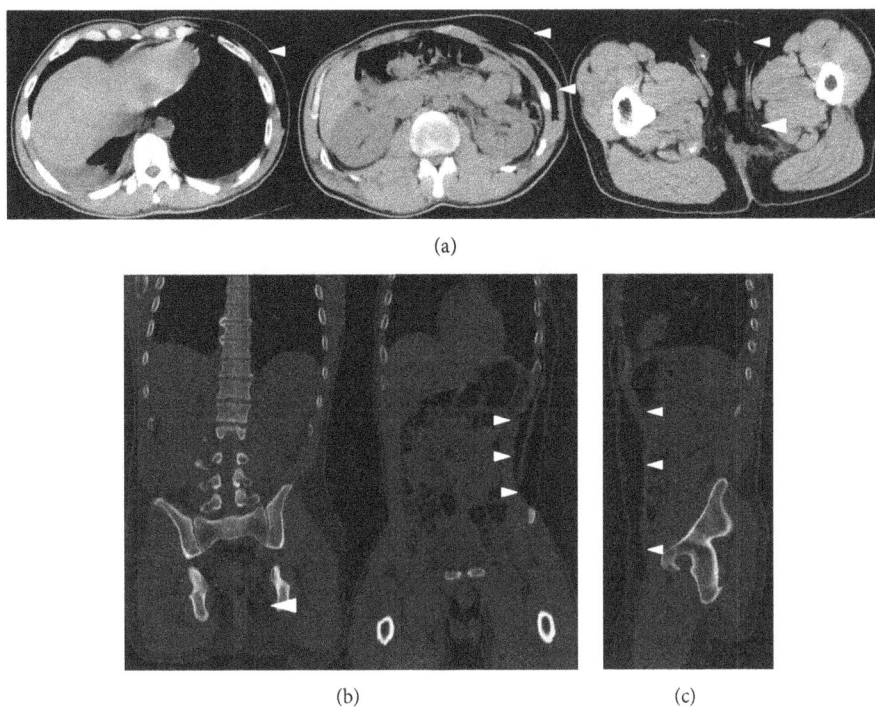

(a)

(b)                                (c)

FIGURE 1: Abdominal CT on admission. Subcutaneous emphysema spreading from the scrotum to the left chest: plain CT (a), frontal section (b), sagittal section (c), and subcutaneous gas (arrow head).

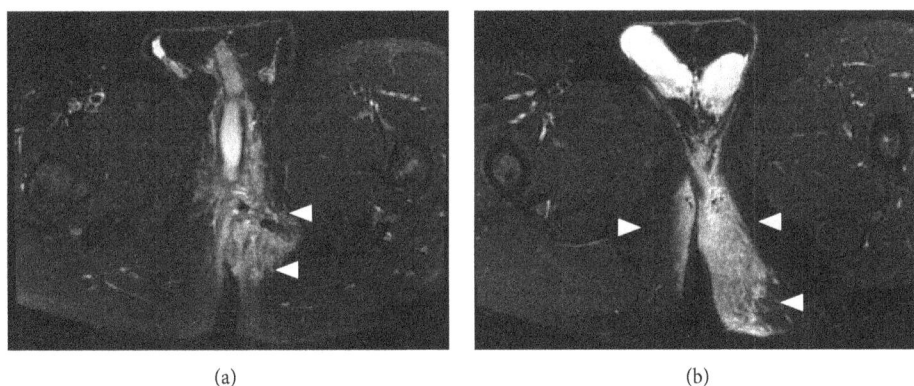

(a)                                          (b)

FIGURE 2: STIR sequence of the MRI showed high intensity around the perineum.

imaging (MRI) showed high intensity around the perineum on short T1 inversion recovery (STIR) sequences, strongly suspicious for necrotizing fasciitis (Figure 2). Additionally, MRI suggested a left anal sphincter injury. We immediately opened the wound and performed an initial debridement and lavage with copious irrigation. On laboratory examination, abnormal values were as follows: white blood cell $11200/\mu L$ (normal range, $3500-9000/\mu L$), platelet $11.8 \times 10^4/\mu L$ (normal range, $14.0-37.9 \times 10^4/\mu L$), aspirate aminotransferase 43 IU/L (normal range, 10–35 IU/L), lactate dehydrogenase 265 IU/L (normal range, 110–225 IU/L), creatinine kinase 1054 IU/L (50–200 IU/L), and C-reactive protein 7.27 mg/dL (0–0.45 mg/dL). Wound cultures showed *Enterobacter cloacae*, *Pseudomonas aeruginosa*, and yeast. After admission

to our hospital, we administered meropenem (2 g/day) and clindamycin (1800 mg/day), kept the patient NPO, and initiated parenteral nutrition. We continued antibiotics and wound lavage until the infection was controlled. Although low grade fever continued for ten days and subcutaneous gas remained in the left flank despite prompt disappearance of emphysema in the scrotum (Figure 3), the inflammation-related laboratory data improved gradually. He resumed oral intake after a week in the hospital. He required no further surgery and was discharged on hospital day 15. The subcutaneous air completely disappeared on abdominal CT two months after the first visit to our hospital. He had no fecal incontinence despite the injury to his sphincter. He is still followed carefully in the ambulatory setting.

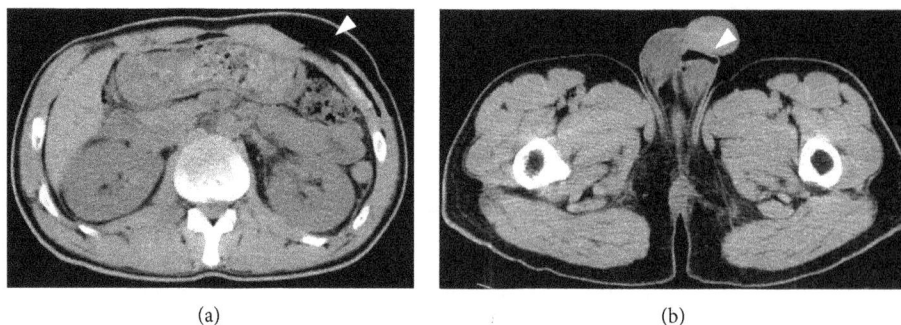

(a)                                    (b)

FIGURE 3: Abdominal CT after 10 days in the hospital. Subcutaneous gas remains in the left flank despite prompt disappearance of emphysema in the scrotum. Subcutaneous gas (arrow head).

## 3. Discussion

In the present case, early diagnosis and treatment prevented the progression of severe NF and led to a favorable clinical outcome. The patient visited our hospital 3 days after primary suture repair for anoperineal trauma. The typical symptoms and signs of NF are as follows: the wound develops tense edema extending beyond the margin of erythema with a wood-like feel, bullae, discoloration progressing to grey and necrotic skin, crepitus, and a broad erythematous tract in the skin along the route of the infection [1, 3, 5, 6]. We would not have suspected NF according to only macroscopic appearance of wound with foul-smelling discharge and white exudate because the appearances of NF in early phase are different. In our case, he did not understand why he had continued general fatigue and was also not aware of the subcutaneous gas with crepitus of his left chest and flank. If he had not suspected a recurrence of a prior inguinal hernia and visited our hospital promptly, his infection may have progressed into a life-threatening condition.

The risk factors for developing NF are skin injuries including insect bites, trauma, and surgical wounds, as well as underlying alcohol abuse, intravenous drug abuse, chronic liver or renal disease, diabetes, malignancies, and immunosuppression [1, 3, 4]. However, our patient had none of these predisposing factors. If primary suture for anoperineal trauma had not been done, he likely would not have suffered from NF because his clinical symptoms were immediately improved by initial debridement, wound irrigation, and open drainage. The laboratory risk indicator for necrotizing fasciitis (LRINEC) score is the most widely adopted scoring system [7]. Moreover, Wall et al. reported that WBC < 15000/$\mu$L and a serum sodium level $\geqq$135 mmol/L had negative predictive value of 99% and 90% sensitivity for detecting NSTIs [8]. However, these criteria could not identify NF in the present case. These criteria are insufficient tools for early diagnosis of NF. Therefore, a detailed history, establishment of the chronology of symptoms, and appropriate studies are important to diagnose early and developing NF.

On MRI, we observed high intensity around the perineum on the STIR sequence (a T2-weighted sequence). STIR reveals the presence of edema as an area with high

intensity compared to the normal tissues [9, 10]. Arslan et al. reported that MRI is not reliable for the diagnosis of NF because while it has been shown to be fairly sensitive, it lacks specificity because tissue enhancement on T2-weighted imaging is frequently seen after trauma and other noninfectious inflammatory processes [11]. However, the evaluation of NF by STIR sequence of MRI may be a helpful tool for diagnosis after a detailed history and physical.

NF of the perineal, genital, or perianal regions is known as Fournier's gangrene (FG), which can spread to the abdominal wall, causing soft tissue necrosis and sepsis [12–14]. In these areas, wound care can be extremely difficult owing to wound contamination from stool. For this reason, patients with FG have often undergone diverting colostomy for infection control. Li et al. have reported that the use of enterostomy could significantly reduce the mortality rate in patients with FG [15]. In the present case, a diverting colostomy was not needed although we considered it upon initial presentation. However, the concurrent use of enterostomy for FG is still controversial [16, 17]. On the other hand, vacuum assisted closure (VAC) has been reported as a useful management for FG, resulting in reducing hospital stay and patient discomfort [18, 19]. In the present case, VAC therapy was not needed because the wound healing was prompt by conventional dressing.

In conclusion, our experience indicates that primary suture for anoperineal injury should not be performed without careful and intensive follow-up due to the potential for developing NF without any predisposing risk factors. Additionally, a less-experienced physician should consult with an experienced physician as to the treatments of anoperineal injury.

## Consent

Written informed consent was obtained from the patient for publication of this case report and any accompanying images.

## Conflict of Interests

Susumu Saigusa and coauthors have no conflict of interests regarding the publication of this paper.

# References

[1] T. Shimizu and Y. Tokuda, "Necrotizing fasciitis," *Internal Medicine*, vol. 49, no. 12, pp. 1051–1057, 2010.

[2] S. Hasham, P. Matteucci, P. R. Stanley, and N. B. Hart, "Necrotising fasciitis," *British Medical Journal*, vol. 330, pp. 830–833, 2005.

[3] T. W. Hakkarainen, N. M. Kopari, T. N. Pham, and H. L. Evans, "Necrotizing soft tissue infections: review and current concepts in treatment, systems of care, and outcomes," *Current Problems in Surgery*, vol. 51, no. 8, pp. 344–362, 2014.

[4] M. S. Morgan, "Diagnosis and management of necrotising fasciitis: a multiparametric approach," *Journal of Hospital Infection*, vol. 75, no. 4, pp. 249–257, 2010.

[5] K. Taviloglu and H. Yanar, "Necrotizing fasciitis: strategies for diagnosis and management," *World Journal of Emergency Surgery*, vol. 2, no. 1, article 19, 2007.

[6] C.-H. Wong and Y.-S. Wang, "The diagnosis of necrotizing fasciitis," *Current Opinion in Infectious Diseases*, vol. 18, no. 2, pp. 101–106, 2005.

[7] C.-H. Wong, L.-W. Khin, K.-S. Heng, K.-C. Tan, and C.-O. Low, "The LRINEC (Laboratory Risk Indicator for Necrotizing Fasciitis) score: a tool for distinguishing necrotizing fasciitis from other soft tissue infections," *Critical Care Medicine*, vol. 32, no. 7, pp. 1535–1541, 2004.

[8] D. B. Wall, C. de Virgilio, S. Black, and S. R. Klein, "Objective criteria may assist in distinguishing necrotizing fasciitis from nonnecrotizing soft tissue infection," *The American Journal of Surgery*, vol. 179, no. 1, pp. 17–21, 2000.

[9] S. D. Wall, M. R. Fisher, E. G. Amparo, H. Hricak, and C. B. Higgins, "Magnetic resonance imaging in the evaluation of abscesses," *American Journal of Roentgenology*, vol. 144, no. 6, pp. 1217–1221, 1985.

[10] J. S. H. Tang, R. H. Gold, L. W. Bassett, and L. L. Seeger, "Musculoskeletal infection of the extremities: evaluation with MR imaging," *Radiology*, vol. 166, no. 1, pp. 205–209, 1988.

[11] A. Arslan, C. Pierre-Jerome, and A. Borthne, "Necrotizing fasciitis: unreliable MRI findings in the preoperative diagnosis," *European Journal of Radiology*, vol. 36, no. 3, pp. 139–143, 2000.

[12] G. L. Smith, C. B. Bunker, and M. D. Dinneen, "Fournier's gangrene," *British Journal of Urology*, vol. 81, no. 3, pp. 347–355, 1998.

[13] M. Sroczyński, M. Sebastian, J. Rudnicki, A. Sebastian, and A. K. Agrawal, "A complex approach to the treatment of Fournier's gangrene," *Advances in Clinical and Experimental Medicine*, vol. 22, no. 1, pp. 131–135, 2013.

[14] N. Eke, "Fournier's gangrene: a review of 1726 cases," *British Journal of Surgery*, vol. 87, no. 6, pp. 718–728, 2000.

[15] Y.-D. Li, W.-F. Zhu, J.-J. Qiao, and J.-J. Lin, "Enterostomy can decrease the mortality of patients with Fournier gangrene," *World Journal of Gastroenterology*, vol. 20, no. 24, pp. 7950–7954, 2014.

[16] O. Estrada, I. Martinez, M. Del Bas, S. Salvans, and L. A. Hidalgo, "Rectal diversion without colostomy in Fournier's gangrene," *Techniques in Coloproctology*, vol. 13, no. 2, pp. 157–159, 2009.

[17] E. Ozturk, Y. Sonmez, and T. Yilmazlar, "What are the indications for a stoma in Fournier's gangrene?" *Colorectal Disease*, vol. 13, no. 9, pp. 1044–1047, 2011.

[18] E. Ozturk, H. Ozguc, and T. Yilmazlar, "The use of vacuum assisted closure therapy in the management of Fournier's gangrene," *The American Journal of Surgery*, vol. 197, no. 5, pp. 660–665, 2009.

[19] G. Cuccia, G. Mucciardi, G. Morgia et al., "Vacuum-assisted closure for the treatment of Fournier's gangrene," *Urologia Internationalis*, vol. 82, no. 4, pp. 426–431, 2009.

# Bilateral Wallerian Degeneration of the Pontocerebellar Tracts

**Azad Hekimoglu,**[1] **Ihsaniye Suer Dogan,**[1] **Aynur Turan,**[1]
**Mehmet Fevzi Oztekin,**[2] **and Baki Hekimoglu**[1]

[1]*Department of Radiology, Diskapi Yildirim Beyazit Training and Research Hospital, Ankara, Turkey*
[2]*Department of Neurology, Diskapi Yildirim Beyazit Training and Research Hospital, Ankara, Turkey*

Correspondence should be addressed to Ihsaniye Suer Dogan; dr.ihsaniye@hotmail.com

Academic Editor: Aristomenis K. Exadaktylos

Wallerian degeneration is the process of progressive demyelination and disintegration of the distal axonal segment following the transection of the axon or damage to the neuron. We report a case of a patient with Wallerian degeneration of the pontocerebellar tracts. She had a history of a pontine infarction 3 months ago. Wallerian degeneration of pontocerebellar tracts is seen bilaterally and symmetrically and is more visible in the middle cerebellar peduncles. Along the middle cerebellar peduncles hyperintense signal was detected on T2 weighted images. Wallerian degeneration of pontocerebellar tracts is a rare entity. It can occur bilaterally after a large pontine infarction. Magnetic resonance imaging seems to be the most effective technique for detection of Wallerian degeneration. In this report we want to mention this rare entity and to prevent wrong diagnosis.

## 1. Introduction

Wallerian degeneration represents a uniform answer to injury within the central and peripheral nervous systems. Infarction is the most common event resulting in WD in the central nervous system. Magnetic resonance imaging seems to be the most effective technique for detection of Wallerian degeneration. Along the affected white matter tractus high signal was detected on both T2 weighted images and fluid-attenuated inversion recovery images.

## 2. Case Presentation

A 73-year-old woman was admitted to emergency service with headache, vertigo, speech difficulties, and right-sided weakness. Patient had no history of arterial hypertension, hypercholesterolemia, and diabetes mellitus.

A transthoracic echocardiogram was performed and findings were normal for her age.

A brain MRI was performed and demonstrated a left, paramedian pontine acute infarct (Figure 1). On T2WI hyperintensities were seen on the left side of the pons (Figure 1(a)). On DWI and ADC maps restricted diffusion (Figures 1(b)-1(c)) was seen which showed the acute infarct.

After 3 months the patient was admitted to the emergency service again with worsening of her symptoms. Speech difficulties, dysarthria, and right hemiparesis on both upper and lower limbs were depicted.

A second brain MRI was performed (Figure 2). On MRI a left sided pons encephalomalacia was seen secondary to pontine infarction (Figure 2(a)). At the same time a new focus of acute infarct was seen on the anterior right side of the pons (Figures 2(e)-2(f)). On T2WI and FLAIR images bilateral and symmetrical hyperintensities along the middle cerebellar peduncles were seen. These lesions were interpreted as WD of pontocerebellar tracts due to previous pontine infarction (Figure 2(b)).

Along the MCPs lesions were hyperintense on both DWI and ADC maps, consistent with T2 shine-through effect (Figures 2(c)-2(d)).

## 3. Discussion

WD represents a uniform answer to injury within the central and peripheral nervous system. In the first days following the injury disintegration of axonal structures occurs, after several weeks infiltration of macrophages and degradation of myelin

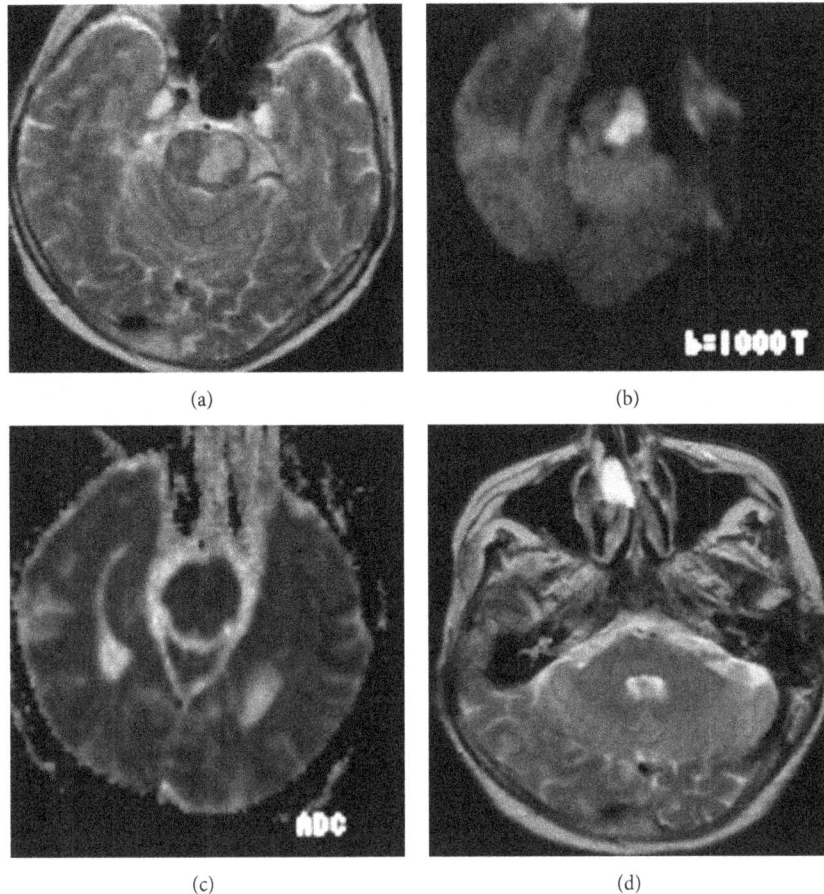

(a)

(b)

(c)

(d)

FIGURE 1: Left paramedian acute pontine infarction: axial T2WI (a) hyperintense signal on the left side of the pons, axial DWI (b) and ADC maps (c) restricted diffusion, and axial T2WI (d) MCPs were normal.

formed, and finally fibrosis and atrophy of the affected fiber tracts appear [1].

WD is most frequently observed in the corticospinal tract following infarction of the motor cortex or internal capsule [2].

Infarction is the most common event resulting in WD in the central nervous system. Also hemorrhage, necrosis, neoplasm, trauma, focal demyelination, white matter disorders, and multisystem atrophy are reported entities that may cause degeneration [3].

After infarction it usually takes two to four weeks before WD can be detected by conventional MRI [1]. Conventional MRI and DWI depict WD when sufficiently large bundles of fibers are involved along the corticospinal tract, the corpus callosum, fibers of the optic radiations, fornices, and cerebellar peduncles [4, 5].

The main finding is a hyperintensity on T2WI and FLAIR images along the affected tracts.

WD of cerebellar peduncles is rarely described. It usually involves the middle ones because they are largest and the main path for pontocerebellar tracts [6]. The MCPs are a massive bundle of fibers connecting the basal portion of the pons with the cerebellum.

WD of the unilateral pontine infarction results in bilateral symmetrical hyperintense lesions secondary to the crossed distribution of the pontocerebellar fibers [7].

Only few reports have described the MR findings of WD in the middle cerebellar peduncles following pontine infarction, hemorrhage, and acute vascular lesions [7, 8].

In our case after a unilateral pontine infarct in the MCPs on T2WI bilateral and symmetrical hyperintense lesions were seen owing to WD.

Bilateral symmetric lesions of the MCPs can also be seen in other conditions, such as central pontine myelinolysis, neurodegenerative disorders, multisystem atrophy, and progressive multifocal leukoencephalopathy. However, clinic and biochemical investigations help in differentiation.

In conclusion the basic understanding required to diagnose WD in the brain is a detailed knowledge of the course of the association fibers.

High signal in the MCPs following a pontine lesion is almost certainly attributable to WD of the pontocerebellar tracts and should not be mistaken for a new infarction.

WD is a secondary lesion and should not be mistaken for a primary, independent lesion.

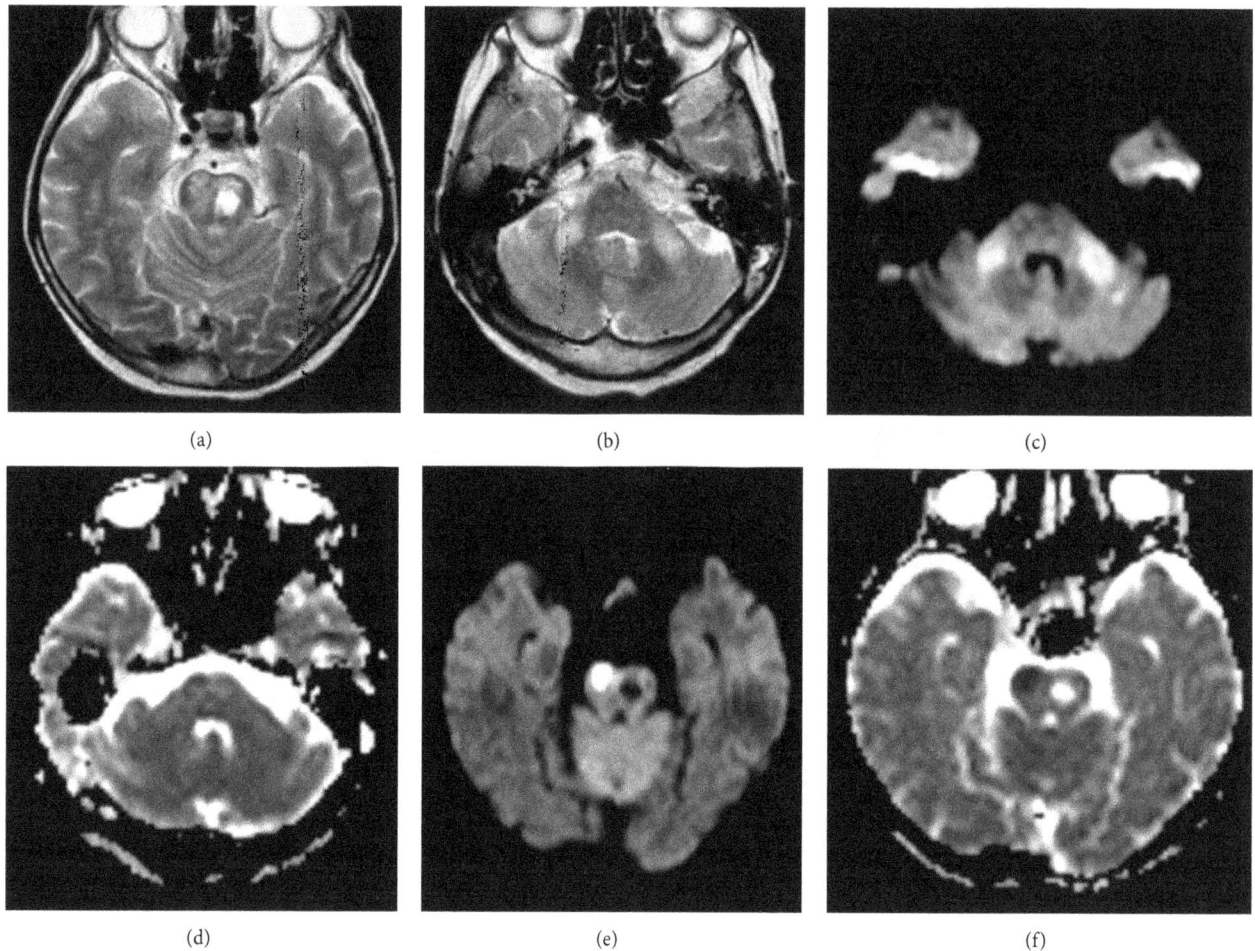

FIGURE 2: 3 months after left paramedian acute pontine infarction. Axial T2WI (a) hyperintense signal in pons due to chronic infarct. Axial T2WI (b) bilateral and symmetrical hyperintense signal in MCPs due to WD. Axial DWI (c) and ADC map (d) shows hyperintense signal. Axial DWI (e) and ADC map (f) shows restricted diffusion due to new acute infarct in the right side of the pons.

## Abbreviations

WD:     Wallerian degeneration
MRI:    Magnetic resonance imaging
MCPs:   Middle cerebellar peduncles
T2WI:   T2 weighted images
DWI:    Diffusion weighted images
ADC:    Apparent diffusion coefficient
FLAIR:  Fluid-attenuated inversion recovery.

## Conflict of Interests

The authors declare that there is no conflict of interests regarding the publication of this paper.

## Authors' Contribution

Azad Hekimoglu contributed to data collection and paper writing. Ihsaniye Suer Dogan contributed to paper writing.

## References

[1] A. C. Johnson, A. R. McNabb, and R. J. Rossiter, "Chemistry of wallerian degeneration; a review of recent studies," *Archives of Neurology & Psychiatry*, vol. 64, no. 1, pp. 105–121, 1950.

[2] M. J. Kuhn, D. J. Mikulis, D. M. Ayoub, B. E. Kosofsky, K. R. Davis, and J. M. Taveras, "Wallerian degeneration after cerebral infarction: evaluation with sequential MR imaging," *Radiology*, vol. 172, no. 1, pp. 179–182, 1989.

[3] R. Musson and C. Romanowski, "Restricted diffusion in Wallerian degeneration of the middle cerebellar peduncles following pontine infarction," *Polish Journal of Radiology*, vol. 75, no. 4, pp. 38–43, 2010.

[4] A. Uchino, A. Sawada, Y. Takase, R. Egashira, and S. Kudo, "Transient detection of early wallerian degeneration on diffusion-weighted MRI after an acute cerebrovascular accident," *Neuroradiology*, vol. 46, no. 3, pp. 183–188, 2004.

[5] K. Yamada, U. Patel, D. A. Shrier, H. Tanaka, J.-K. Chang, and Y. Numaguchi, "MR imaging of CNS Tractopathy: wallerian and transneuronal degeneration," *American Journal of Roentgenology*, vol. 171, no. 3, pp. 813–818, 1998.

[6] M. Mejdoubi, I. Catalaa, C. Cognard, and C. Manelfe, "Bilateral Wallerian degeneration of the middle cerebellar peduncles due to unilateral pontine infarction: a morphologic and spectroscopic study," *Journal of Neuroradiology*, vol. 33, no. 4, pp. 263–265, 2006.

[7] T. O'Uchi, "Wallerian degeneration of the pontocerebellar tracts after pontine hemorrhage," *International Journal of Neuroradiology*, vol. 4, pp. 171–177, 1998.

[8] K. Okamoto, S. Tokiguchi, T. Furusawa et al., "MR features of diseases involving bilateral middle cerebellar peduncles," *The American Journal of Neuroradiology*, vol. 24, no. 10, pp. 1946–1954, 2003.

# 54

# The Great Imitator Strikes Again: Syphilis Presenting as "Tongue Changing Colors"

**Jessica Swanson and Janna Welch**

*University of Texas Dell School of Medicine, Austin, TX 78701, USA*

Correspondence should be addressed to Janna Welch; drjannawelch@gmail.com

Academic Editor: Serdar Kula

Syphilis is known as the great imitator, making its diagnosis in the emergency department difficult. A 29-year-old male presented with the chief complaint of "my tongue is changing colors." A syphilis rapid plasma reagin (RPR) test resulted as positive. In primary syphilis, the chancre is the characteristic lesion. While chancres are frequently found on the external genitalia or anus, extragenital chancres arise in 2% of patients. With oral involvement, the chancre is commonly found on the lip or tongue. The patient was treated for secondary syphilis with 2.4 million units of long acting penicillin intramuscularly. On follow-up a month later, the patient's symptoms had resolved.

## 1. Case Presentation

A 29-year-old male presented to the emergency department with the chief complaint of "my tongue is changing colors." The symptoms had been present for the past week. He denied any pain or history of similar symptoms in the past. On review of systems, his only other complaint was arthralgias, primarily located in his hips and knees bilaterally. Of note, he denied any recent rashes, weight loss, hair loss, or genital lesions. His past medical history was significant only for a chlamydia infection five years previously, which had been treated. On social history, he denied any alcohol or illicit drug use, including any intravenous drugs. He did endorse having sex with men, and his most recent new sexual partner was 2 months ago.

On physical exam, he was found to be afebrile with normal vital signs. Overall, he was a thin, well appearing male. Head and neck exam revealed three shallow, nonpainful erosions covered with a grayish membrane on the posterior aspect of his tongue (Figure 1). There was no cervical lymphadenopathy. Exam of his hips and knees was unimpressive; there was no swelling, redness, or pain with palpation or range of motion. There were no lesions or rashes on the skin.

There is a broad differential diagnosis for pigmented macules of the oropharynx, which includes autoimmune, viral, mycotic causes as well as hereditary syndromes, heavy metal ingestion, cigarette use, and medication related cause. In addition to taking a thorough history, we performed basic screening complete blood count, metabolic panel, and erythrocyte sedimentation rate, which were normal. We did not order a lead level but kept heavy metal in the differential in cases the syphilis testing was negative. A screening syphilis qualitative RPR test was ordered, which came back positive. The confirmatory microhemagglutination assay, (MTA-TPS) which recognizes treponema to rule out false positives, also indicated syphilis. The patient was treated for secondary syphilis with 2.4 million units of long acting penicillin intramuscularly. Of note, the patient declined HIV testing in the emergency department. On follow-up a month later, the patient's symptoms had resolved.

## 2. Discussion

Syphilis, known as the great imitator, can present in a variety of ways, making its diagnosis in the emergency department difficult. As emergency medicine practitioners, we must keep syphilis on our differential list as its incidence continues to rise, particularly among men who have sex with men (MSM). In 2013, there were 56,471 new reported syphilis

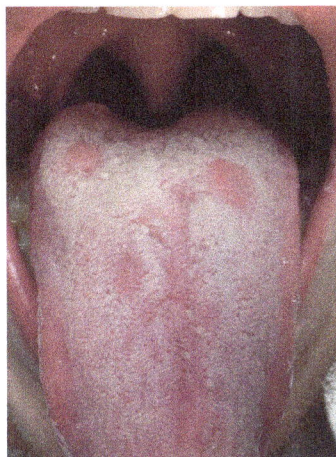

FIGURE 1

TABLE 1: The oral manifestations of syphilis.

| Disease stage | Oral manifestations |
| --- | --- |
| Primary syphilis | Chancre: painless or painful |
| Secondary syphilis | Mucosal patches |
| | Ulcerations: solitary or multiple |
| | Leukoplakia-like plaques |
| | Maculopapular lesions |
| | Aphthous lesions |
| | Pseudomembranous lesions |
| | Condyloma lata |
| Tertiary syphilis | Gumma |
| | Atrophic glossitis |
| | Syphilitic leukoplakia |

cases in the US. According to the Center for Disease Control, between 2012 and 2013, the number of reported primary and secondary syphilis cases increased by 10.9%, with 75% of these cases in MSM. Men aged 20–29 had the highest incidence of primary and secondary syphilis, followed by women 20–24 years old (CDC).

Characteristic skin findings are found in all stages of syphilis. Oral manifestations are significantly less common than those of the skin but can be seen in all stages of syphilis (Table 1). Only one case (from 1978) was found in the author's literature search in which a patient with secondary syphilis presented solely with complaints of changes to the tongue [1]. A PubMed literature review performed by Leuci et al. looked at the oral involvement of syphilis over a 61-year time period. Their literature review found only 34 patients with reports of oral involvement. In addition, they also reported a retrospective, multicenter case series of 12 patients that had presented with oral manifestations of syphilis in all stages of disease. Of those with secondary syphilis, most had some other manifestation of the disease aside from oral involvement.

In primary syphilis, the chancre is the characteristic lesion. It develops at the site of inoculation, beginning as a papule that progresses to ulceration. Chancres are generally painless, solitary lesions, although they can be multiple. While chancres are most frequently found on the external genitalia or anus, extragenital chancres arise in 2% of patients [2]. Of the extragenital sites, the mouth is the site in 40–70% of [3]. When the mouth is involved, the chancre is most commonly found on the lip and occasionally the tongue. Rarely, the pharynx or tonsils may be involved. The upper lip is more commonly affected in males and the lower lip in females. Cervical lymphadenopathy generally accompanies the chancre [4]. Regardless of location, the chancre typically regresses, regardless of treatment, after 2–8 weeks [5].

Secondary syphilis is characterized by a variety of nonspecific, flu-like symptoms, including fever, malaise, headache, sore throat, and arthralgias. A disseminated, symmetric rash occurs in 75% of patients [3]. The morphology of the rash varies greatly, from macular to maculopapular to nodular. It characteristically involves the palms of the hands and soles of the feet. Additional symptoms may include ocular manifestations, condyloma lata, hepatitis, arthritis, and neurologic involvement [5].

Approximately, 30% of patients with secondary syphilis have involvement of the oral cavity. However, oral findings are rarely the only manifestation [6]. The primary oral manifestations of secondary syphilis are mucus patches (as seen in this patient) and maculopapular lesions, although nodules may be found as well. The mucous patches are typically slightly raised and covered with a grayish white pseudomembrane. Macular lesions are generally found on the hard palate, while mucus patches are most commonly found on, but not limited to, the tongue [6].

Tertiary syphilis can present with neurosyphilis or cardiovascular syphilis or as gummatous syphilis. The gumma is granulomatous lesion, often found on the skin, bone, or liver. However, gummas can involve any organ [7]. In the oral cavity, it is most commonly seen as a swelling on the tongue or hard palate, which eventually ulcerates. Gumma complications include bone erosion, palatal perforation, and oronasal fistulas [8].

When a diagnosis of syphilis is suspected, serological testing should be performed. Nontreponemal and treponemal tests are the standard for diagnosing syphilis in the US in all stages of the disease [9]. Generally, nontreponemal tests are performed first, the most common of which are the VDRL or RPR tests. These tests become positive 6 weeks after exposure and 1–4 weeks after appearance of the primary lesion. In the case of a positive test result, it should be confirmed with a treponemal test [8]. As received by the patient in this case, 2.4 million units of benzathine penicillin is the treatment of choice for patients diagnosed with primary, secondary, or early latent syphilis [10].

When a diagnosis of syphilis is made, it is important to consider testing for HIV as well. While our patient declined an HIV test in the emergency department, we educated him on how to obtain HIV testing should he change his mind. As of 2002, incidence of syphilis in HIV infected patients has been reported as 77 times higher when compared to the general population [11]. Syphilis appears to increase the transmission of HIV due to local immunological and bacteriological reactions that occur at the site of chancre formation (CDC). In patients coinfected with HIV, syphilis may present even more subtly than in non-HIV patients. Finally, syphilis serology tests may result in false negatives in HIV infected patients [5].

## 3. Conclusion

Oftentimes, due to issues with access to medical care, the emergency physician must also take on the role of primary care doctor. Thus, it is important to keep a wide differential diagnosis, even with seemingly benign complaints. Syphilis, the great imitator, should remain at the back of our minds. A detailed history, with an emphasis on sexual history, can aid in making the diagnosis. In patients diagnosed with syphilis, HIV testing should be strongly encouraged, as the two diseases are often cotransmitted.

## Conflict of Interests

The authors declare that there is no conflict of interests regarding the publication of this paper.

## References

[1] N. J. Fiumara, D. J. Grande, and J. L. Giunta, "Papular secondary syphilis of the tongue," *Oral Surgery, Oral Medicine, Oral Pathology*, vol. 45, no. 4, pp. 540–542, 1978.

[2] B. Neville, J. Bouquot, D. Damm, and C. Allen, *Oral and Maxillofacial Pathology*, Saunders, Elsevier, St. Louis, Mo, USA, 3rd edition, 2009.

[3] L. A. Dourmishev and A. L. Dourmishev, "Syphilis: uncommon presentations in adults," *Clinics in Dermatology*, vol. 23, no. 6, pp. 555–564, 2005.

[4] N. J. Fiumara and M. Berg, "Primary syphilis in the oral cavity," *British Journal of Venereal Diseases*, vol. 50, no. 6, pp. 463–464, 1974.

[5] G. Ficarra and R. Carlos, "Syphilis: the renaissance of an old disease with oral implications," *Head and Neck Pathology*, vol. 3, no. 3, pp. 195–206, 2009.

[6] J. C. Leão, L. A. Gueiros, and S. R. Porter, "Oral manifestations of syphilis," *Clinics*, vol. 61, no. 2, pp. 161–166, 2006.

[7] R. H. Kampmeier, "The late manifestations of syphilis: skeletal, visceral and cardiovascular," *Medical Clinics of North America*, vol. 48, pp. 667–697, 1964.

[8] S. Leuci, S. Martina, D. Adamo et al., "Oral syphilis: a retrospective analysis of 12 cases and a review of the literature," *Oral Diseases*, vol. 19, no. 8, pp. 738–746, 2013.

[9] M. R. Golden, C. M. Marra, and K. K. Holmes, "Update on syphilis: resurgence of an old problem," *The Journal of the American Medical Association*, vol. 290, no. 11, pp. 1510–1514, 2003.

[10] K. A. Workowski, "Sexually transmitted infections and HIV: diagnosis and treatment," *Topics in Antiviral Medicine*, vol. 20, no. 1, pp. 11–16, 2012.

[11] H. W. Chesson, J. D. Heffelfinger, R. F. Voigt, and D. Collins, "Estimates of primary and secondary syphilis rates in persons with HIV in the United States, 2002," *Sexually Transmitted Diseases*, vol. 32, no. 5, pp. 265–269, 2005.

# 55

# An Unusual Case of Spontaneous Esophageal Rupture after Swallowing a Boneless Chicken Nugget

**Zeenia Aga,**[1] **Jackie Avelino,**[2] **Gail E. Darling,**[3] **and Jo Jo Leung**[2]

[1]*Faculty of Medicine, University of Toronto, Toronto, ON, Canada M5S 1A8*
[2]*Department of Emergency Medicine, University Health Network, Toronto, ON, Canada M5G 2C4*
[3]*Division of Thoracic Surgery, University Health Network, Toronto, ON, Canada M5G 2C4*

Correspondence should be addressed to Jo Jo Leung; jojo.leung@uhn.ca

Academic Editor: Aristomenis K. Exadaktylos

A 25-year-old previously healthy man presented to our Emergency Department with shortness of breath and epigastric pain after swallowing a boneless chicken nugget one hour prior to presentation. Physical examination revealed epigastric rigidity and tenderness. Serology was normal except for mildly elevated bilirubin and amylase. Computed tomography (CT) scan of the chest revealed a distal esophageal rupture with accompanying pneumomediastinum and left-sided pleural effusion. Treatment was initiated with administration of intravenous fluids and broad-spectrum antibiotics. Subsequently, an esophageal stent was inserted endoscopically in addition to VATS (Video-Assisted Thoracoscopic Surgery) drainage of the left-sided pleural space. This case illustrates an unusual presentation of Boerhaave's syndrome: a rare and life-threatening form of noniatrogenic esophageal rupture most often preceded by forceful vomiting. Our case demonstrates that physicians should maintain an index of suspicion for spontaneous esophageal rupture in patients presenting with shortness of breath and epigastric pain even in the absence of preceding vomiting, cough, or seizure. Additionally, ingestion of boneless, shell-less foods may be sufficient to cause rupture in individuals without underlying esophageal pathology. CT scan of the thorax and upper abdomen should be performed in these patients to rule out this rare and life-threatening diagnosis.

## 1. Introduction

Esophageal rupture is most commonly caused by accidental endoscopic perforation [1–4]. Rarely, spontaneous perforation of the esophagus can occur due to a rapid rise in intraluminal pressure after forceful vomiting in a phenomenon known as Boerhaave's syndrome. This occurs most often in the lateral, lower 1/3 of the esophagus [5, 6] and is associated with a mortality rate of 20–75% [7–9]. Many patients present with symptoms such as chest pain, shock, or respiratory distress and physical exam findings are often nonspecific (tachycardia, tachypnea, or fever). As a result of these nonspecific findings, Boerhaave's syndrome is often misdiagnosed as an aortic emergency, pericarditis, myocardial infarction, pulmonary embolus, spontaneous pneumothorax, perforated peptic ulcer, or pancreatitis [10–12]. Delayed diagnosis is one of the major differences in the management of iatrogenic esophageal rupture versus spontaneous rupture and may be

responsible for the higher mortality rate in the latter. To our knowledge, this is the first published case of esophageal rupture following ingestion of a boneless, soft food item in the absence of any underlying esophageal pathology or food impaction [13], with only eight cases worldwide of spontaneous esophageal rupture without a preceding episode of vomiting, seizure, or prolonged cough [14]. We outline the case of a 25-year-old man, who presented to the ED with shortness of breath and epigastric pain starting immediately after swallowing a boneless chicken nugget. We will discuss the clinical presentation, appropriate diagnostic steps, and treatment strategies of this rare but potentially life-threatening condition.

## 2. Case Presentation

A 25-year-old previously healthy male presented to our Emergency Department with shortness of breath and epigastric

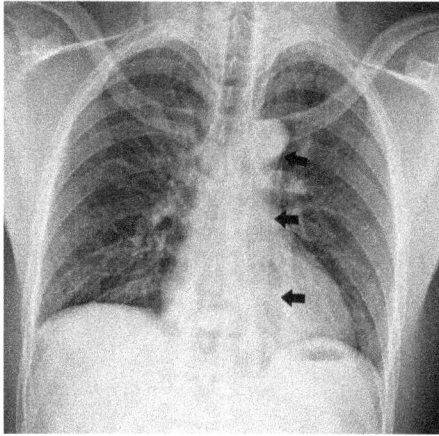

FIGURE 1: Chest X-ray displaying pneumomediastinum (indicated by black arrows) and left-sided pleural effusion.

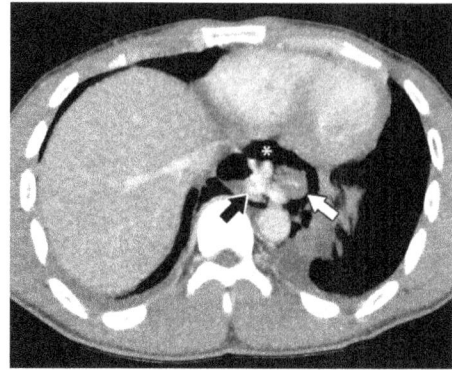

FIGURE 2: Chest computed tomography (CT) scan revealing a distal esophageal rupture with an oral contrast leak (indicated by the black arrow) from the ruptured esophagus (indicated by the white arrow), in addition to pneumomediastinum (asterisk) and left-sided pleural effusion.

pain that started immediately after swallowing a boneless chicken nugget one hour prior to presentation. He had no antecedent history of marked vomiting prior to symptom onset and denied any foreign body sensation. He had no significant past medical history with the exception of 2-3-week duration of mild gastroesophageal reflux. Our patient was not taking any medications at the time of presentation.

At admission, he was afebrile with a pulse of 64 beats/min, blood pressure of 134/87 mmHg, and oxygen saturation of 100%. He was alert and oriented with facial pallor and appeared uncomfortable on the stretcher. Physical examination revealed a tender, rigid abdomen (predominantly in the epigastric region) with voluntary guarding (2+) but no signs of peritonitis. On respiratory examination equal air entry was auscultated bilaterally with no adventitious sounds, no signs of subcutaneous air or tracheal deviation. He was able to speak clearly. Heart sounds were normal (S1, S2, and no murmurs) and no evidence of previous surgeries was found. The rest of the physical examination was unremarkable.

Blood work was normal at the time of presentation (CBC, calcium, phosphate, magnesium, sodium, chloride, bicarbonate, anion gap, AST/ALT/ALP, and albumin) except for slight elevations of WBC ($14.0 \times 10^9$ cells/L), bilirubin ($28 \mu$mol/L), and amylase (185 U/L). Lactate was tested six hours later, revealing an elevated level of 4.1 mmol/L. Chest X-ray was suggestive of mediastinal air (Figure 1) and revealed a left-sided pleural effusion. There was no evidence of foreign objects in the esophagus or free air in the abdomen. A computed tomography (CT) scan of the chest revealed a rupture in the distal esophagus with oral contrast leaking from the rupture, a pneumomediastinum, and left-sided pleural effusions (Figure 2).

Treatment began with cessation of oral intake, administration of IV fluids, morphine, and intravenous broad-spectrum antibiotics, and repeat blood work. As the patient was clinically well and did not require emergent surgery, he was admitted under the Thoracic Surgery Team and transferred to a step-down unit. Esophageal gastroscopy was performed revealing a mucosal tear at 40 cm into

the esophagus, extending just to the gastroesophageal junction. An esophageal stent was positioned to cover the perforation. Video-Assisted Thoracoscopic Surgery (VATS) drainage of the pleural space was conducted with samples taken for culture. Intercostal nerve blocks were placed and a right-angle chest tube was inserted on the left side.

After 5 days, he developed a fever with increasing chest pain and leukocytosis whilst still on antibiotics. CT scan of the chest showed a mediastinal abscess and right pleural collection. He underwent VATS drainage of the abscess and decortication of the right pleural space. After three weeks, his esophageal stent was removed and the esophageal tear was observed to have healed nicely.

## 3. Discussion

The nonspecific physical exam findings and the lack of any classical symptoms of Boerhaave's syndrome often result in delayed and misdiagnosis of this rare and lethal form of noniatrogenic esophageal rupture. As such, it has a significant mortality rate estimated between 20 and 75% [7, 8]. "Mackler's Triad," consisting of repeated vomiting (79%), lower chest pain (83%), and subcutaneous emphysema (27%), is only present in a minority of patients, and approximately half of all cases of Boerhaave's syndrome are atypical [10, 12, 15, 16]. Mediastinitis, sepsis, and shock are frequently seen late in the course of the illness, which further confuses the diagnostic picture. Given the low incidence of noniatrogenic esophageal rupture (less than 10%), it is unlikely for physicians to have a high index of suspicion for esophageal rupture compared to more common causes of chest pain, shortness of breath, and vomiting.

We report the case of a 25-year-old, previously healthy patient who developed a distal esophageal rupture and left-sided pleural effusion shortly after swallowing a boneless chicken nugget, during which he felt a sharp, scratching sensation. Importantly, our patient had no antecedent history of forceful vomiting (or similar esophageal strain through coughing, laughing, or seizure) which is typically associated with noniatrogenic rupture of the esophagus. At presentation, he showed nonspecific symptoms of dyspnea and epigastric pain and physical examination revealed a tender, rigid abdomen. Blood work was predominantly normal at presentation. It was only after a chest X-ray and CT scan of the chest that we were able to make a clear diagnosis of esophageal rupture. Importantly, there was no radiological evidence of an esophageal foreign body or food impaction, which can also cause spontaneous esophageal rupture [13].

This case demonstrates two salient teaching points for physicians and emergency responders. Firstly, noniatrogenic, life-threatening esophageal rupture can occur in the absence of any preceding history of vomiting, seizure, or chronic cough in patients without underlying esophageal pathology. Boerhaave's syndrome is classically described as a spontaneous transmural perforation of the esophagus associated with repetitive vomiting and is distinguished from a Mallory-Weiss tear based on the depth of esophageal damage. However, this case demonstrates that physicians should maintain an index of suspicion for Boerhaave's syndrome in patients presenting with shortness of breath and epigastric pain, even in the absence of a preceding history of strain through either vomiting, seizure, parturition, or chronic coughing and laughing. To our knowledge, this unique presentation has never been described in Canadian literature, with only eight published cases in the English literature [14, 17]. In these patients, CT of the chest and abdomen should be performed to rule out esophageal rupture. Second, and most unique to our case, is that even ingestion of boneless, shell-less, soft food items such as a chicken nugget may be sufficient to raise intraluminal pressure to the point of perforation in patients with no underlying esophageal pathology. To our knowledge, this is the first published case worldwide demonstrating esophageal rupture after swallowing a boneless, shell-less food item in a healthy esophagus without any radiological evidence of food impaction. Chicken nuggets have the consistency of many commonly eaten foods that are not typically associated with esophageal perforation (i.e., foods that are boneless and flexible and without sharp edges). Thus, physicians and emergency responders should not rule out esophageal perforation based on the consistency of the last meal and patients with suspicious findings for perforation including new epigastric pain or shortness of breath should be sent for radiological assessment.

The management of Boerhaave's syndrome, regardless of the specific cause, begins with cessation of oral intake, administration of intravenous fluids and broad-spectrum antibiotics followed by surgical or endoscopic treatment of the tear [18–21]. An isolated nonoperative approach can only be taken in a minority of patients who have radiologic findings showing lack of mediastinal or pleural contamination and no systemic symptoms of infection at the time of presentation [9, 11, 22, 23].

## 4. Conclusion

Our case illustrates the need for emergency physicians to consider the rare but life-threatening diagnosis of spontaneous esophageal rupture in patients presenting with epigastric pain and shortness of breath without a preceding history of forceful vomiting or persistent cough. Additionally, physicians should consider the possibility of esophageal perforation induced by forcefully swallowing food items, even in the case of boneless, shell-less, soft foods in patients with no underlying esophageal disease.

## Conflict of Interests

The authors declare that there is no conflict of interests regarding the publication of this paper.

## Acknowledgment

Special thanks are due to Dr. Stephen Lyen, MBBS, FRCR (Division of Radiology, University Health Network, Toronto, Ontario, Canada), for his assistance and expertise with the radiographic images.

## References

[1] H. Vidarsdottir, S. Blondal, H. Alfredsson, A. Geirsson, and T. Gudbjartsson, "Oesophageal perforations in Iceland: a whole population study on incidence, aetiology and surgical outcome," *The Thoracic and Cardiovascular Surgeon*, vol. 58, no. 8, pp. 476–480, 2010.

[2] A. Merchea, D. C. Cullinane, M. D. Sawyer et al., "Esophagogastroduodenoscopy-associated gastrointestinal perforations: a single-center experience," *Surgery*, vol. 148, no. 4, pp. 876–882, 2010.

[3] N. M. Gupta and L. Kaman, "Personal management of 57 consecutive patients with esophageal perforation," *The American Journal of Surgery*, vol. 187, no. 1, pp. 58–63, 2004.

[4] M. R. Bladergroen, J. E. Lowe, and R. W. Postlethwait, "Diagnosis and recommended management of esophageal perforation and rupture," *The Annals of Thoracic Surgery*, vol. 42, no. 3, pp. 235–239, 1986.

[5] J. P. De Schipper, A. F. Pull Ter Gunne, H. J. M. Oostvogel, and C. J. H. M. Van Laarhoven, "Spontaneous rupture of the oesophagus: Boerhaave's syndrome in 2008. Literature review and treatment algorithm," *Digestive Surgery*, vol. 26, no. 1, pp. 1–6, 2009.

[6] A. G. Hill, A. T. Tiu, and I. G. Martin, "Boerhaave's syndrome: 10 years experience and review of the literature," *ANZ Journal of Surgery*, vol. 73, no. 12, pp. 1008–1010, 2003.

[7] K. J. Janjua, "Boerhaave's syndrome," *Postgraduate Medical Journal*, vol. 73, no. 859, pp. 265–270, 1997.

[8] C. L. Connelly, P. J. Lamb, and S. Paterson-Brown, "Outcomes following Boerhaave's syndrome," *Annals of the Royal College of Surgeons of England*, vol. 95, no. 8, pp. 557–560, 2013.

[9] S. Wahed, B. Dent, R. Jones, and S. M. Griffin, "Spectrum of oesophageal perforations and their influence on management," *British Journal of Surgery*, vol. 101, no. 1, pp. e156–e162, 2014.

[10] G. van der Weg, M. Wikkeling, M. van Leeuwen, and E. ter Avest, "A rare case of oesophageal rupture: Boerhaave's syndrome," *International Journal of Emergency Medicine*, vol. 7, no. 1, article 27, 2014.

[11] L. Granel-Villach, C. Fortea-Sanchis, D. Martínez-Ramos et al., "Boerhaave's syndrome: a review of our experience over the last 16 years," *Revista de Gastroenterología de México*, vol. 79, no. 1, pp. 67–70, 2014.

[12] J. A. Henderson and A. M. Péloquin, "Boerhaave revisited: spontaneous esophageal perforation as a diagnostic masquerader," *The American Journal of Medicine*, vol. 86, no. 5, pp. 559–567, 1989.

[13] R. M. Aronberg, S. R. Punekar, S. I. Adam, B. L. Judson, S. Mehra, and W. G. Yarbrough, "Esophageal perforation caused by edible foreign bodies: a systematic review of the literature," *The Laryngoscope*, vol. 125, no. 2, pp. 371–378, 2015.

[14] M. Kamiyoshihara, S. Kakinuma, T. Kusaba et al., "Occult Boerhaave's syndrome without vomiting prior to presentation. Report of a case," *The Journal of Cardiovascular Surgery*, vol. 39, no. 6, pp. 863–865, 1998.

[15] N. S. Blencowe, S. Strong, and A. D. Hollowood, "Spontaneous oesophageal rupture," *British Medical Journal*, vol. 346, Article ID f3095, 2013.

[16] T. Lemke and L. Jagminas, "Spontaneous esophageal rupture: a frequently missed diagnosis," *The American Surgeon*, vol. 65, no. 5, pp. 449–452, 1999.

[17] J. A. Søreide and A. Viste, "Esophageal perforation: diagnostic work-up and clinical decision-making in the first 24 hours," *Scandinavian Journal of Trauma, Resuscitation and Emergency Medicine*, vol. 19, article 66, 2011.

[18] B. Sepesi, D. P. Raymond, and J. H. Peters, "Esophageal perforation: surgical, endoscopic and medical management strategies," *Current Opinion in Gastroenterology*, vol. 26, no. 4, pp. 379–383, 2010.

[19] K. Ben-David, K. Behrns, S. Hochwald et al., "Esophageal perforation management using a multidisciplinary minimally invasive treatment algorithm," *Journal of the American College of Surgeons*, vol. 218, no. 4, pp. 768–774, 2014.

[20] C. D. Mavroudis and J. C. Kucharczuk, "Acute management of esophageal perforation," *Current Surgery Reports*, vol. 2, no. 1, pp. 1–8, 2014.

[21] M. Schweigert, R. Beattie, N. Solymosi et al., "Endoscopic stent insertion versus primary operative management for spontaneous rupture of the esophagus (Boerhaave syndrome): an international study comparing the outcome," *The American Surgeon*, vol. 79, no. 6, pp. 634–640, 2013.

[22] G.-J. Zhao, J.-Y. Cheng, S.-C. Zhi, X. Jin, and Z.-Q. Lu, "Conservative management of esophageal perforation due to external air-blast injury: a case report and literature review," *Therapeutic Advances in Gastroenterology*, vol. 8, no. 4, pp. 234–238, 2015.

[23] A. Peng, Y. Li, Z. Xiao, and W. Wu, "Study of clinical treatment of esophageal foreign body-induced esophageal perforation with lethal complications," *European Archives of Oto-Rhino-Laryngology*, vol. 269, no. 9, pp. 2027–2036, 2012.

# Pentobarbital Toxicity after Self-Administration of Euthasol Veterinary Euthanasia Medication

**Steven Jason Crellin and Kenneth D. Katz**

*Department of Emergency Medicine, Lehigh Valley Hospital and Health Network, USF MCOM,*
*Cedar Crest Boulevard and I-78, Allentown, PA 18103, USA*

Correspondence should be addressed to Kenneth D. Katz; katzkd1@gmail.com

Academic Editor: Chih Cheng Lai

Suicide attempt via sodium pentobarbital is uncommon. A 48-year-old woman with a history of depression and prior suicide attempt was found unresponsive by her veterinarian spouse near a syringe containing pink solution. Upon EMS' arrival, the patient was experiencing apnea, hypoxemia, and miotic pupils; her blood glucose level measured 73 mg/dL. She was bradycardic and administered atropine with transient improvement in heart rate and transported to an emergency department; 2 mg of intravenous naloxone was administered without effect. She was endotracheally intubated via rapid sequence intubation. Rapid urine drug screening detected both benzodiazepines and barbiturates. The patient was transferred to an intensive care unit where she demonstrated a nearly absent radial pulse. Emergent fasciotomy to the left forearm and carpal tunnel was performed for acute compartment syndrome; "Euthasol" had been self-administered into the antecubital fossa. Expanded toxicological analysis via liquid chromatography/mass spectroscopy detected caffeine, atropine, 7-aminoclonazepam, phenytoin, citalopram, and naproxen. The patient's coma resolved over 48 hours and she was successfully extubated without complication. Emergency physicians must closely monitor patients exposed to veterinary euthanasia agents who develop central nervous system and respiratory depression, hypothermia, bradycardia, hypotension, or skin injury. Consultation with a regional poison center and medical toxicologist is recommended.

## 1. Introduction

Suicide attempt via self-administration of sodium pentobarbital is extremely uncommon but may occur in those who have access to veterinary medications. The dramatic presentations of barbiturate-associated poisoning are often accompanied by characteristic history and physical findings that can facilitate early identification and treatment of these potentially lethal overdoses. A unique case of a patient suffering from sodium pentobarbital toxicity after intravenous injection is described.

## 2. Case Presentation

A 48-year-old woman with a history of depression and prior suicide attempt who was prescribed clonazepam and citalopram was found by her veterinarian spouse unresponsive at home at approximately 10:30 pm. Cardiopulmonary resuscitation was initiated by the husband due to observed apnea while awaiting EMS' arrival. A syringe containing a pink solution with a needle attached was found adjacent to the patient and appeared to have been used to inject the patient's left antecubital fossa. A suicide note and an empty bottle of 2 mg clonazepam tablets were also found at the scene. Upon EMS' arrival, the patient had a Glasgow Coma Scale (GCS) score of "3" with apnea, hypoxemia, and miotic pupils. Her blood glucose level measured 73 mg/dL. She was bradycardic and was administered atropine on scene with transient improvement in heart rate.

The patient was rapidly transported to a local emergency department. Her vital signs on arrival included a heart rate of 46 beats per minute, blood pressure 99/53 mmHg, agonal respirations, temperature 94.6°F, and room air pulse oximetry of 78%. Physical examination revealed a GCS of "3," pupils measuring 3 mm and being sluggishly reactive, and a taught, "dusky" left forearm with delayed capillary refill distal to a left antecubital vein injection site. Two milligrams of intravenous naloxone was administered without effect, and she was then endotracheally intubated via rapid sequence intubation. Computed tomography of her head demonstrated no hemorrhage, mass, or ischemic change. Serum creatinine phosphokinase and ethanol measured 806 U/L and 58 mg/dL, respectively. Complete metabolic panel, serum salicylate, and acetaminophen levels were unremarkable. Rapid urine drug screening detected both benzodiazepines and barbiturates. The patient was then transferred to a local tertiary care facility for further management.

Upon arrival to the intensive care unit (ICU), the patient was evaluated by the surgical service. After clinical examination with a nearly absent radial pulse on Doppler examination, she underwent emergent fasciotomy of the left forearm and carpal tunnel for acute compartment syndrome. Contemporaneous discussion with her spouse revealed that the pink solution found in the syringe, which had been transported with the patient, was Euthasol (390 mg/mL pentobarbital and 50 mg/mL phenytoin; see Figure 1) and had been stolen from his on-site, secured pharmacy. The previously unused 100 mg vial was missing approximately 8 mL of solution.

Serum pentobarbital and phenytoin levels were drawn on arrival at the ICU and measured 12.6 $\mu$g/mL (1.0–5.0 $\mu$g/mL) and 2.5 $\mu$g/mL (10–20 $\mu$g/mL), respectively. Serum cell counts with differential, electrolytes, renal function, and liver enzymes were all within normal limits. Serum creatinine phosphokinase measured 1057 U/L (26–192 U/L). Expanded toxicological screening at the receiving hospital via liquid chromatography/mass spectroscopy detected caffeine, atropine, 7-aminoclonazepam, phenytoin, citalopram, and naproxen.

The patient's coma resolved over the following 48 hours, and she was successfully extubated on hospital day three. Serum pentobarbital levels declined to 8.6 (at 12 hours), 6.4 (at 24 hours), and 2.1 $\mu$g/mL (at 48 hours) at time of extubation. Serum creatinine phosphokinase peaked at 4727 U/L. The plastic surgery service was consulted to repair the fasciotomy surgical wounds. The patient was ultimately evaluated by a psychiatrist, who made the diagnoses of mood disorder not otherwise specified, suicide attempt secondary to mood disorder, and alcohol use disorder. She was discharged to an inpatient facility in good condition on hospital day thirteen without neurologic sequelae.

## 3. Discussion

Pentobarbital is a short-acting barbiturate currently utilized to initiate and maintain medically induced coma, as well as for management of elevated intracranial pressure, particularly in the setting of traumatic brain injury [1]. In the United States' judicial system, the drug is utilized as a means of lethal injection in humans. Veterinarians administer pentobarbital most frequently for euthanasia purposes.

Barbiturates are derivatives of barbituric acid and are classified as either short- or long-acting. The short-acting barbiturates (e.g., pentobarbital) when compared to long-acting agents differ by more rapid onset, higher pKa values,

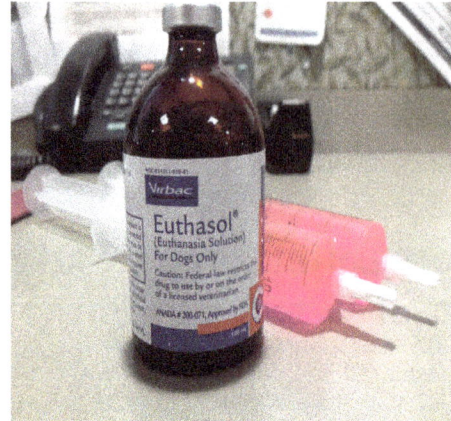

FIGURE 1: Euthasol bottle and syringes.

are more protein bound and lipid soluble, have a shorter duration of action, and undergo more hepatic metabolism. Pentobarbital possesses a duration of action of three to four hours and a variable elimination half-life of 15 to 48 hours [2]. These generalizations, however, may be misleading in overdose as the severity and time course following barbiturate overdose vary greatly, and toxicokinetics are encountered rather than expected pharmacokinetics [1].

There are several distinguishing physical examination and historical features regarding barbiturate toxicity. Cutaneous manifestations of barbiturate toxicity are not uncommon and include barbiturate blisters or bullae and dermal discoloration with necrosis [3–5]. These can result from extravascular injection or prolonged external compression, both of which may be accompanied by rhabdomyolysis [6, 7]. Other well-described clinical features of barbiturate overdose are hypothermia and cardiovascular collapse, with bradycardia and refractory hypotension [8]. Furthermore, respiratory depression or embarrassment may be evident in the barbiturate-poisoned patient unlike other sedative-hypnotic medications, such as benzodiazepines. Historical clues that suggest barbiturate toxicity include access to professional veterinary euthanasia agents, as illustrated in this case [9–11]. Delayed complications of barbiturate toxicity in survivors include aspiration with and without pneumonia, pulmonary edema, cerebral edema and infarct, and multiorgan failure [1].

Concentrated solutions of sodium pentobarbital are routinely used for the purposes of animal euthanasia because of rapid onset of action and efficacy (see Table 1) [12]. Solutions often contain greater than 300 mg/mL sodium pentobarbital. Intravenous injection in humans and animals results in rapid coma, respiratory depression, hypotension, bradycardia, and hypothermia. These effects lead to prompt induction of asystole and death. While the majority of these agents are administered intravenously, they are also efficacious via oral, intramuscular, or intraperitoneal routes. It has been reported that oral doses of sodium pentobarbital as little as 100 mg can induce hypnosis in adults, which substantially increases the lethality of unsecured concentrated veterinary formulations [10].

TABLE 1: Pentobarbital-containing veterinary euthanasia solutions [12].

| Pentobarbital-containing veterinary euthanasia solutions | | |
|---|---|---|
| | Concentrations | Trade names | Veterinary uses |
| Pentobarbital sodium powder | 392 mg/mL when reconstituted in 250 mL | *Fatal-Plus Powder* (Vortech) *Pentasol Powder* (Virbac) | Approved for all warm-blooded animals |
| Pentobarbital sodium for injection | 260 mg/mL in 100 mL bottles | *Sleepaway* (Fort Dodge) | Approved for use in dogs and cats |
| | 389 mg/mL in 100 mL or 250 mL vials | *Socumb-6 gr* (Butler) *Somlethal* (Webster) | Approved for use in dogs and cats |
| | 390 mg/mL in 250 mL vials | *Fatal-Plus* Solution (Vortech) | Approved for use in dogs and cats |
| Pentobarbital sodium/ phenytoin sodium | 390 mg/mL pentobarbital sodium and 50 mg/mL phenytoin sodium in 100 mL vials | *Beuthanasia-D Special* (Schering-Plough) *Euthasol* (Virbac) | Approved for use in dogs |

Concentrated veterinary solutions (and lower-dose formulations utilized for human use) often contain chemical vehicles, which—while facilitating administration of the medication—can also have significant side effects. These diluents are often alcohol derivatives, for instance, isopropanol, ethanol, and propylene glycol. Side effects of these additives include potentiation of the sedative-hypnotic effects of the barbiturate and metabolic derangements such as lactic acidosis documented from propylene glycol additives [13].

Several formulations of pentobarbital-containing veterinary euthanasia agents have varying types of Vaughan-Williams Class-Ib antiarrhythmics, most frequently phenytoin sodium. According to the Euthasol package insert, the rapid administration of these agents reportedly produces cardiotoxic effects during the anesthesia stage of euthanasia by "hastening the cessation of electrical activity of the heart" via interference with myocardial sodium channel function. In this patient, the clinical toxicity observed stemmed directly from sedative-hypnotic toxicity and likely very little from the phenytoin.

Similar to other medications in the sedative-hypnotic class, the treatment for barbiturate overdose remains primarily supportive. If toxic amounts were ingested orally, activated charcoal could be considered, but, given the potential for significant CNS depression and subsequent aspiration, the benefit appears small [14]. Pentobarbital metabolism occurs primarily via hydroxylation and glucuronidation in the liver, and excretion occurs primarily in the kidneys. Alkaline diuresis does not enhance excretion because of the high pKa of the short-acting barbiturates [10]. Hemodialysis appears to be less effective for the short-acting agents compared to long-acting ones and is described as "moderately dialyzable" [2, 10, 15]. The patient described in this case report improved spontaneously with meticulous supportive care and maintained normal renal function, so hemodialysis was deemed unnecessary.

Pentobarbital poisoning is extremely uncommon but still can be lethal. Emergency physicians must be cognizant of patients who develop CNS and respiratory depression, hypothermia, bradycardia, hypotension, or skin injury, especially in the setting of exposure to veterinary euthanasia agents. Meticulous intensive care is the mainstay of treatment with attention to respiratory and cardiovascular support, and high flux hemodialysis may enhance elimination in severe, refractory cases. Consultation with both a regional poison center and a medical toxicologist is recommended.

## Conflict of Interests

The authors have no outside support information, conflicts, or financial interest to disclose.

## References

[1] D. J. Greenblatt, D. Allen, J. S. Harmatz, B. J. Noel, and R. I. Shader, "Overdosage with pentobarbital and secobarbital: assessment of factors related to outcome," *Journal of Clinical Pharmacology*, vol. 19, no. 11-12, pp. 758–768, 1979.

[2] R. Mactier, M. Laliberté, J. Mardini et al., "Extracorporeal treatment for barbiturate poisoning: recommendations from the EXTRIP workgroup," *American Journal of Kidney Diseases*, vol. 64, no. 3, pp. 347–358, 2014.

[3] G. W. Beveridge, "Bullous lesions in poisoning," *British Medical Journal*, vol. 4, no. 779, pp. 116–117, 1971.

[4] C. Dunn, J. L. Held, J. Spitz, D. N. Silver, M. E. Grossman, and S. R. Kohn, "Coma blisters: report and review," *Cutis*, vol. 45, no. 6, pp. 423–426, 1990.

[5] D. Gröschel, A. R. Gerstein, and J. M. Rosenbaum, "Skin lesions as a diagnostic aid in barbiturate poisoning," *The New England Journal of Medicine*, vol. 283, no. 8, pp. 409–410, 1970.

[6] Oak Pharmaceuticals, *Nembutal Sodium Solution (Pentobarbital Sodium Injection): Prescribing Information*, Oak Pharmaceuticals, Lake Forest, Ill, USA, 2012, http://akorn.com/documents/catalog/package_inserts/76478-501-20.pdf.

[7] G. K. McEvoy, Ed., *AHFS Drug Information 2007. Barbiturates General Statement*, American Society of Health-System Pharmacists, Bethesda, Md, USA, 2007.

[8] R. H. Fell, A. J. Gunning, K. D. Bardhan, and D. R. Triger, "Severe hypothermia as a result of barbiturate overdose complicated by cardiac arrest," *The Lancet*, vol. 1, no. 7539, pp. 392–394, 1968.

[9] N. Romain, C. Giroud, K. Michaud, and P. Mangin, "Suicide by injection of a veterinarian barbiturate euthanasia agent: report of a case and toxicological analysis," *Forensic Science International*, vol. 131, no. 2-3, pp. 103–107, 2003.

[10] W. H. Cordell, S. C. Curry, R. B. Furbee, and D. L. Mitchell-Flynn, "Veterinary euthanasia drugs as suicide agents," *Annals of Emergency Medicine*, vol. 15, no. 8, pp. 939–943, 1986.

[11] S. Hangartner, J. Steiner, F. Dussy, R. Moeckli, K. Gerlach, and T. Briellmann, "A suicide involving intraperitoneal injection of pentobarbital," *International Journal of Legal Medicine*, 2015.

[12] D. C. Plumb, *Plumb's Veterinary Handbook*, Wiley-Blackwell Publishing, Hoboken, NJ, USA, 5th edition, 2005.

[13] M. A. Miller, A. Forni, and D. Yogaratnam, "Propylene glycol-induced lactic acidosis in a patient receiving continuous infusion of pentobarbital," *Annals of Pharmacotherapy*, vol. 42, no. 10, pp. 1502–1506, 2008.

[14] P. A. Chyka and D. Seger, "Position paper: single-dose activated charcoal," *Journal of Toxicology*, vol. 43, no. 2, pp. 61–87, 2005.

[15] D. Wermeling, K. Record, R. Bell, W. Porter, and R. Blouin, "Hemodialysis clearance of pentobarbital during continuous infusion," *Therapeutic Drug Monitoring*, vol. 7, no. 4, pp. 485–487, 1985.

# 57

# Spontaneous Arachnoid Cyst Rupture with Subdural Hygroma in a Child

**Muhammad Faisal Khilji,[1] Niranjan Lal Jeswani,[1] Rana Shoaib Hamid,[2] and Faisal Al Azri[2]**

[1]Department of Emergency Medicine, Sultan Qaboos University Hospital, Al-Khod, P.O. Box 38, 123 Muscat, Oman
[2]Department of Radiology, Sultan Qaboos University Hospital, Muscat, Oman

Correspondence should be addressed to Muhammad Faisal Khilji; faisalkhilji@yahoo.com

Academic Editor: Vasileios Papadopoulos

Arachnoid cyst of the brain is common in children but its association with spontaneous subdural hygroma is rare. A case of a nine-year-old boy, without any preceding history of trauma, is presented here who came to the emergency department of a tertiary care hospital with complaints of headache, nausea, and vomiting for the last two weeks but more for the last two days. Examination showed a young, fully conscious oriented boy with positive Cushing's reflex and papilledema of left eye. MRI (magnetic resonance imaging) of the brain showed left temporal extra-axial cystic lesion of 5.40 × 4.10 cm in size, representing arachnoid cyst, with bilateral frontoparietal subdural hygromas. Cyst was partially drained through left temporal craniectomy and subdural hygromas were drained through bilateral frontal burr holes. Postoperatively the child recovered uneventfully and was discharged on the seventh postoperative day. Histopathology proves it to be arachnoid cyst of the brain with subdural CSF (cerebrospinal fluid) collection or hygroma.

## 1. Introduction

Arachnoid cysts are common childhood developmental anomalies, but their association with spontaneous subdural hygroma is rare [1–3]. They are benign lesions and may be associated with complications such as subdural hematoma, subdural hygroma, and intracystic hemorrhage. Minor head injury is known to result in subdural hygroma or hematoma due to rupture of arachnoid cyst; however spontaneous rupture of arachnoid cyst may occur rarely [3]. Most of these cysts are in middle cranial fossa where they are likely to be symptomatic if they are large. Chances of expansion are greatest in middle cranial fossa [1]. They are more common in males as compared to females [3, 4]. In children they are frequently associated with seizures and cranial deformity [1, 5, 6].

## 2. Case Report

We present a case of a nine-year-old, previously healthy boy, presenting to the emergency department of a tertiary care hospital with complaints of severe frontal headache for the last two weeks but more for the last two days. Headache was associated with nausea, vomiting, photophobia, and pain in both eyes. There was no history of fever, jerking movements, or trauma. The child had no past medical or surgical history. He achieved all developmental milestones normally and was doing well at school. His examination revealed a fully conscious and oriented child with a heart rate of 77 per minute and blood pressure of 159/112 mm Hg. Power was 5/5 on both sides, all cranial nerves were intact, and no sensory loss was observed. There were no meningeal signs but there was right side papilledema. The rest of the exam was normal. His blood investigations, including blood glucose, full blood count, serum creatinine, and electrolytes, were normal. MRI of the brain was done, after initial symptomatic management. MRI showed left temporal, extra-axial collection measuring 5.40 × 4.10 cm of CSF-like intensity compatible with arachnoid cyst and bilateral frontoparietal subdural enlargement compatible with subdural hygroma (Figure 1).

Within an hour of ED admission the child's frequency of vomiting increased along with mild drowsiness. At that

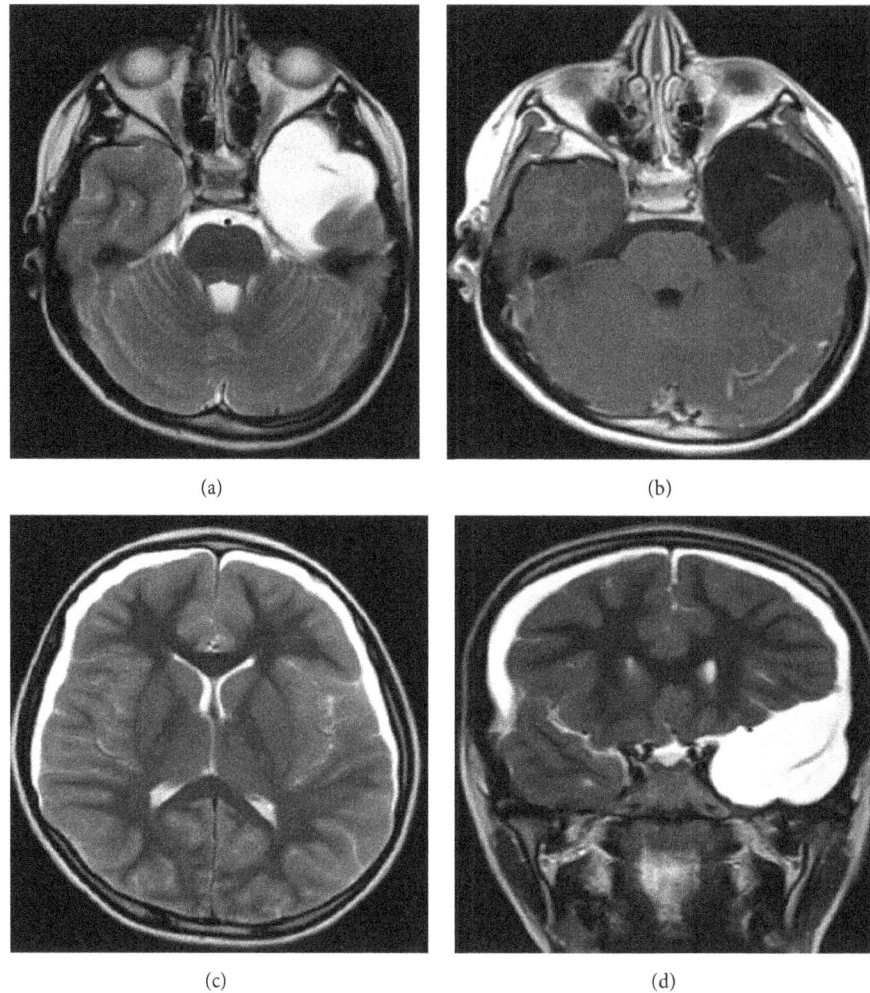

FIGURE 1: MRI brain axial T2 and T1 weighted postcontrast images (a) and (b) showing an extra-axial fluid signal intensity lesion in the left temporal region without any solid component or abnormal enhancement. Axial and coronal T2 weighted images show bilateral frontoparietal crescent shaped subdural fluid collections.

point Cushing's reflex was positive with heart rate was 64/minute and blood pressure of 177/110 mm Hg. The child was referred to the neurosurgery team and the subdural hygromas were drained through bilateral frontal burr holes. Left temporal arachnoid cyst was partially drained through left temporal craniotomy. A left subdural-peritoneal shunt was placed for drainage of any future collection. Drained CSF was xanthochromic and negative for malignant cells. CSF culture showed no growth. Histopathology of cyst confirmed radiological diagnosis of arachnoid cyst. Final diagnosis of left temporal arachnoid cyst with spontaneous subdural hygroma was made as the child presented symptomatically in the absence of any history of trauma. Postoperatively the child recovered uneventfully and was discharged on the 7th postoperative day. Any medium term CT scan was not performed.

## 3. Discussion

Arachnoid cysts are CSF collections between the two layers of arachnoid membrane and are mainly benign lesions. About 1% of intracranial space occupying lesions is arachnoid cysts. They usually grow slowly and occasionally disappear without treatment [1, 7]. Arachnoid cysts complicated, with cystic expansion, intracystic hemorrhage, subdural hematoma, and subdural hygroma, are usually symptomatic. Their association with subdural hygroma is rare [8–10]. In 1924 Naffziger postulated, for the first time, the possible mechanism of subdural hygroma formation [11], according to which a tear in the arachnoid membrane resulting in one-way valve mechanism with accumulation of CSF is thought to be responsible for subdural hygromas [12]. Tears of outer cyst membrane are the main cause of subdural hygroma in arachnoid cyst patients. The rupture is either traumatic, due to surgical manipulation, or rarely spontaneous [13]. Raised intracranial pressure with Valsalva maneuver is another possible cause of cyst rupture leading to hygroma. Most of the cases present with symptoms of raised intracranial pressure like nausea, vomiting, headache, and rarely diplopia from VI nerve palsy. Parsch et al. reported subdural hemorrhage in 2.43% and subdural hygroma in 0.46% of patients with arachnoid cyst reported on MRI [6]. Mild head injury is the most common cause of arachnoid cyst rupture; however rarely do they rupture spontaneously [8]. Gradual increase in size of hygroma is due to the continuous transudation of cerebrospinal fluid in the ruptured cyst. CSF itself is less expansive and compressive than blood due to its low osmotic and hydrostatic pressure [8]. Patients with arachnoid cyst may have complications by subdural hematoma as they are predisposed to it [8]. Different treatment options of arachnoid cyst are controversial. Surgical treatment of symptomatic cysts is generally acceptable. Craniotomy and fenestration of cyst, subdural evacuation, and CSF derivation are procedures performed in arachnoid cyst rupture depending upon the size, location, and clinical presentation [1]. CSF derivation is the preferred procedure in patients with raised intracranial pressure [3]. Di Rocco et al. demonstrated the usefulness of prolonging preoperative intracranial pressure recording [14]. Craniotomy and fenestration is adopted to treat well-circumscribed cysts. Cyst either decreases or disappears after subdural evacuation [13]. Prophylactic surgical treatment is not recommended.

## 4. Conclusion

Spontaneous subdural hygroma should be suspected in symptomatic arachnoid cyst patients without any history of head injury. Symptomatic hygroma is not an absolute indication of surgical treatment; however most of such patients need surgical treatment.

## Conflict of Interests

The authors declare that there is no conflict of interests regarding the publication of this paper.

## References

[1] A. Rajesh, V. Bramhaprasad, and A. K. Purohit, "Traumatic rupture of arachnoid cyst with subdural hygroma," *Journal of Pediatric Neurosciences*, vol. 7, no. 1, pp. 33–35, 2012.

[2] J. W. Donaldson, M. Edwards-Brown, and T. G. Luerssen, "Arachnoid cyst rupture with concurrent subdural hygroma," *Pediatric Neurosurgery*, vol. 32, no. 3, pp. 137–139, 2000.

[3] F. C. Albuquerque and S. L. Giannotta, "Arachnoid cyst rupture producing subdural hygroma and intracranial hypertension: case reports," *Neurosurgery*, vol. 41, no. 4, pp. 951–956, 1997.

[4] R. N. Sener, "Arachnoid cysts associated with post-traumatic and spontaneous rupture into the subdural space," *Computerized Medical Imaging and Graphics*, vol. 21, no. 6, pp. 341–344, 1997.

[5] M. Choux, C. Raybaud, N. Pinsard, J. Hassoun, and D. Gambarelli, "Intracranial supratentorial cysts in children excluding tumor and parasitic cysts," *Child's Brain*, vol. 4, no. 1, pp. 15–32, 1978.

[6] C. S. Parsch, J. Krauss, E. Hofmann, J. Meixensberger, and K. Roosen, "Arachnoid cysts associated with subdural hematomas and hygromas: analysis of 16 cases, long-term follow-up, and review of the literature," *Neurosurgery*, vol. 40, no. 3, pp. 483–490, 1997.

[7] R. L. Dodd, P. D. Barnes, and S. L. Huhn, "Spontaneous resolution of a prepontine arachnoid cyst: case report and review of the literature," *Pediatric Neurosurgery*, vol. 37, no. 3, pp. 152–157, 2002.

[8] A.-L. M. L. Poirrier, I. Ngosso-Tetanye, M. Mouchamps, and J.-P. Misson, "Spontaneous arachnoid cyst rupture in a previously asymptomatic child: a case report," *European Journal of Paediatric Neurology*, vol. 8, no. 5, pp. 247–251, 2004.

[9] E. Cakir, Kayhankuzeyli, O. C. Sayin, B. Peksoylu, and G. Karaarslan, "Arachnoid cyst rupture with subdural hygroma: case report and literature review," *Neurocirugia*, vol. 15, no. 1, pp. 72–75, 2004.

[10] C. Offiah, W. S. C. Forbes, and J. Thorne, "Non-haemorrhagic subdural collection complicating rupture of a middle cranial fossa arachnoid cyst," *British Journal of Radiology*, vol. 79, no. 937, pp. 79–82, 2006.

[11] H. C. Naffziger, "Subdural fluid accumulations following head injury," *The Journal of the American Medical Association*, vol. 82, no. 22, pp. 1751–1752, 1924.

[12] C. Çokluk, A. Şenel, F. Çelik, and H. Ergür, "Spontaneous disappearance of two asymptomatic arachnoid cysts in two different locations," *Minimally Invasive Neurosurgery*, vol. 46, no. 2, pp. 110–112, 2003.

[13] K. Mori, T. Yamamoto, N. Horinaka, and M. Maeda, "Arachnoid cyst is a risk factor for chronic subdural hematoma in Juveniles: twelve cases of chronic subdural hematoma associated with arachnoid cyst," *Journal of Neurotrauma*, vol. 19, no. 9, pp. 1017–1027, 2002.

[14] C. Di Rocco, G. Tamburrini, M. Caldarelli, F. Velardi, and P. Santini, "Prolonged ICP monitoring in Sylvian arachnoid cysts," *Surgical Neurology*, vol. 60, no. 3, pp. 211–218, 2003.

# 58

# Ischemic Left Ventricular Perforation Covered by a Thrombus in a Patient Presenting with Cerebral Ischemia: Importance of Time-Sensitive Performance and Adequate Interpretation of Bedside Transthoracic Echography

**A. J. Fischer,[1] P. Lebiedz,[2] M. Wiaderek,[3] M. Lichtenberg,[4] D. Böse,[5] S. Martens,[6] and F. Breuckmann[5]**

[1]*Department of Cardiovascular Medicine, Division of Electrophysiology, University of Münster, 48149 Münster, Germany*
[2]*Department of Cardiovascular Medicine, University of Münster, 48149 Münster, Germany*
[3]*Department of Neurology, Arnsberg Medical Center, 59759 Arnsberg, Germany*
[4]*Department of Angiology, Arnsberg Medical Center, 59759 Arnsberg, Germany*
[5]*Department of Cardiology, Arnsberg Medical Center, 59759 Arnsberg, Germany*
[6]*Department of Cardiothoracic Surgery, Division of Cardiac Surgery, University of Münster, 48149 Münster, Germany*

Correspondence should be addressed to F. Breuckmann; f.breuckmann@klinikum-arnsberg.de

Academic Editor: Aristomenis K. Exadaktylos

If myocardial infarction remains silent, only clinical signs of complications may unveil its presence. Life-threatening complications include myocardial rupture, thrombus formation, or arterial embolization. In the presented case, a 76-year-old patient was admitted with left-sided hemiparesis. In duplex sonography, a critical stenosis of the right internal carotid artery was identified and initially but retrospectively incorrectly judged as the potential cause for ischemia. During operative thromboendarterectomy, arterial embolism of the right leg occurred coincidentally, more likely pointing towards a cardioembolic origin. Percutaneous interventions remained unsuccessful and local fibrinolysis was applied. Delayed bedside echocardiography by an experienced cardiologist demonstrated a discontinuity of the normal myocardial texture of the left ventricular apex together with an echodense, partly floating structure merely attached by a thin bridge not completely sealing the myocardial defect, accompanied by pericardial effusion. The patient was immediately transferred to emergency cardiac surgery with extirpation of the thrombus, aortocoronary bypass graft placement, and aneurysmectomy. This didactic case reveals decisive structural shortcomings in patient's admission and triage processes and underlines, if performed timely and correctly, the value of transthoracic echocardiography as a noninvasive and cost-effective tool allowing immediate decision-making, which, in this case, led to the correct but almost fatally delayed diagnosis.

## 1. Introduction

Myocardial infarction is one of the major causes of death in the industrialized world. It is characterized as an ischemic necrosis of cardiac cells in a clinical setting consistent with acute myocardial ischemia [1]. Patients with myocardial infarction may present with different symptoms ranging from epigastric pain to typical left thoracic chest pain. As little as 40% of patients present with typical clinical signs of myocardial infarction [2]. Therefore, diagnosis is often delayed as to the time patients present with clinical signs of complications of myocardial infarction only. There are several severe complications worsening the overall prognosis. Myocardial rupture that can appear in the acute setting with laceration of the myocardium represents a main life-threatening complication. Fibrinolytic agents should not be administered as it has been shown that cardiac rupture may be accelerated by thrombolytic therapy, especially in case a thrombus seals the perforated myocardium by adherence to the pericardium [3]. Another serious complication is left

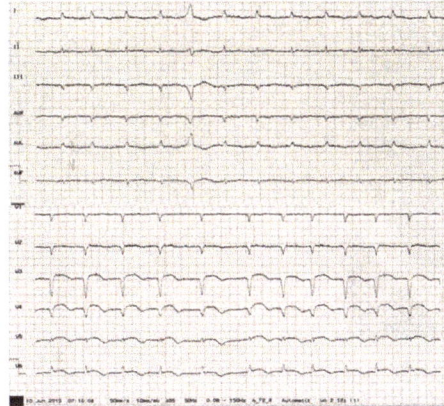

FIGURE 1: Initial twelve-lead ECG demonstrating atrial fibrillation and ST-segment elevation of the anterior leads.

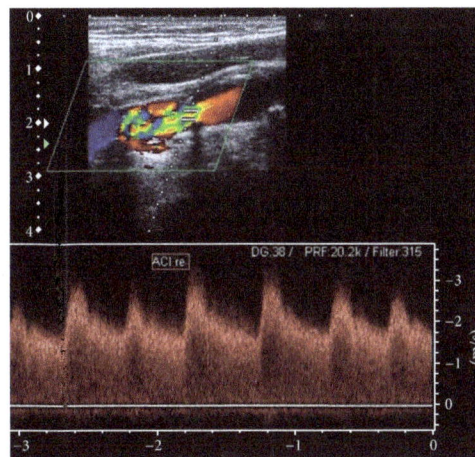

FIGURE 2: Doppler ultrasound assessment of the right internal cerebral artery showing a critical stenosis with a systolic maximal flow velocity of >3 m/s.

ventricular thrombus formation. After myocardial infarction, wall motion abnormalities may lead to stagnated blood flow and thus ventricular thrombus formation. After confirmation of a left ventricular thrombus, systemic anticoagulation is the treatment of choice in addition to antiplatelet therapy, reducing the incidence of embolism [1, 4, 5].

If performed and adequately interpreted, transthoracic echocardiography is an adequate diagnostic tool to visualize ventricular thrombi [4, 6]. However, especially if myocardial infarction remains silent within the acute setting, only ventricular thrombus embolization unveils its presence.

## 2. Case Presentation

A 76-year-old patient presented with left-sided hemiparesis to our neurologic department. Clinical assessment revealed a NIH Stroke Scale of eight. Electrocardiogram at admission showed atrial fibrillation concomitant with ST elevation in the anterior leads V3–V6 (Figure 1). The initial native cranial computed tomography (CT) did not show significant changes. As the patient reported that symptoms persisted since the day before presentation, potential lysis therapy was

not an option and additional contrast-enhanced scans were omitted. Instead, because of a positive history of vascular disease, early carotid as well as transcranial duplex was performed. A stenosis of the right internal carotid artery of about 80% was diagnosed and considered as origin for the acute cerebral ischemia (Figure 2). As to progressive left-sided hemiparesis, it was decided to perform operative thromboendarterectomy of the right carotid artery immediately. During surgery, coincident embolization of the right leg occurred. Bedside transthoracic echocardiography by a nonprofessional observer disclosed signs of chronic myocardial infarction and a suspicious, partly free-floating echodense structure attached to the thinned anterior wall. Retrospectively, cardioembolic stroke due to atrial fibrillation or left ventricular thrombus was now assumed. Repeated cranial CT confirmed ischemia in the posterior flow area and pointed towards simultaneous ischemic brain stem stroke (Figure 3). Duplex sonography of the right leg revealed an occlusion of the femoral artery. Therefore, the patient was subsequently transferred to percutaneous transluminal angioplasty (Figure 4). Up to this point, only unfractionated heparin was administered for anticoagulation. As during

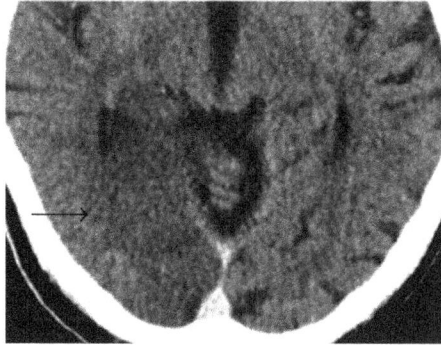

FIGURE 3: Contrast-enhanced cranial computed tomographic scan showing an insult of the right posterior region with hypodensity of the parafalcine parenchyma as well as loss of grey/white matter differentiation (black arrow).

the interventional procedure perfusion of the leg remained impaired, local fibrinolysis was applied as bail-out. Due to persisting insufficient perfusion, operative popliteopedal bypass surgery had to be performed finally. In the intensive care unit, an experienced cardiologist repeated postinterventional transthoracic echocardiography. Imaging showed a severely impaired left ventricular function accompanied by a discontinuity of the normal myocardial texture of the apex together with an echodense, partly floating structure merely attached by a thin bridge, not completely sealing the assumed myocardial defect anymore. Simultaneously, a progression of the pericardial effusion had occurred. Transesophageal echocardiography confirmed transthoracic suspicion (Figure 5). Imminent myocardial rupture was feared and urgent cardiac surgery was planned, accepting an elevated risk of secondary cerebral bleeding. Preoperative coronary catheterization showed a complete occlusion of the proximal left anterior descending artery (Figure 6). Cardiac CT imaging showed a thrombus with exophytic components into the left ventricle adherent to a postischemic anterior aneurysm with extremely thinned myocardium (Figure 7). Surgery validated a perforated left ventricle partly covered by a thrombus. An extirpation of the thrombus and coronary bypass graft were performed (Figure 8). The apical aneurysm was resected. Endomyocardial biopsies revealed thrombotic material along with fibrosis.

In the following days, the perfusion of the right leg remained critically impaired despite reoperation. Ultimately, an amputation of the right lower limb got necessary. A hemiparesis persisted. Transthoracic echocardiographic follow-up before discharge revealed that the patients' left ventricular ejection fraction had improved without any more thrombus formation.

## 3. Discussion

Often, clinical signs of myocardial infarction are unspecific, particularly in females, elderly, diabetics, and patients with dementia or suffering from chronic renal disease [1, 7]. As a consequence, patients may present in a subacute setting with clinical signs of complications as in the presented case.

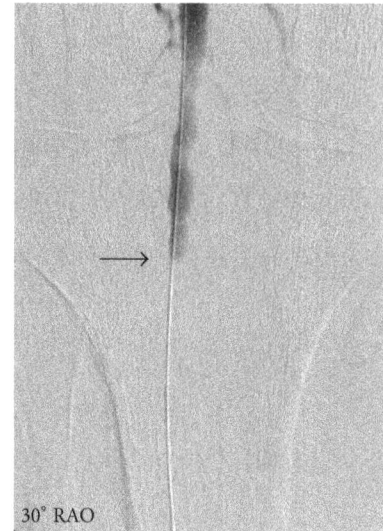

FIGURE 4: Percutaneous transluminal angiography demonstrating the occlusion of the right popliteal artery (black arrow).

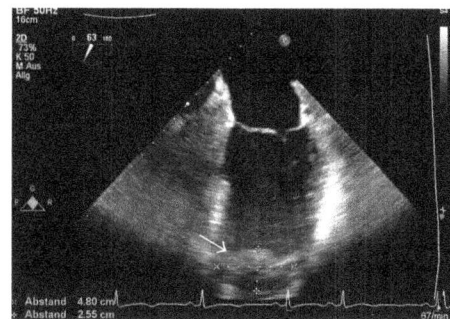

FIGURE 5: Transesophageal echocardiographic assessment of the left ventricular thrombus in the two-chamber view. The thrombus is marked with a white arrow.

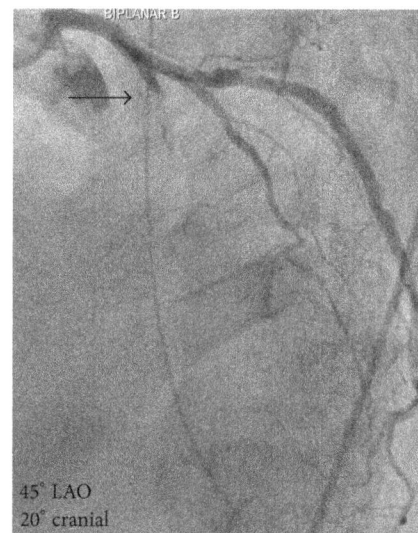

FIGURE 6: Coronary angiography revealing a complete occlusion of the left anterior descending coronary artery marked with the black arrow.

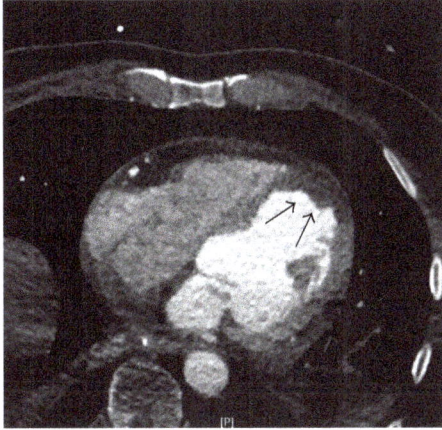

Figure 7: Contrast enhanced ECG-gated chest computed tomographic scan showing loosening of the myocardial anteroapical wall as well as thrombus formation (black arrow).

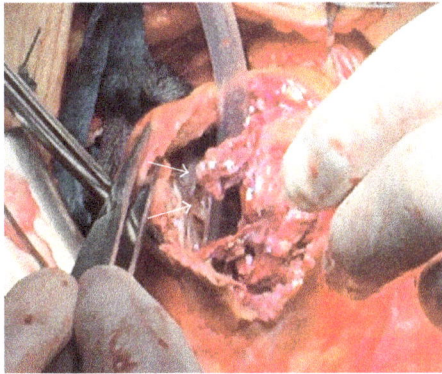

Figure 8: Intraoperative situs showing an ischemic myocardial perforation of the left ventricle.

Particularly, myocardial infarction of the anterior wall can lead to thrombus formation because of apical aneurysm and, thus, stagnant blood flow in the apex. In a multicenter trial on patients after acute myocardial infarction who were considered in low to medium risk for left ventricular thrombi, in 5.1%, a thrombus could be diagnosed within predischarge echocardiogram. In anterior myocardial infarction, there was even an incidence of 11.5% [8]. If the thrombus is free-floating within the left ventricle, there is a considerable risk of arterial embolism. In fact, the risk for cardioembolic events is fivefold higher in patients after myocardial infarction with detected thrombus formation as compared to patients without echocardiographic signs of thrombus formation [5]. Even though these cardioembolic events are well known, early bedside transthoracic echocardiogram is, as in our case, not yet implemented in clinical practice. Our case, which can be considered as a teaching case, demonstrates the value of transthoracic echocardiography as a noninvasive and cost-effective tool for immediate decision-making, at least within experts' hands. At initial presentation of the patient, an ECG was performed where atrial fibrillation as a potential cause for thromboembolism and ST elevation of the anterior leads as a sign for myocardial ischemia or myocardial aneurysm were detected. Because of structural failures in a common setting without central interdisciplinary emergency department but in case of leading neurological symptoms direct admission to the stroke unit, neurological work-up was overweighed and the ECG was not given sufficient attention. Even though it has been shown that particularly in patients with intracerebral hemorrhage but also with ischemic stroke ECG changes such as ST-segment elevation can be present, however, an echocardiography directly at admission or prior to surgery performed by an experienced physician may have led to much earlier diagnosis of imminent myocardial rupture, preventing unnecessary surgery of the internal carotid artery and further systemic embolization [9]. Most dramatically, orientating echocardiography by a noncardiologist even was performed within the clinical work-up; however, the information gathered was misinterpreted or not correctly weighted, particularly when local fibrinolysis was applied in the later course. Even though anticoagulation is the adequate treatment for prevention of thromboembolic events when left ventricular thrombus has been detected, thrombolytic therapy should not be administered [1, 4]. In the presented case, inadequate application of fibrinolytic agents resulted in an almost fatal rupture of the myocardium.

Nonetheless, it would be inappropriate to blame rescue fibrinolytic therapy initiating this sort of medical nightmare. By contrast, the presented case initiated internal discussions and review of procedural shortcomings in the aforementioned common patient population, thereby helping us to improve processes in our hospital. We learned that echocardiography has to be performed early in the clinical course in patients with seemingly unrelated clinical symptoms and integrated early ECG and echocardiography assessment within our stroke unit protocols. Even in acute and urgent cases, where a delay of operative treatment may potentially lead to more neurological damage, at least a short cardiologic consultation should be prompted whenever there are hints for a cardioembolic origin. Otherwise, potentially life-threatening illnesses may be missed.

## Conflict of Interests

The authors declare that there is no conflict of interests regarding the publication of this paper.

## References

[1] M. Roffi, C. Patrono, J.-P. Collet et al., "2015 ESC Guidelines for the management of acute coronary syndromes in patients presenting without persistent ST-segment elevation: task force for the management of acute coronary syndromes in patients presenting without persistent ST-segment elevation of the European Society of Cardiology (ESC)," *European Heart Journal*, vol. 37, no. 3, pp. 267–315, 2015.

[2] U. Keil, "The Worldwide WHO MONICA Project: results and perspectives," *Gesundheitswesen*, vol. 67, supplement 1, pp. S38–S45, 2005.

[3] R. C. Becker, J. M. Gore, C. Lambrew et al., "A composite view of cardiac rupture in the United States National Registry

of Myocardial Infarction," *Journal of the American College of Cardiology*, vol. 27, no. 6, pp. 1321–1326, 1996.

[4] L. L. Cregler, "Antithrombotic therapy in left ventricular thrombosis and systemic embolism," *American Heart Journal*, vol. 123, no. 4, part 2, pp. 1110–1114, 1992.

[5] P. T. Vaitkus and E. S. Barnathan, "Embolic potential, prevention and management of mural thrombus complicating anterior myocardial infarction: a meta-analysis," *Journal of the American College of Cardiology*, vol. 22, no. 4, pp. 1004–1009, 1993.

[6] J. R. Stratton, G. W. Lighty Jr., A. S. Pearlman, and J. L. Ritchie, "Detection of left ventricular thrombus by two-dimensional echocardiography: sensitivity, specificity, and causes of uncertainty," *Circulation*, vol. 66, no. 1, pp. 156–166, 1982.

[7] M. R. Gimenez, M. Reiter, R. Twerenbold et al., "Sex-specific chest pain characteristics in the early diagnosis of acute myocardial infarction," *JAMA Internal Medicine*, vol. 174, no. 2, pp. 241–249, 2014.

[8] F. Chiarella, E. Santoro, S. Domenicucci, A. Maggioni, and C. Vecchio, "Predischarge two-dimensional echocardiographic evaluation of left ventricular thrombosis after acute myocardial infarction in the GISSI-3 study," *American Journal of Cardiology*, vol. 81, no. 7, pp. 822–827, 1998.

[9] G. Khechinashvili and K. Asplund, "Electrocardiographic changes in patients with acute stroke: a systematic review," *Cerebrovascular Diseases*, vol. 14, no. 2, pp. 67–76, 2002.

# 59

# Atraumatic Subdural Hematoma in a Third-Trimester Gravid Patient

## D. C. Traficante, A. Marin, and A. Catapano

*Department of Emergency Medicine, St. Joseph's Regional Medical Center, Paterson, NJ 07503, USA*

Correspondence should be addressed to D. C. Traficante; david.traficante@gmail.com

Academic Editor: Chih Cheng Lai

Acute atraumatic subdural hematoma is a rare occurrence and there exist few case studies which describe suspected cases and causes for this condition. We present a case of a 36-year-old female at 32-week gestation who initially presented to the emergency department for evaluation of lower extremity cellulitis but had acute neurologic change while being in the ED. Computed tomography revealed a right subdural hematoma with midline shift and mass effect. The primary cause for the patient's subdural hematoma is unknown; however, this patient had several risk factors for developing an atraumatic subdural hematoma.

## 1. Introduction

Acute atraumatic, or nontraumatic, subdural hematoma is a rare condition and much of the literature regarding this pathology is limited to case reports. Some described causes of atraumatic SDH include ruptured aneurysm, arteriovenous malformations, preeclampsia, cocaine abuse, and severe coagulopathy. The authors present a case of a third-trimester gravid patient with an acute atraumatic subdural hematoma.

## 2. Case Report

A 36-year-old female $G_6P_{2032}$ at 32-week gestation presented to the emergency department for evaluation of bilateral lower extremity rash and leg pain. The patient reported that she was recently hospitalized for similar symptoms. Chart review showed that the patient was admitted to the hospital 8 weeks priorly for endocarditis, severe sepsis, and lower extremity cellulitis; however, she signed out against medical advice after approximately 2 weeks of treatment. The patient stated that she was noncompliant with her prenatal care and with the antibiotics prescribed to her when she signed out AMA approximately 6 weeks priorly. Past medical history was significant for Hepatitis C, IV drug abuse, and chronic lower extremity cellulitis. She admitted injecting heroin and cocaine into her right antecubital fossa prior to arrival in the hospital.

Physical exam on arrival revealed blood pressure of 103/53, pulse 117, respiratory rate 16, temperature 98.6 degrees Fahrenheit, and oxygen saturation of 97% on room air. The patient appeared older than her stated age, gravid, unkempt, and obviously ill. Her pupils were equal, round, and reactive to light and extraocular muscles were intact. Oral mucosa was dry, with stomatitis. Systolic 3/6 heart murmur was present, and she was tachycardic at a rate of ~120 bpm. She was alert and oriented to person, place, time, and situation; GCS was 15. In addition, she followed commands but was somewhat slow to respond. Skin exam revealed Janeway lesions and Osler nodes on the right and left hand. There were also bilateral lower extremity swelling and well demarcated erythema extending from the ankles to midcalf with scattered superficial ulcerations. There were no obvious outward signs of trauma.

Laboratories were obtained, along with three sets of blood cultures. Labs returned with WBC of 7.4, but with moderate bandemia of 23 bands. Hgb and Hct were 9.0 and 26.5, respectively. Platelets were 71,000. CMP revealed $CO_2$ of 16, Cr of 1.74, and mildly elevated liver function tests. Urinalysis was grossly positive with large leukocyte esterase, too many WBC, and proteinuria >100. A troponin-I was obtained as patient had been complaining of chest pain, which returned to be elevated at 0.392. Chest X-ray was unremarkable. EKG showed sinus tachycardia without ischemic changes. A bedside ultrasound showed a positive intrauterine pregnancy

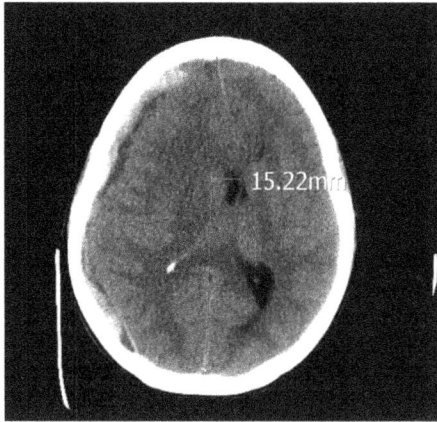

FIGURE 1: Computed tomography axial image showing right subdural hematoma with midline shift.

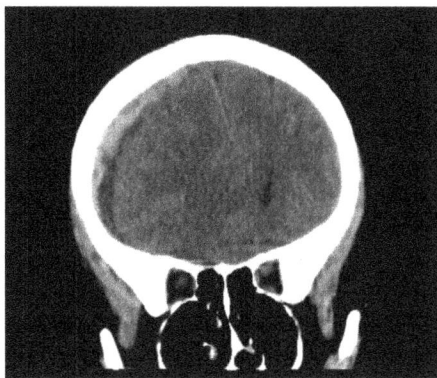

FIGURE 2: Computed tomography coronal image showing right subdural hematoma with midline shift.

consistent with 32-week gestation, positive fetal movement, and a fetal heart rate of 142 bpm.

The patient was started on a course of IV antibiotics and received 2L NS during the ED course. After approximately two hours in the department, the patient developed an acute change in mental status. She was less responsive, slurring her words, and found to have a right sided blown pupil. A stat CT scan revealed an acute right subdural hematoma with midline shift and mass effect (Figures 1 and 2). During the CT scan, the patient developed apnea and, therefore, was intubated for airway protection. She was given a bolus of mannitol and emergent consults were placed with neurosurgery and OB/GYN. She was immediately transferred to the operating room where she underwent simultaneous emergent cesarean section and right hemicraniectomy.

The patient's family decided to withdraw care and she died on day 3 in the surgical ICU, likely secondary to extensive cerebral infarcts and herniation. The patient's baby girl was discharged from the hospital into child protection custody on day 21.

## 3. Discussion

A subdural hematoma is a collection of blood between the dura and arachnoid membrane layers of the meninges. It is

the most common type of intracranial mass lesion, seen in approximately 5–25% of patients with severe head injuries, and is associated with high morbidity and mortality rates [1]. The most common cause of acute subdural hematoma is trauma. Causes of atraumatic subdural hematoma, which are much less common, include aneurysm rupture, ruptured cortical artery, hypertensive cerebral hemorrhage, arteriovenous malformations and dural arteriovenous fistula, neoplasms, hematological disorders, anticoagulant and thrombolytic therapy, cerebral amyloid angiopathy, acquired immunodeficiency syndrome, cocaine abuse, moyamoya disease, preeclampsia, HELLP syndrome, and severe coagulopathy. In addition, the pregnant patient undergoes physiological hormonally mediated changes in circulation, vascular tissue structure, and coagulability, all of which can contribute to further increased risk of stroke and bleeds [2, 3].

Prognosis is typically poor for patients with subdural hematomas, with the amount of associated direct brain damage and the damage resulting from the mass effect of the hematoma dictating the ultimate outcome. Mortality rates range from 16% to over 60% in some studies, with certain prognostic factors increasing the rate. These factors include increased age, time from injury to treatment, GCS on admission, immediate coma or lucid interval, CT findings (hematoma volume, degree of midline shift, associated intradural lesion, and compression of basal cisterns), postoperative ICP, and the type of surgery the patient underwent [4, 5]. Also several studies have shown increased mortality in patients with the presence of pupillary abnormalities, which was seen acutely in our patient. Koç et al. reported that patients with acute SDH who presented with bilateral or unilateral nonreactive pupils had mortality rates of 97% and 81%, respectively [6].

In our case, likely the combination of thrombocytopenia, preeclampsia, early HELLP syndrome, cocaine use, and disseminated intravascular coagulation secondary to severe sepsis may have all contributed to some extent to the development of an acute atraumatic subdural hematoma. Alternative causes in our patient's case could also include showered septic emboli secondary to her known recent history of endocarditis or ruptured mycotic aneurysm.

## 4. Conclusion

Subdural hematomas are a relatively common finding in patients who present with severe head trauma. When there are no outward signs of trauma but there is a focal neurological sign or change, it is important to consider atraumatic subdural hematoma as a potential diagnosis. In our case, there was likely a multifactorial cause that ultimately resulted in the acute subdural hematoma with thrombocytopenia, early HELLP syndrome, sepsis, cocaine use, and possible preeclampsia all contributing to her condition. Acute subdural hematomas carry significant mortality in the pregnant patient. As this situation affects two patients, mother and fetus, care must be taken to detect these early and treat them effectively. In cases where the pregnant patient is unstable, it is important to weigh the risk of fetal compromise and to act quickly to deliver the baby if needed.

## Conflict of Interests

The authors do not have any conflict of interests to declare.

## References

[1] S. Ichimura, T. Horiguchi, S. Inoue, and K. Yoshida, "Nontraumatic acute subdural hematoma associated with the myelodysplastic/myeloproliferative neoplasms," *Journal of Neurosciences in Rural Practice*, vol. 3, no. 1, pp. 98–99, 2012.

[2] S. K. Feske, "Stroke in pregnancy," *Seminars in Neurology*, vol. 27, no. 5, pp. 442–452, 2007.

[3] H. Yokota, K. Miyamoto, K. Yokoyama, H. Noguchi, K. Uyama, and M. Oku, "Spontaneous acute subdural haematoma and intracerebral haemorrhage in patient with HELLP syndrome: case report," *Acta Neurochirurgica*, vol. 151, no. 12, pp. 1689–1692, 2009.

[4] F. Servadei, "Prognostic factors in severely head injured adult patients with acute subdural haematoma's," *Acta Neurochirurgica*, vol. 139, no. 4, pp. 279–285, 1997.

[5] C. G. Ryan, R. E. Thompson, N. R. Temkin, P. K. Crane, R. G. Ellenbogen, and J. G. Elmore, "Acute traumatic subdural hematoma: current mortality and functional outcomes in adult patients at a Level I trauma center," *Journal of Trauma and Acute Care Surgery*, vol. 73, no. 5, pp. 1348–1353, 2012.

[6] R. K. Koç, H. Akdemir, I. S. Öktem, M. Meral, and A. Menkü, "Acute subdural hematoma: outcome and outcome prediction," *Neurosurgical Review*, vol. 20, no. 4, pp. 239–244, 1997.

# 60

# A Tuboovarian Abscess Associated with a Ruptured Spleen

### Jennifer S. Li and Johnathan Michael Sheele

*Department of Emergency Medicine, University Hospitals Case Medical Center and Case Western Reserve University, 11100 Euclid Avenue, B-517, Cleveland, OH 44139, USA*

Correspondence should be addressed to Jennifer S. Li; jennifer.li@uhhospitals.org

Academic Editor: Aristomenis K. Exadaktylos

We report the first case of a tuboovarian abscess complicated by a ruptured spleen. Our patient was a 27-year-old female with human immunodeficiency virus (HIV) who presented to the emergency department (ED) with complaints of urinary symptoms and diarrhea. After being diagnosed with a tuboovarian abscess (TOA), she received antibiotics and was admitted to the gynecology service. Shortly thereafter she developed hemorrhagic shock, necessitating a splenectomy and salpingooophorectomy from a ruptured spleen.

## 1. Introduction

A TOA is an inflammatory mass involving the fallopian tube and ovary. It is one of the most common causes of a pelvic mass in reproductive age women, with approximately 66,000 cases in the United States annually [1]. Risk factors for TOA include multiple sexual partners, not using contraceptives, and a history of pelvic inflammatory disease (PID) [2]. Up to 46% of patients with TOAs report a prior history of PID, and TOA is a complication of 15% of patients with PID [3, 4].

TOA can be a potentially life-threatening condition leading to sepsis or a ruptured abscess, with 15% of cases requiring aggressive medical and surgical intervention [1]. In postmenopausal women, TOAs have been associated with a high risk of malignancy [5]. Other possible complications of tuboovarian abscesses include infertility, ectopic pregnancy, pelvic thrombophlebitis, chronic pelvic pain, and ovarian vein thrombosis [1].

We report a case of a surgically confirmed tuboovarian abscess in a HIV-positive female with an intrauterine device (IUD) who presented to the ED with urinary symptoms and diarrhea. A spontaneously ruptured spleen leading to hemorrhagic shock and an emergent splenectomy and salpingooophorectomy complicated her inpatient clinical course. A ruptured spleen previously has not been reported as a complication of a TOA.

## 2. Case Presentation

We present a case of a G1P1001 27-year-old female with HIV on highly active antiretroviral therapy (HAART) with an unknown CD4 count and an undetectable viral load who had a single episode of gonorrhea treated nine years ago. She had a Mirena intrauterine device (IUD) placed several years ago and was in a year-long monogamous relationship with a female partner. The patient presented for her first ED visit with complaints of dysuria, abdominal pain, and constipation. She was diagnosed with a urinary tract infection and prescribed seven days of double-strength trimethoprim/sulfamethoxazole before being discharged home. She presented to our ED one month later for her second visit with complaints of dysuria, urinary frequency, and diarrhea. She reported nonbloody diarrhea and intermittent, bilateral abdominal, and lower back pains. In the ED, the patient's temperature was 38.7°C. Her abdomen was diffusely tender with no guarding or CVA tenderness. Pelvic exam revealed white vaginal discharge but no cervical motion or adnexal tenderness. Her urine pregnancy test was negative. Her urinalysis showed 1+ leukocyte esterase but no nitrites, and microscopic urinalysis showed 3 white blood cells, 2 squamous cells, and 4+ bacteria. The patient had a leukocytosis of $16.1 \times 10^3$, but her hepatic function panel and lipase were normal. Wet prep was negative for *Trichomonas vaginalis*,

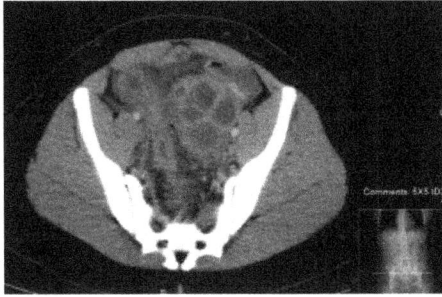

FIGURE 1: CT scan showing a large multicystic left ovarian mass measuring 6 × 9 cm.

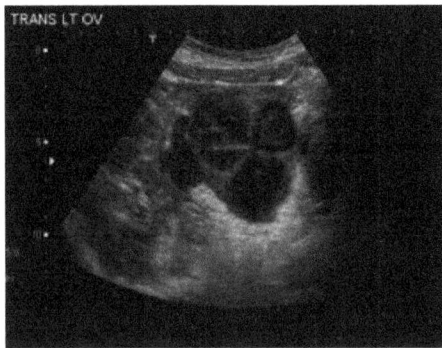

FIGURE 2: Ultrasound image showing large, complex cystic mass in the left adnexa measuring 5.9 × 8.4 × 5.5 cm in dimensions.

clue cells, or yeast. A computed tomography (CT) scan of the abdomen and pelvis with intravenous (IV) contrast showed a large, multicystic left ovarian mass measuring approximately 6 × 9 cm (Figure 1).

The patient was treated with IV doxycycline and ampicillin-sulbactam for a TOA and admitted on the gynecology service. During her hospitalization, she was managed with IV cefoxitin (2 grams every 6 hours), doxycycline (100 mg twice a day), and metronidazole (500 mg twice a day). Gonorrhea, chlamydia, hepatitis B, and syphilis tests were negative. After an infectious diseases consult she was discharged from hospital day #7 with a two-week course of oral ciprofloxacin and amoxicillin-clavulanic.

One month later the patient returned for a third ED visit complaining of abdominal pain and chills. The patient was afebrile with a white blood cell count of $10.5 \times 10^3$. Physical exam showed diffuse abdominal tenderness, guarding, and both cervical and bilateral adnexal tenderness. Wet mount was positive for Trichomonas vaginalis and clue cells. Pelvic ultrasound showed a complex cystic mass in the left adnexa measuring 5.9 × 8.4 × 5.5 cm (Figure 2) suggesting a persistent, left-sided TOA.

The patient was treated with intramuscular ceftriaxone (250 mg), IV doxycycline, and metronidazole in the ED and readmitted to the gynecology service where she was started on IV ampicillin (1 gram every 6 hours), clindamycin (900 mg every 8 hours), and gentamicin (400 mg every 24 hours). On hospital day #2, she underwent ultrasound (US) and

computed tomography- (CT-) guided transvaginal drainage of her left tuboovarian abscess by interventional radiology (IR), and 35 mL of frank pus was drained. The gram stain showed 4+ mixed bacteria with no predominant organism. Cultures from the drainage showed no growth aerobically or anaerobically.

On hospital day #4, the patient acutely decompensated with tachycardia, hypotension, anuria, abdominal pain, and a drop in her hemoglobin from 12 to 6 g/dL. She received an emergent exploratory laparotomy and was found to have massive hemoperitoneum due to a ruptured spleen. There was no evidence of short gastric vessels to the spleen. The patient required five units of packed red blood cells, four units of fresh frozen plasma, a splenectomy, and a left salpingooophorectomy. She was discharged home on postop day #6 with a two-week course of oral doxycycline and metronidazole.

The pathology report of the spleen noted acute inflammation involving the splenic capsule and focal evidence of remote hemorrhage and possible splenic tear in the hilar region. The operative report also noted inflammation in the upper abdomen. It is possible that infectious material from the TOA extended superiorly, causing adhesion with the spleen leading to the splenic rupture. There were no complications reported by IR during the US- and CT-guided drainage of the TOA.

## 3. Discussion

Wandering spleen is a rare condition involving laxity of the splenic ligament. It is found in less than 0.25% of the patients who require splenectomy [6]. One-third of patients with wandering spleen are children under the age of 10 [6]. In adults, a wandering spleen usually presents between the ages of 20 and 40 years and is ten times more common in females than males. Wandering spleen can be detected on ultrasound or CT, but there were no radiographic reports of the condition on her previous imaging studies [7]. The definitive management for a wandering spleen is splenectomy.

TOAs are most commonly polymicrobial aerobic, facultative, and anaerobic organisms including Escherichia coli, aerobic streptococci, Bacteroides fragilis, Prevotella, and anaerobic Peptostreptococcus. It is thought that normal vaginal flora or a sexually transmitted organism invades the fallopian tube epithelium, resulting in tissue damage and necrosis. This area of ischemia provides an environment for anaerobes to flourish. The bacteria produce an inflammatory response that spreads outside the fallopian tubes to the other adnexal structures. The body attempts to localize the inflammatory process by enclosing the abscess [1]. The abscess may cause abdominal or pelvic pain, fevers and chills, vaginal discharge, or change in bowel habits [1, 4]. Laboratory studies are nonspecific but may include a leukocytosis, elevated erythrocyte sedimentation rate, or elevated C-reactive protein [4]. Broad-spectrum antibiotics are effective in clearing 70% of TOAs. If patients do not respond to medical management within 48–72 hours then drainage or surgical procedures (hysterectomy or oophorectomy) should be considered [1].

Case reports have shown associations between patients with IUDs and unilateral TOAs [8]. Women infected with HIV are at increased risk of developing a TOA and are more likely to have a complicated clinical course compared with those uninfected with HIV. There is no data supporting early surgical intervention for HIV-infected women with a TOA [9].

US is the primary imaging modality for evaluating patients with suspected TOA. On pelvic ultrasound, TOAs appear as adnexal or retrouterine masses that may be cystic, solid, or complex in nature. Additionally, there may be septations, free fluid in the cul-de-sac, or indistinct uterine margins [10]. Ultrasound accurately identifies a mass in almost all of surgically confirmed TOAs [4].

The most common appearance of TOAs on CT is tubular or spherical cystic adnexal masses with internal septations, relatively uniform wall thickening, and loss of fat planes between the mass and adjacent organs [11]. The presence of internal gas bubbles is the most specific radiologic finding suggestive of TOA, but this is rarely seen [10].

Medical management with broad-spectrum antibiotic therapy is effective in resolving approximately 70% of all TOA cases. One study showed a 72% success rate in patients treated with clindamycin and an aminoglycoside ($n = 101$) compared to an 82% success rate in patients treated with cefoxitin or cefotetan and doxycycline ($n = 62$), but the differences were not statistically significant [1]. Other published studies have also supported the safety and use of these two antibiotic regimens in treatment of TOAs.

Penicillin-based antibiotic therapy is less efficacious in the treatment of TOAs compared with alternative regimens. One study showed only a 42% response rate in patients with TOAs treated with penicillin and aminoglycoside [12]. Ampicillin, which was used in our patient, occasionally is added to antibiotic regimens containing aminoglycoside and either clindamycin or metronidazole to provide sufficient coverage against enterococci. The use of metronidazole, which has bactericidal activity against anaerobes, is less studied in the management of TOAs. If patients do not respond to medical management within 48–72 hours, drainage or surgical procedures (such as hysterectomy or oophorectomy) should be considered [1].

Interventional radiology in the management of TOAs is increasingly being used. A retrospective study in California showed a steady increase in the proportion of hospitalizations associated with drainage procedures, with an increase from 2.6% in 1991 to 7.6% in 2001 [13]. In one study, a combination of antibiotic therapy and ultrasound-guided percutaneous drainage of TOAs was found to be successful in 95% of patients [14]. Transvaginal drainage of TOAs has been shown to be effective with limited complications. The use of either percutaneous or transvaginal drainage of TOAs decreases the need for surgical intervention and prevents associated surgical complications.

Some studies have demonstrated that more aggressive treatment with early drainage of TOAs can improve patient outcome and decrease morbidity, length of hospital stay, and cost. A randomized controlled study of 40 patients by Perez-Medina et al. found that 90% of patients who received a combination of antibiotics and early transvaginal drainage of an unruptured TOA responded successfully to treatment. In contrast, 65% of patients in the control group who received only antibiotic treatment had a favorable outcome [15]. A retrospective study of 302 cases by Gjelland et al. looked at patients who underwent combined antibiotic treatment and transvaginal drainage of a TOA. It found that 93% of the patients did not need surgery or have major complications [16]. While the drainage of TOAs can be effective, up to 25% of all patients with a TOA may still require surgical intervention [1].

A TOA's size helps dictate management and clinical care. A retrospective study by DeWitt et al. found that TOAs with a maximum diameter greater than 8 cm were associated with a higher risk of complications, including increased need for drainage or surgery when compared to smaller abscesses (35% versus 9%, resp., $p < 0.01$) [17]. The study showed a 43% failure rate when only medical management was used for abscesses >8 cm [17]. A study by Reed et al. showed a 35% failure rate for abscesses between 7 and 9 cm and a 60% failure rate for abscesses ≥10 cm [3]. Every 1 cm increase in abscess size has been associated with an increase in hospital stay by 0.4 days per average length of hospitalization of $4.9 \pm 1.6$ days [17]. There was no difference between the average lengths of hospital stay in patients with TOAs who required readmission within ninety days when compared to those who were not readmitted [13].

We report a complicated case of a TOA requiring percutaneous drainage after failing conservative management with antibiotics. The patient suffered a ruptured spleen leading to hemorrhagic shock and splenectomy and salpingooophorectomy.

## Conflict of Interests

The authors declare that there is no conflict of interests regarding the publication of this paper.

## References

[1] H. C. Wiesenfeld and R. L. Sweet, "Progress in the management of tuboovarian abscesses," *Clinical Obstetrics and Gynecology*, vol. 36, no. 2, pp. 433–444, 1993.

[2] A. E. Washington, S. O. Aral, P. Wølner-Hanssen, D. A. Grimes, and K. K. Holmes, "Assessing risk for pelvic inflammatory disease and its sequelae," *The Journal of the American Medical Association*, vol. 266, no. 18, pp. 2581–2586, 1991.

[3] S. D. Reed, D. V. Landers, and R. L. Sweet, "Antibiotic treatment of tuboovarian abscess: comparison of broad-spectrum $\beta$-lactam agents versus clindamycin-containing regimens," *American Journal of Obstetrics and Gynecology*, vol. 164, no. 6, part 1, pp. 1556–1562, 1991.

[4] D. V. Landers and R. L. Sweet, "Tubo-ovarian abscess: contemporary approach to management," *Reviews of Infectious Diseases*, vol. 5, no. 5, pp. 876–884, 1983.

[5] M. Hoffman, K. Molpus, W. S. Roberts, G. H. Lyman, and D. Cavanagh, "Tubo-ovarian abscess: contemporary approach to management," *Reviews of Infectious Diseases*, vol. 5, no. 5, pp. 876–884, 1983.

[6] A. Ben Ely, E. Seguier, G. Lotan, S. Strauss, and G. Gayer, "Familial wandering spleen: a first instance," *Journal of Pediatric Surgery*, vol. 43, no. 5, pp. e23–e25, 2008.

[7] A. A. Nemcek Jr., F. H. Miller, and S. W. Fitzgerald, "Acute torsion of a wandering spleen: diagnosis by CT and duplex Doppler and color flow sonography," *American Journal of Roentgenology*, vol. 157, no. 2, pp. 307–309, 1991.

[8] M. Y. Dawood and S. J. Birnbaum, "Unilateral tubo-ovarian abscess and intrauterine contraceptive device," *Obstetrics and Gynecology*, vol. 46, no. 4, pp. 429–432, 1975.

[9] C. R. Cohen, S. Sinei, M. Reilly et al., "Effect of human immunodeficiency virus type 1 infection upon acute salpingitis: a laparoscopic study," *Journal of Infectious Diseases*, vol. 178, no. 5, pp. 1352–1358, 1998.

[10] A. C. Wilbur, R. I. Aizenstein, and T. E. Napp, "CT findings in tuboovarian abscess," *American Journal of Roentgenology*, vol. 158, no. 3, pp. 575–579, 1992.

[11] J. H. Ellis, I. R. Francis, M. Rhodes, N. M. Kane, and K. Fechner, "CT findings in tuboovarian abscess," *Journal of Computer Assisted Tomography*, vol. 15, no. 4, pp. 589–592, 1991.

[12] L. R. Manara, "Management of tubo-ovarian abscess," *Journal of the American Osteopathic Association*, vol. 81, no. 7, pp. 476–480, 1982.

[13] C. K. Paik, L. E. Waetjen, G. Xing, J. Dai, and R. L. Sweet, "Hospitalizations for pelvic inflammatory disease and tuboovarian abscess," *Obstetrics and Gynecology*, vol. 107, no. 3, pp. 611–616, 2006.

[14] N. J. Worthen and J. E. Gunning, "Percutaneous drainage of pelvic abscesses: management of the tubo-ovarian abscess," *Journal of Ultrasound in Medicine*, vol. 5, no. 10, pp. 551–556, 1986.

[15] T. Perez-Medina, M. A. Huertas, and J. M. Bajo, "Early ultrasound-guided transvaginal drainage of tubo-ovarian abscesses: a randomized study," *Ultrasound in Obstetrics and Gynecology*, vol. 7, no. 6, pp. 435–438, 1996.

[16] K. Gjelland, E. Ekerhovd, and S. Granberg, "Transvaginal ultrasound-guided aspiration for treatment of tubo-ovarian abscess: a study of 302 cases," *American Journal of Obstetrics & Gynecology*, vol. 193, no. 4, pp. 1323–1330, 2005.

[17] J. DeWitt, A. Reining, J. E. Allsworth, and J. F. Peipert, "Tuboovarian abscesses: is size associated with duration of hospitalization & complications?" *Obstetrics and Gynecology International*, vol. 2010, Article ID 847041, 5 pages, 2010.

# 61

# Retained Products of Conception: An Atypical Presentation Diagnosed Immediately with Bedside Emergency Ultrasound

**Kristin Adkins,[1] Joseph Minardi,[2] Erin Setzer,[2] and Debra Williams[2]**

[1]*West Virginia University School of Medicine, Morgantown, WV, USA*
[2]*Department of Emergency Medicine, West Virginia University, 7413B HSS, 1 Medical Center Drive, Morgantown, WV 26506, USA*

Correspondence should be addressed to Joseph Minardi; jminardi@hsc.wvu.edu

Academic Editor: Aristomenis K. Exadaktylos

*Background.* Retained products of conception is an important diagnosis to consider in patients presenting with postpartum complaints. Bedside ultrasound is a rapid, accurate, noninvasive modality to evaluate these patients. *Objective.* To report an atypical case of retained products of conception diagnosed with bedside ultrasound in the emergency department. *Case Report.* A 27-year-old female who was 1-month postpartum presented with vaginal bleeding, pelvic pain, and no fever. At the time of initial H&P, bedside ultrasound revealed echogenic material within the endometrial cavity with blood flow seen by color Doppler consistent with retained products of conception. The bedside ultrasound rapidly narrowed the differential and allowed a definitive diagnosis immediately. Ob/Gyn was consulted and dilation and curettage was performed in the operating room. *Conclusions.* Retained products of conception is an important diagnosis for the emergency physician to consider in at-risk patients. The sonographic findings are easily obtained and interpreted by emergency physicians. Earlier diagnosis of this disease process should lead to more focused patient evaluations and management.

## 1. Introduction

Postpartum complaints are common in the emergency department. Retained products of conception (RPOC) is one of the most important differential considerations in these patients. RPOC should be suspected if a postpartum patient presents with symptoms of endometritis or hemorrhage, specifically pelvic pain, vaginal discharge or bleeding, and possibly fever [1]. The presentation can be variable. Traditionally, ultrasound is ordered to evaluate these complaints, but radiology ultrasound is frequently only available during limited hours. The common application of bedside ultrasound by emergency physicians should translate well to evaluating this diagnosis. The typical sonographic findings are relatively easy to identify. Emergency physicians should be capable of recognizing these findings leading to more rapid diagnosis, decreased use of other resources, and more expeditious management. Although this diagnosis is commonly made by obstetrician/gynecologists and radiologists, to the authors' knowledge, there have been no descriptions of this diagnosis and its findings by emergency physicians using bedside ultrasound.

## 2. Case Report

A 27-year-old female presented to the emergency department with excessive vaginal bleeding and an episode of syncope. She was approximately one-month postpartum from a vaginal delivery. She reported heavy bleeding during delivery but had been asymptomatic until three days prior to presentation when she noticed some vaginal spotting. Approximately 30 minutes prior to presentation, she experienced a syncopal episode and reported heavy vaginal bleeding associated with mild suprapubic pain. She denied other symptoms. Her past medical and surgical histories were otherwise unremarkable.

Initial vital signs were BP 118/70, pulse 103, respirations 18, temp. 36.6, and pulse ox 100%. On physical examination, she appeared anxious and pale with small abrasion over the bridge of her nose. Her abdomen was tender to deep palpation over the pubic area, and her uterus was not

(a)                                                                (b)

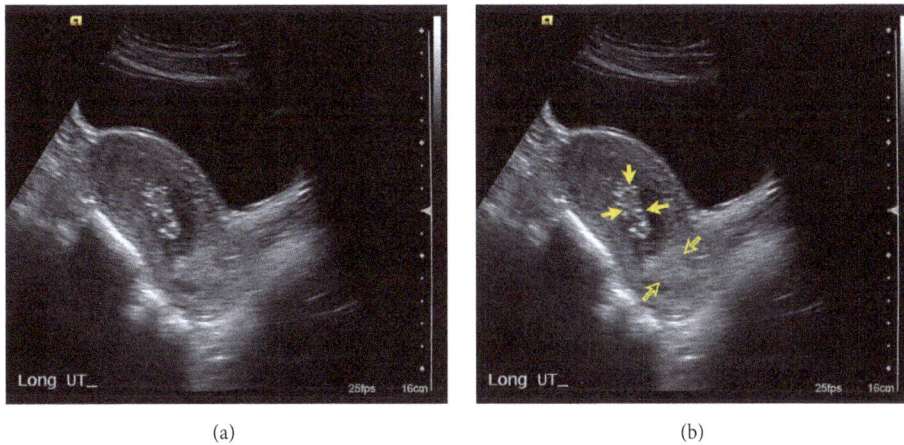

Figure 1: (a) *TA Sag Uterus*. Transabdominal sagittal view of the uterus shows thickened, heterogeneous, and hyperechoic material within the endometrial cavity. There is also echogenic material located in the lower uterine segment. (b) Opaque arrows indicate heterogeneous echogenic endometrial tissue. Open arrows indicate echogenic material in the lower uterine segment near the cervical os.

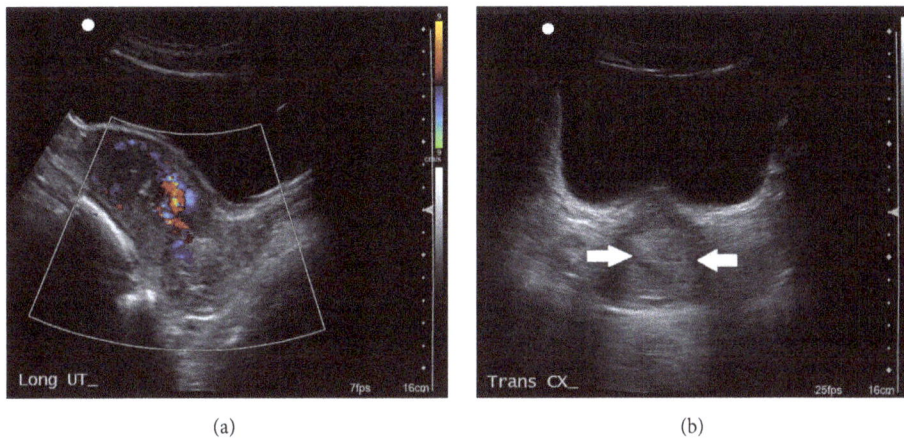

(a)                                                                (b)

Figure 2: (a) *TA Sag Uterus, Color*. Transabdominal uterus showing blood flow within the echogenic intraendometrial tissue, making retained products highly likely. (b) *TA Trans Uterus*. Transabdominal transverse view of the uterus showing echogenic material within the lower endometrial cavity (arrows).

palpable. Pelvic exam revealed blood and clots in the vagina, initially occluding the view of the cervix. The blood returned after suctioning. Cervical os was closed. The remainder of her physical examination was unremarkable.

Differential diagnoses included retained products of conception, uterine rupture, ectopic pregnancy, spontaneous abortion, and dysfunctional uterine bleeding.

Bedside transabdominal ultrasound was performed by the emergency physician revealing heterogeneous and echogenic material within the endometrial cavity (as seen in Figure 1). Internal blood flow was demonstrated by color Doppler (as seen in Figure 2). The adnexa were unremarkable and there was no significant intraperitoneal free fluid. These findings were felt consistent with retained products of conception. Serum human chorionic gonadotropin level was negative and hemoglobin returned normal.

Ob/Gyn was consulted and the patient was taken for dilation and curettage, where placental tissue was removed from the cervical os and the uterus. Pathology confirmed that the

tissue was chorionic villi and decidua. The patient tolerated the procedure well and had an unremarkable postoperative course.

## 3. Discussion

Retained products of conception is one of the most common reasons for readmission postpartum [2]. RPOC may be found after 1% of term pregnancies [3]. In one study, the median period from delivery to presentation was 11 days [2]. The diagnosis of RPOC should be considered in postpartum women who present with vaginal bleeding, fever, foul-smelling discharge, and abdominal or pelvic pain. This presentation is nonspecific, and clinical diagnosis alone has a high false-positive rate, up to 40% [4]. Dilation and curettage, the treatment of choice for RPOC, carries a risk of serious complications including uterine bleeding, perforation, infection, adhesions, and infertility. Because of this, it is important to rule out other diagnoses such as ectopic pregnancy, uterine rupture, or hematometra, to avoid the complications of unnecessary D&C. Ultrasonography is the diagnostic test of choice for evaluation of febrile postpartum patients due to its safety, accessibility, and cost benefits. However, the availability of radiology can be limited in emergency departments and the common use of bedside ultrasound by emergency physicians should translate well to this application. Typical sonographic findings include hyperechoic, intrauterine material with internal vascularity observed with color Doppler and high-velocity, low-resistance flow by spectral Doppler. Blood products may have a similar echogenic appearance but no internal flow [5]. According to Kamaya et al., the presence of any vascularity has a 96% positive predictive value for RPOC [6]. If RPOC is suspected, uterine evacuation may be necessary. This can be accomplished with sharp or suction curettage. If the bedside US exam is equivocal, antibiotics and close monitoring may be adequate. If there is an excellent response to antibiotics in the first 24 hours, surgical intervention may be avoided [7].

In summary, we report a case of retained products of conception, presenting atypically, rapidly and accurately diagnosed at the bedside by an emergency physician using clinical ultrasound. The clinical and sonographic findings are ones that all emergency physicians should recognize. Clinicians with a baseline skill set in clinical ultrasound can readily recognize the findings of this diagnosis.

## 4. Why an Emergency Physician Should Know about This

Retained POC is one of the more important diagnoses to be considered in the symptomatic postpartum ED patient. The typical sonographic findings are relatively straightforward and can be recognized by emergency physicians with existing skills in bedside ultrasound of the female pelvis. Making this diagnosis at the bedside may expedite management and limit the need for other investigations and consultations, particularly when radiology ultrasound is not immediately available.

## Conflict of Interests

The authors are not aware of any personal or financial conflict of interests that are associated with this study.

## References

[1] S. M. Durfee, M. C. Frates, A. Luong, and C. B. Benson, "The sonographic and color Doppler features of retained products of conception," *Journal of Ultrasound in Medicine*, vol. 24, no. 9, pp. 1181–1186, 2005.

[2] R. Matijevic, M. Knezevic, O. Grgic, and L. Zlodi-Hrsak, "Diagnostic accuracy of sonographic and clinical parameters in the prediction of retained products of conception," *Journal of Ultrasound in Medicine*, vol. 28, no. 3, pp. 295–299, 2009.

[3] I. Wolman, E. Altman, G. Faith et al., "Combined clinical and ultrasonographic work-up for the diagnosis of retained products of conception," *Fertility and Sterility*, vol. 92, no. 3, pp. 1162–1164, 2009.

[4] O. Sadan, A. Golan, O. Girtler et al., "Role of sonography in the diagnosis of retained products of conception," *Journal of Ultrasound in Medicine*, vol. 23, no. 3, pp. 371–374, 2004.

[5] S. L. Laifer-Narin, E. Kwak, H. Kim, E. M. Hecht, and J. H. Newhouse, "Multimodality imaging of the postpartum or posttermination uterus: evaluation using ultrasound, computed tomography, and magnetic resonance imaging," *Current Problems in Diagnostic Radiology*, vol. 43, no. 6, pp. 374–385, 2014.

[6] A. Kamaya, I. Petrovitch, B. Chen, C. E. Frederick, and R. B. Jeffrey, "Retained products of conception: spectrum of color Doppler findings," *Journal of Ultrasound in Medicine*, vol. 28, no. 8, pp. 1031–1041, 2009.

[7] D. A. Carusi, *Retained Products of Conception*, J. Steinauer and S. J. Falk, Eds., Waltham, Mass, USA, UpToDate, 2015.

# 62

# Diagnosis of Mondor's Disease in the Emergency Department with Bedside Ultrasound

**J. Michael O'Neal,[1] Erik Castleberg,[1] and Vi Am Dinh[1,2]**

[1]Department of Emergency Medicine, Loma Linda University, 11234 Anderson Street, A-108, Loma Linda, CA 92354, USA
[2]Division of Critical Care, Department of Internal Medicine, Loma Linda University, 11234 Anderson Street, A-108, Loma Linda, CA 92354, USA

Correspondence should be addressed to Vi Am Dinh; vadinh@llu.edu

Academic Editor: Michael J. Ramdass

Mondor's disease is a rare condition characterized by a superficial thrombophlebitis that can occur in the thoracoabdominal and genital areas. Findings with ultrasound in penile Mondor's disease are readily measurable: a noncompressible penile vein without flow and absence of tears of the corpus cavernosum or tunica albuginea, hematoma, or evidence of fracture of the penis. We present a case of Mondor's disease, diagnosed with bedside ultrasound, in the emergency department. Ultrasonography is readily available within the emergency department, and we suggest its use in aiding diagnosis of genitourinary disorders such as Mondor's disease.

## 1. Introduction

Mondor's disease is a relatively uncommon disease, first described by Mondor in 1939 referring to the superficial thrombophlebitis in the thoracoabdominal wall [1]. Manifestations of the disease have subsequently been noted on the penis, groin, axilla, antecubital fossa, abdominal wall, and posterior cervical region [1].

The true incidence of Mondor's disease is unknown, but one series showed an incidence of 18 of 1296 (1.39%) patients in a sexually transmitted disease clinic over a 12-year period [2]. The study demonstrated an association with several sexual behaviors in the patients, including a history of vigorous sex after a period of abstinence in 17 of the 18 patients, which is consistent with the presentation of the patient presented here.

## 2. Case Presentation

A 24-year-old previously healthy male presented to the emergency department complaining of five days of painful penile swelling after experiencing a "popping" sensation during intercourse. The swelling was described as being at the base of the penis and extending down the shaft. The patient reported intermittent swelling of the penile shaft lasting between four and five days for the past three to four months. He described vigorous intercourse preceding these events. The patient otherwise denied trauma, dysuria, hematuria, difficulty with erection, multiple sexual partners, or attempted intercourse since the "popping" sensation was noted.

Upon presentation, the patient was normotensive (138/83) with a normal heart (100) and respiratory (18) rate and was afebrile (36.8°C). Physical examination revealed a well-developed male in no distress without palpable hernias. Genitourinary exam revealed an uncircumcised penis and a palpable cord on the right dorsal side of the penis. Mild tenderness of the penile shaft was noted and testicular exam revealed no swelling or pain on palpation.

Ultrasound of the penis using an Ultrasonix Sonix-TOUCH (Vancouver, British Columbia) machine, with a high frequency linear probe (L15-5) on the small parts setting, demonstrated a noncompressible, hypoechoic right lateral superficial dorsal vein (Figures 1 and 2). The uncompressed vein did not exhibit a reduction in caliber compared to additional superficial dorsal vein identified. Color Doppler ultrasonography demonstrated a lack of flow compared to the deep dorsal vein and dorsal arteries (Figure 3). The arteries and soft tissues of the penis were otherwise unremarkable.

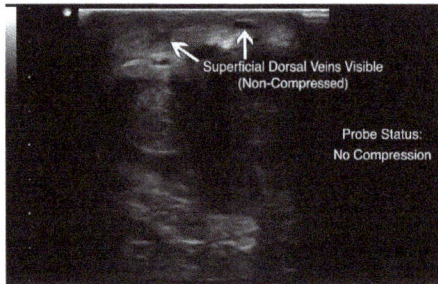

FIGURE 1: Noncompressed view of superficial dorsal veins with hypoechoic right sided vessel, suggesting superficial thrombophlebitis (depth set at 4 cm).

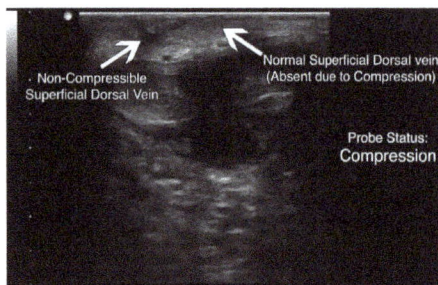

FIGURE 2: Compressed view of superficial dorsal veins showing noncompressible right superficial dorsal vein (depth set at 4 cm).

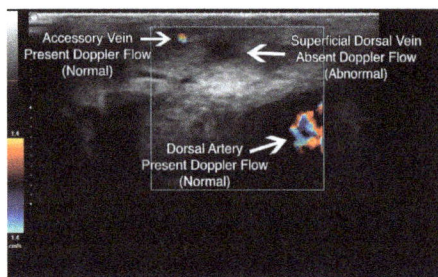

FIGURE 3: Color Doppler ultrasonography showing absent flow in right superficial vein when compared to accessory vein and dorsal artery, which both demonstrate normal flow (depth set at 2 cm).

Urology was consulted, and the patient was diagnosed with superficial thrombophlebitis (Mondor's disease) of the right lateral superficial dorsal vein without evidence of penile fracture. Conservative management with NSAIDs was recommended with outpatient follow-up to ensure the resolution of symptoms, which was expected to take up to 4 weeks. The patient was contacted by phone 8 weeks later and reports his symptoms had resolved within 4 weeks with ibuprofen treatment and cessation of intercourse.

## 3. Discussion

Ultrasound has been shown to have consistent features in Mondor's disease, including noncompressible veins and lack of venous color Doppler flow [1, 3, 4]. Other signs of thrombus include vein lumen size and thrombus echogenicity

where a chronic thrombus has a smaller lumen size and increased echogenicity (i.e., hyperechoic) [5]. In this particular case, the vessel was noncompressible, lacked venous color Doppler flow, had a normal size lumen, and had decreased echogenicity (i.e., hypoechoic). These constellations of findings are consistent with an acute phase of Mondor's disease. These described findings are also found with Mondor's disease in other areas, such as the breast [1, 6]. Hye et al. additionally found weak flow and high resistance in nearby arteries using pulsed Doppler in examining Mondor's disease of the penis [7].

Mondor's disease can be diagnosed clinically with the findings of a palpable cord in the affected area without other significant findings beyond swelling [1, 3]. However, the disease is rare enough that many emergency providers may have some hesitancy in diagnosing the condition without supporting diagnostic evidence given that penile fracture is also an emergent condition in the differential for penile trauma. Kervancioglu et al. demonstrated the findings that would support the diagnosis of penile fracture on ultrasound, such as tears of the corpus cavernosum and tunica albuginea, as well as the presence of hematomas. Vascular injuries to the superficial dorsal vein, deep dorsal vein, dorsal artery, and deep cavernous artery may also be seen sonographically in penile fractures [8]. The absence of these additional sonographic findings can be used by the emergency providers to support the benign diagnosis, such as in this case.

Further imaging studies have been used for the diagnosis of superficial thrombophlebitis. For the cases of the disease occurring in the breast, mammography is commonly used, showing densities along the affected area [1, 9]. MRI angiography can also demonstrate thrombus and be used to evaluate extension of the thrombus, even into areas difficult or impossible to image with ultrasound or presence of hematoma; however, MRI is expensive and adds little to the clinical management of the disease [10]. Belleflamme et al. have suggested ultrasound be the confirmatory imaging modality of choice [11].

A case series by Al-Mwalad et al. [3] covered 25 patients over a six-year period with Mondor's disease of the penis with symptoms of feeling of tension in various locations of the penis without pain [3]. Improvement with conservative treatment was shown in 23 of 25 patients, with the remainder requiring surgical intervention, demonstrating that Mondor's disease of the penis is a relatively benign condition. Causative factors for Mondor's disease have not been definitively identified, though trauma, tumors, and surgery are considered risk factors [3]. One case study suggested urogenital infection and muscular strain as possible causes [12]. Immunohistochemistry demonstrated thrombophlebitis as the underlying pathology in most cases of Mondor's disease with occasional lymphangitis as a cause [13].

Proper identification of Mondor's disease assisted by ultrasonography allows for proper management of the disease. Patients diagnosed in the emergency department should be given proper follow-up, which may include testing for protein C and protein S or antithrombin III deficiencies [3], evaluation for other thrombophilic conditions [11], and possible search for occult malignancy [1, 11]. Treatment in the interim should consist of NSAIDs and cessation of inter-course [1, 3].

## 4. Conclusion

Ultrasound has been shown to be an effective means of supporting the diagnosis of Mondor's disease of the penis. Findings on ultrasound are a noncompressible penile vein without flow and absence of tears of the corpus cavernosum or tunica albuginea, hematoma, or evidence of fracture of the penis. Its use has been validated and accepted by specialties outside of the emergency department. Given the availability and low cost of the modality within the ED, familiarity with the sonographic findings can lead to the fact that emergency providers are able to quickly diagnose this rare condition at bedside with relative certainty.

## Conflict of Interests

None of the authors identify any conflict of interests.

## Acknowledgment

The authors acknowledge the Loma Linda Emergency Medicine Research Division.

## References

[1] H. Álvarez-Garrido, A. A. Garrido-Ríos, C. Sanz-Muñoz, and A. Miranda-Romero, "Mondor's disease," *Clinical and Experimental Dermatology*, vol. 34, no. 7, pp. 753–756, 2009.

[2] B. Kumar, T. Narang, B. D. Radotra, and S. Gupta, "Mondor's disease of penis: a forgotten disease," *Sexually Transmitted Infections*, vol. 81, no. 6, pp. 480–482, 2005.

[3] M. Al-Mwalad, H. Loertzer, A. Wicht, and P. Fornara, "Subcutaneous penile vein thrombosis (Penile Mondor's Disease): pathogenesis, diagnosis, and therapy," *Urology*, vol. 67, no. 3, pp. 586–588, 2006.

[4] A. Ozel, F. Issayev, S. M. Erturk, A. M. Halefoglu, and Z. Karpat, "Sonographic diagnosis of penile mondor's disease associated with absence of a dorsal penile artery," *Journal of Clinical Ultrasound*, vol. 38, no. 5, pp. 263–266, 2010.

[5] V. F. Tapson, B. A. Carroll, B. L. Davidson et al., "The diagnostic approach to acute venous thromboembolism. Clinical practice guideline. American Thoracic Society," *The American Journal of Respiratory and Critical Care Medicine*, vol. 160, no. 3, pp. 1043–1066, 1999.

[6] B. Yanik, I. Conkbayir, Ö. Öner, and B. Hekimoğlu, "Imaging findings in Mondor's disease," *Journal of Clinical Ultrasound*, vol. 31, no. 2, pp. 103–107, 2003.

[7] Y. H. Hye, J. C. Dong, W. K. Kum, and M. H. Cheol, "Pulsed and color Doppler sonographic findings of penile Mondor's disease," *Korean Journal of Radiology*, vol. 9, no. 2, pp. 179–181, 2008.

[8] S. Kervancioglu, A. Ozkur, and M. M. Bayram, "Color Doppler sonographic findings in penile fracture," *Journal of Clinical Ultrasound*, vol. 33, no. 1, pp. 38–42, 2005.

[9] A. Adeniji-Sofoluwe and O. Afolabi, "Mondor's disease: classical imaging findings in the breast," *BMJ Case Reports*, vol. 2011, 2011.

[10] R. Boscolo-Berto, M. Iafrate, G. Casarrubea, and V. Ficarra, "Magnetic resonance angiography findings of penile Mondor's disease," *Journal of Magnetic Resonance Imaging*, vol. 30, no. 2, pp. 407–410, 2009.

[11] M. Belleflamme, A. Penaloza, M. Thoma, P. Hainaut, and F. Thys, "Mondor disease: a case report in ED," *The American Journal of Emergency Medicine*, vol. 30, no. 7, pp. 1325.e1–1325.e3, 2012.

[12] L. Girardi, "Mondor's disease affecting the superficial dorsal vein of the penis," *VASA—Journal of Vascular Diseases*, vol. 41, no. 3, pp. 233–235, 2012.

[13] A. Ichinose, A. Fukunaga, H. Terashi et al., "Objective recognition of vascular lesions in Mondor's disease by immunohistochemistry," *Journal of the European Academy of Dermatology and Venereology*, vol. 22, no. 2, pp. 168–173, 2008.

# Permissions

# List of Contributors

**Francesca Gatti, Marco Spagnoli, Simone Maria Zerbi and Mario Landriscina**
Anaesthesia and Intensive Care Unit 2, Sant'Anna Hospital, San Fermo della Battaglia, 22020 Como, Italy

**Dario Colombo**
Anaesthesia and Intensive Care Unit 1, Sant'Anna Hospital, San Fermo della Battaglia, 22020 Como, Italy

**Fulvio Kette**
Bergamo 118 Operative Dispatch Center, Azienda Regionale Emergenza Urgenza (AREU), Via Campanini 6, 20124 Milan, Italy

**Christian T. Braun, David S. Srivastava and Aristomenis K. Exadaktylos**
Department of Emergency Medicine, Inselspital, University Hospital Bern, Freiburgstrasse, 3010 Bern, Switzerland

**Bianca Maria Engelhardt**
Department of Surgery, Inselspital, University Hospital Bern, Freiburgstrasse, 3010 Bern, Switzerland

**Gregor Lindner**
Department of Respiratory and Critical Care Medicine, OttoWagner Hospital, Baumgartner Höhe 1, 1140 Vienna, Austria

**Ryan Yu**
Department of Pathology and Molecular Medicine, McMaster University, Hamilton, ON, Canada L8S 4L8

**Melanie Ferri**
Department of Diagnostic Imaging, Juravinski Hospital and Cancer Centre and McMaster University, Hamilton, ON, Canada L8V 5C2

**Shalini Koppisetty and Alton G. Smith**
Department of Radiology, Beaumont Health System, Grosse Pointe, MI 48230, USA

**Ravneet K. Dhillon**
Emergency Medicine, Henry Ford Health System, West Bloomfield, MI 48322, USA

**Emily Charlotte Ironside and Andrew James Hotchen**
Oxford University Hospitals, Headley Way, Headington, Oxford OX3 9DU, UK

**M. Yger, C. Zavanone and Y. Samson**
Unité Neurovasculaire, Hôpital de la Pitie-Salpetrière, APHP, 75013 Paris, France
Université Pierre et Marie Curie, 75006 Paris, France
Service de Rééducation Neurologique, Hôpital de la Pitie-Salpetrière, APHP, 75013 Paris, France

**F. Clarençon and S. Dupont**
Université Pierre et Marie Curie, 75006 Paris, France
Service de Rééducation Neurologique, Hôpital de la Pitie-Salpetrière, APHP, 75013 Paris, France
Neuroradiologie, Hôpital de la Pitie-Salpetrière, APHP, 75013 Paris, France
Service d'Épilpeptologie, Hôpital de la Pitie-Salpetrière, APHP, 75013 Paris, France

**L. Abdennour and W. Koubaa**
Unité de Réanimation Neurologique, Hôpital de la Pitie-Salpetrière, APHP, 75013 Paris, France

**Sarah White, Janna Welch and Lawrence H. Brown**
Dell School of Medicine, University of Texas at Austin, USA

**Birdal Yildirim, Ethem Acar and Halil Beydilli**
Department of Emergency Medicine, Muğla Sıtkı Koçman University Medical Faculty, Orhaniye Mahallesi Haluk Ozsoy Caddesi, 48000 Mugla, Turkey

**Ulku Karagoz and Omer Dogan Alatas**
Emergency Clinic, Muğla Sıtkı Koçman University Training and Investigation Hospital, Orhaniye Mahallesi Haluk Ozsoy Caddesi, 48000 Mugla, Turkey

**Emine Nese Yeniceri**
Department of Family Medicine, Muğla Sıtkı Koçman University Medical Faculty, Orhaniye Mahallesi Haluk Ozsoy Caddesi, 48000 Mugla, Turkey

**Ozgur Tanriverdi**
Department of Internal Medicine and Medical Oncology, Muğla Sıtkı Koçman University Medical Faculty, Orhaniye Mahallesi Haluk Ozsoy Caddesi, 48000 Mugla, Turkey

**Fükrü Kasap**
Clinic of Plastic and Reconstructive Surgery, Muğla Sıtkı Koçman University Training and Investigation Hospital, Orhaniye Mahallesi Haluk Ozsoy Caddesi, 48000 Mugla, Turkey

**Konstantinos Bouliaris, Grigorios Christodoulidis, Dimitrios Symeonidis, Alexandros Diamantis and Konstantinos Tepetes**
Surgical Department, University Hospital of Larissa, Mezurlo, 4110 Larissa, Greece

**Hassan Tahir and Vistasp Daruwalla**
Department of Internal Medicine, Temple University/ Conemaugh Memorial Hospital, 1086 Franklin Street, Johnstown, PA 15905, USA

**Basheer Tashtoush, Jonathan Schroeder, Roya Memarpour, Eduardo Oliveira, Anas Hadeh, Jose Ramirez and Laurence Smolley**
Department of Pulmonary and Critical Care Medicine, Cleveland Clinic Florida, Weston, FL, USA

**Michael Medina**
Department of Otolaryngology, Cleveland Clinic Florida, Weston, FL, USA

**Casey Chiu and Johnathan Michael Sheele**
Department of Emergency Medicine, University Hospitals Case Medical Center and Case Western Reserve University, Cleveland, OH 44106, USA

**Manan Parikh, Abhinav Agrawal, Braghadheeswar Thyagarajan and Sayee Sundar Alagusundaramoorthy**
Department of Internal Medicine, Monmouth Medical Center, Long Branch, NJ 07740, USA

**James Martin**
Department of Emergency Medicine, Monmouth Medical Center, Long Branch, NJ 07740, USA

**Carlo Brembilla, Luigi Andrea Lanterna, Emanuele Costi, Gianluigi Dorelli, Elena Moretti and Claudio Bernucci**
Department of Neurosurgery, Pope John XXIII Hospital, OMS Square No. 1, 24100 Bergamo, Italy

**Paolo Gritti**
Department of Anesthesia and Intensive Care, Pope John XXIII Hospital, OMS Square No. 1, 24100 Bergamo, Italy

**Christian T. Braun, Meret E. Ricklin, Aristomenis K. Exadaktylos and Carmen A. Pfortmueller**
Department of Emergency Medicine, Inselspital, University Hospital Bern, Freiburgstrasse 10, 3010 Bern, Switzerland
Department of General Anesthesiology, Intensive Care and Pain Management, Medical University of Vienna, Waehringerguertel 18-22, 1090 Vienna, Austria

**Andreina Pauli and Daniel Ott**
University Institute of Diagnostic, Interventional and Pediatric Radiology, Inselspital, University Hospital Bern, Freiburgstrasse 10, 3010 Bern, Switzerland

**Tuğba Atmaca Temrel, Alp Şener, Ferhat Eçme, Gül Pamukçu GünaydJn, Yavuz Otal and Gülhan Kurtoğlu Çelik**
Department of Emergency Medicine, Ankara Atatürk Training and Research Hospital, Üniversiteler Mahallesi Bilkent Caddesi No. 1, Çankaya, 06800 Ankara, Turkey

**Fervan Gökhan and Ayhan Özhasenekler**
Department of Emergency Medicine, Faculty of Medicine, Yildirim Beyazit University, Üniversiteler Mahallesi Bilkent Caddesi No. 1, Çankaya, 06800 Ankara, Turkey

**Eleni Paschou**
Department of Family Medicine, General Hospital of Pella, 58200 Edessa, Greece

**Eleni Gavriilaki and Asterios Kalaitzoglou**
Medical School, Aristotle University of Thessaloniki, 54124 Thessaloniki, Greece

**Maria Mourounoglou**
Department of General Surgery, General Hospital of Pella, 58200 Edessa, Greece

**Nikolaos Sabanis**
Nephrological Department, General Hospital of Pella, 58200 Edessa, Greece

**H. Ben Ghezala, S. Snouda, J. Ouali and M. Kaddour**
Teaching Department of Emergency and Intensive Care Medicine, Regional Hospital of Zaghouan, Street of Republic, 1100 Zaghouan, Tunisia

**N. Chaouali, I. Gana, A. Nouioui, I. Belwaer, W. Masri, D. Ben Salah, D. Amira, H. Ghorbal and A. Hedhili**
Research Laboratory of Toxicology-Environment LR12SP07, Laboratory of Toxicology, Center for Emergency Medical Assistance, Montfleury, 1008 Tunis, Tunisia

**Joshua Strommen**
Department of Emergency Medicine, Carl R Darnall Army Medical Center, 36000 Darnall Loop, Fort Hood, TX 76554, USA

**Farshad Shirazi**
Arizona Poison & Drug Information Center (APDIC), University of Arizona College of Pharmacy, Tucson, AZ 85721, USA
Arizona Emergency Medicine Research Center, University of Arizona College of Medicine, Tucson, AZ 85721, USA

**Gökhan Aksel, Tanju TaGyürek and Febnem Eren Çevik**
Umraniye Training and Research Hospital, Emergency Medicine Clinic, Istanbul, Turkey

**Özlem Güneysel and Ergül Kozan**
Dr. Lutfi Kirdar Kartal Education and Research Hospital, Emergency Medicine Clinic, Istanbul, Turkey

**Tolga Dinc, Selami Ilgaz Kayilioglu and Faruk Coskun**
Department of General Surgery, Ankara Numune Training and Research Hospital, Anafartalar Mah, Talatpasa Boulevard No. 5, Genel Cerrahi AD, 2. Kat B216, Altındağ, 06100 Ankara, Turkey

**Daniel Solomin, Stephen W. Borron and Susan H. Watts**
Department of Emergency Medicine, Paul Foster School of Medicine, Texas Tech University Health Sciences Center at El Paso, El Paso, TX 79905, USA

**Gultekin Gulbahar and Ahmet Gokhan Gundogdu**
Division of Thoracic Surgery, Dr. Nafiz Korez Sincan State Hospital, Ankara, Turkey

**Tevfik Kaplan and Serdar Han**
Department of Thoracic Surgery, Ufuk University School of Medicine, Ankara, Turkey

**Hatice Nurdan Baran**
Division of Anesthesiology and Reanimation, Dr. Nafiz Korez Sincan State Hospital, Ankara, Turkey

**Burak Kazanci**
Department of Neurosurgery, Ufuk University School of Medicine, Ankara, Turkey

**Bulent Kocer**
Division of Thoracic Surgery, Ankara Numune Teaching and Research Hospital, Ankara, Turkey

**T. Evans and M. Rocker**
Department of General Surgery, Royal Glamorgan Hospital, Llantrisant CF72 8XR, UK

**S. Roy**
Department of Orthopaedic Surgery, Royal Glamorgan Hospital, Llantrisant CF72 8XR, UK

**Ahmet Rencuzogullari, Kubilay Dalci and Orcun Yalav**
Department of General Surgery, Cukurova University Medical Faculty, 01330 Adana, Turkey

**M. Hedaiaty, N. Eizadi-Mood and A. M. Sabzghabaee**
Clinical Toxicology Department, Isfahan Clinical Toxicology Research Center, Noor Hospital, Isfahan University of Medical Sciences, Isfahan 81458-31451, Iran

**Eiji Mitate and Seiji Nakamura**
Section of Oral and Maxillofacial Oncology, Division of Maxillofacial Diagnostic and Surgical Sciences, Faculty of Dental Science, Kyushu University, 3-1-1 Maidashi, Higashi-ku, Fukuoka 812-8582, Japan
Emergency and Critical Care Center, Kyushu University Hospital, 3-1-1 Maidashi, Higashi-ku, Fukuoka 812-8582, Japan

**Kensuke Kubota, Rumi Inoue, Kenta Momii and Yoshihiko Maehara**
Emergency and Critical Care Center, Kyushu University Hospital, 3-1-1 Maidashi, Higashi-ku, Fukuoka 812-8582, Japan

**Kenji Ueki**
Department of Integrated Therapy for Chronic Kidney Disease, Faculty of Medical Sciences, Kyushu University, 3-1-1 Maidashi, Higashi-ku, Fukuoka 812-8582, Japan

**Ryosuke Inoue**
Special Patient Oral Care Unit, Kyushu University Hospital, 3-1-1 Maidashi, Higashi-ku, Fukuoka 812-8582, Japan

**Hiroshi Sugimori**
Cerebrovascular Center, Saga-Ken Medical Centre Koseikan, 400 Oaza Nakabaru, Kasemachi, Saga 840-8571, Japan

**Charles W. Hwang and F. Eike Flach**
Department of Emergency Medicine, University of Florida College of Medicine, 1329 SW16th Street, P.O. Box 100186, Gainesville, FL 32610-0186, USA

**Saileswar Goswami**
Department of Otolaryngology, Calcutta National Medical College, Kolkata, West Bengal 700014, India

**Choitali Goswami**
Department of General Emergency, Medical College, Kolkata, West Bengal 700073, India

**Thomas M. Nappe, Anthony M. Pacelli and Kenneth Katz**
Department of Emergency Medicine, Lehigh Valley Hospital/USF Morsani College of Medicine, Cedar Crest Boulevard and Interstate 78, Allentown, PA 18103, USA

**Paul B. McBeth, Perseus I.Missirlis, Harry Brar and Vinay Dhingra**
Division of Critical Care Medicine, University of British Columbia, Vancouver General Hospital, Vancouver, BC, Canada V5Z 1M9

**Zeljko Vucicevic**
Department of Internal Medicine, Intensive Care Unit, School of Medicine, "Sestre Milosrdnice" University Hospital Centre, University of Zagreb, Vinogradska Cesta 29, 10000 Zagreb, Croatia

**Joanna M. Janczak and Ulrich Beutner**
Department of General, Visceral and Transplantation Surgery, Kantonsspital St. Gallen, Rorschacherstrasse 95, 9007 St. Gallen, Switzerland

**Karin Hasler**
Emergency Department, Kantonsspital St. Gallen, Rorschacherstrasse 95, 9007 St. Gallen, Switzerland

**Melissa Joseph, Marissa Camilon and Tarina Kang**
Department of Emergency Medicine, LAC+USC Medical Center, 1200 N. State Street, Los Angeles, CA 90033, USA

**D. Amin, T. McCormick and T. Mailhot**
Department of Emergency Medicine, Los Angeles County-University of Southern California, Los Angeles, CA 90033, USA

**Gul Pamukcu Gunaydin and Gulhan Kurtoglu Celik**
Ankara Ataturk Training and Research Hospital, Bilkent Yolu 3 Km., Ankara, Turkey

**Nurettin Ozgur Dogan**
Department of Emergency Medicine, Faculty of Medicine, Kocaeli University, Umuttepe Kampüsü, Kocaeli, Turkey

**Sevcan Levent**
Bilecik State Hospital, Gazipaşa Mahallesi Tevfikbey Caddesi No. 4, Bilecik, Turkey

**Ghan-Shyam Lohiya**
Occupational Medicine & Toxicology, Royal Medical Group, 1120 W. Warner Avenue, Santa Ana, CA 92707, USA

**Sapna Lohiya**
University of Washington, Seattle, WA 98104, USA

**Sunita Lohiya**
Royal Medical Group, 1120W. Warner Avenue, Santa Ana, CA 92707, USA

**Vijay Krishna**
MidMichigan Medical Center, Midland, MI 48640, USA

**C. Meier and P. Lebiedz**
Department of Cardiovascular Medicine, University Hospital Münster, 48149 Münster, Germany

**M. Lichtenberg**
Department of Angiology, Arnsberg Medical Center, 59759 Arnsberg, Germany

**F. Breuckmann**
Department of Cardiology, Arnsberg Medical Center, 59759 Arnsberg, Germany

**Gultekin Gulbahar**
Division of Thoracic Surgery, Dr. Nafiz Korez Sincan State Hospital, Ankara, Turkey

**Hasan Bozkurt Turker**
Division of Orthopedics and Traumatology, Dr. Nafiz Korez Sincan State Hospital, Ankara, Turkey

**Ahmet Gokhan Gundogdu**
Division of Thoracic Surgery, Arnavutkoy State Hospital, Istanbul, Turkey

**Christine Hall, David Levy and Steven Sattler**
Emergency Medicine Residency Program, Good Samaritan Hospital Medical Center, West Islip, NY 11795, USA

**Gül Pamukçu GünaydJn, Hatice Duygu Çiftçi Sivri, Yavuz Otal and Gülhan Kurtoğlu Çelik**
Department of Emergency Medicine, Ankara Atatürk Training and Research Hospital, Çankaya, 06800 Ankara, Turkey

**Serkan Sivri**
Department of Cardiology, Ankara Atatürk Training and Research Hospital, Çankaya, 06800 Ankara, Turkey

**Ayhan Özhasenekler**
Department of Emergency Medicine, Faculty of Medicine, Yıldırım Beyazıt University, Çankaya, Ankara, Turkey

**Gerard O'Connor**
Department of Emergency Medicine, Mater Misericordiae University Hospital, Eccles Street, Dublin 7, Ireland

**Gareth Fitzpatrick, Ayman El-Gammal and Peadar Gilligan**
Department of Emergency Medicine, Beaumont Hospital, Beaumont Road, Dublin 9, Ireland

**Shamir O. Cawich, Fawwaz Mohammed, Richard Spence and Vijay Naraynsingh**
Department of Clinical Surgical Sciences, University of the West Indies, St. Augustine Campus, St. Augustine, Trinidad and Tobago

**Matthew Albert**
The Center for Colon and Rectal Surgery, 661 East Altamonte Drive, Altamonte Springs, FL 32701, USA

**Evelyn Lee**
LAC+USC Medical Center, 1200 North State Street 1060H, Los Angeles, CA 90033, USA

**Jan Shoenberger and Jonathan Wagner**
LAC+USC Medical Center, Keck School of Medicine of USC, Los Angeles, CA, USA

**Georgios F. Giannakopoulos**
Department of Trauma Surgery, VU University Medical Centre, P.O. Box 7057, 1007 MB Amsterdam, Netherlands

**Udo J. L. Reijnders**
Department of Forensic Medicine, Public Health Service, P.O. Box 2200, 1000 CE Amsterdam, Netherlands

**Christopher K. J. O'Neill, Richard J. Napier, Owen J. Diamond, Seamus O'Brien and David E. Beverland**
Primary Joint Unit, Musgrave Park Hospital, Stockmans Lane, Belfast BT9 7JB, UK

**Anna Sarah Messmer, Christian Hans Nickel and Dirk Bareiss**
Department of Emergency Medicine, University Hospital Basel, Petersgraben 2, 4031 Basel, Switzerland

**David Migneault**
Department of Emergency Medicine, Vancouver General Hospital, University of British Columbia, Room 3300 910, West 10th Avenue, Vancouver, BC, Canada V5Z 1M9

**Zachary Levine and François de Champlain**
Emergency Department, Montreal General Hospital, McGill University Health Centre, 1650 Cedar Avenue, Room B2.117, Montreal, QC, Canada H3G 1A4

**Khalida Itriyeva**
Department of Pediatrics, Cohen Children's Medical Center of New York, 269-01 76th Avenue, New Hyde Park, NY 11040, USA

**Matthew Harris, Joshua Rocker and Robert Gochman**
Pediatric Emergency Medicine, Cohen Children's Medical Center of New York, 269-01 76th Avenue, New Hyde Park, NY 11040, USA

**Erdal Gursul, Ercan Aksit and Basak Ugurlu**
Biga State Hospital, Kibris Sehitleri Street, Biga, 17200 Canakkale, Turkey

**Serdar Bayata**
Katip Celebi University Ataturk Training and Research Hospital, Izmir, Turkey

**Susumu Saigusa, Masaki Ohi, Hiroki Imaoka, Ryo Uratani, Minako Kobayashi and Yasuhiro Inoue**
Department of Surgery, Wakaba Hospital, 28-13 Minami-Chuo, Tsu, Mie 514-0832, Japan
Department of Gastrointestinal and Pediatric Surgery, Mie University Graduate School of Medicine, 2-174 Edobashi, Tsu, Mie 514-8507, Japan

**Azad Hekimoglu, Ihsaniye Suer Dogan, Aynur Turan and Baki Hekimoglu**
Department of Radiology, Diskapi Yildirim Beyazit Training and Research Hospital, Ankara, Turkey

**Mehmet Fevzi Oztekin**
Department of Neurology, Diskapi Yildirim Beyazit Training and Research Hospital, Ankara, Turkey

**Jessica Swanson and Janna Welch**
University of Texas Dell School of Medicine, Austin, TX 78701, USA

**Zeenia Aga**
Faculty of Medicine, University of Toronto, Toronto, ON, Canada M5S 1A8

**Jackie Avelino and Jo Jo Leung**
Department of Emergency Medicine, University Health Network, Toronto, ON, Canada M5G 2C4

**Gail E. Darling**
Division of Thoracic Surgery, University Health Network, Toronto, ON, Canada M5G 2C4

**Steven Jason Crellin and Kenneth D. Katz**
Department of Emergency Medicine, Lehigh Valley Hospital and Health Network, USF MCOM, Cedar Crest Boulevard and I-78, Allentown, PA 18103, USA

**Muhammad Faisal Khilji and Niranjan Lal Jeswani**
Department of Emergency Medicine, Sultan Qaboos University Hospital, Al-Khod, P.O. Box 38, 123 Muscat, Oman

**Rana Shoaib Hamid and Faisal Al Azri**
Department of Radiology, Sultan Qaboos University Hospital, Muscat, Oman

**A. J. Fischer**
Department of Cardiovascular Medicine, Division of Electrophysiology, University of Münster, 48149 Münster, Germany

**P. Lebiedz**
Department of Cardiovascular Medicine, University of Münster, 48149 Münster, Germany

**M. Wiaderek**
Department of Neurology, Arnsberg Medical Center, 59759 Arnsberg, Germany

**M. Lichtenberg**
Department of Angiology, Arnsberg Medical Center, 59759 Arnsberg, Germany

**D. Böse and F. Breuckmann**
Department of Cardiology, Arnsberg Medical Center, 59759 Arnsberg, Germany

**S. Martens**
Department of Cardiothoracic Surgery, Division of Cardiac Surgery, University of Münster, 48149 Münster, Germany

**D. C. Traficante, A. Marin and A. Catapano**
Department of Emergency Medicine, St. Joseph's Regional Medical Center, Paterson, NJ 07503, USA

**Jennifer S. Li and Johnathan Michael Sheele**
Department of Emergency Medicine, University Hospitals Case Medical Center and Case Western Reserve University, 11100 Euclid Avenue, B-517, Cleveland, OH 44139, USA

**Kristin Adkins**
West Virginia University School of Medicine, Morgantown, WV, USA

**Joseph Minardi, Erin Setzer and Debra Williams**
Department of Emergency Medicine, West Virginia University, 7413B HSS, 1 Medical Center Drive, Morgantown, WV 26506, USA

**J. Michael O'Neal and Erik Castleberg**
Department of Emergency Medicine, Loma Linda University, 11234 Anderson Street, A-108, Loma Linda, CA 92354, USA

**Vi Am Dinh**
Department of Emergency Medicine, Loma Linda University, 11234 Anderson Street, A-108, Loma Linda, CA 92354, USA
Division of Critical Care, Department of Internal Medicine, Loma Linda University, 11234 Anderson Street, A-108, Loma Linda, CA 92354, USA

www.ingramcontent.com/pod-product-compliance
Lightning Source LLC
Chambersburg PA
CBHW080515200326
41458CB00012B/4220